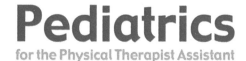

Pediatrics
for the Physical Therapist Assistant

Pediatrics
for the Physical Therapist Assistant

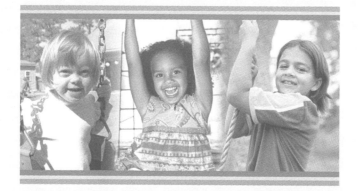

Roberta Kuchler O'Shea, PT, PhD

Associate Professor
Physical Therapy Department
Governors State University
University Park, Illinois

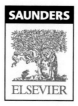

SAUNDERS

ELSEVIER

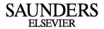

11830 Westline Industrial Drive
St. Louis, Missouri 63146

PEDIATRICS FOR THE PHYSICAL THERAPIST ASSISTANT   978-1-4160-4750-6
Copyright © 2009 by Saunders, an imprint of Elsevier Inc.

Notice

Knowledge and best practice in this field are constantly changing. As new research and experience broaden our knowledge, changes in practice, treatment and drug therapy may become necessary or appropriate. Readers are advised to check the most current information provided (i) on procedures featured or (ii) by the manufacturer of each product to be administered, to verify the recommended dose or formula, the method and duration of administration, and contraindications. It is the responsibility of the practitioner, relying on their own experience and knowledge of the patient, to make diagnoses, to determine dosages and the best treatment for each individual patient, and to take all appropriate safety precautions. To the fullest extent of the law, neither the Publisher nor the Authors assume any liability for any injury and/or damage to persons or property arising out of or related to any use of the material contained in this book.

The Publisher

Library of Congress Cataloging-in-Publication Data

O'Shea, Roberta Kuchler.
   Pediatrics for the physical therapist assistant / Roberta Kuchler O'Shea.
      p. ; cm.
   Includes bibliographical references and index.
   ISBN 978-1-4160-4750-6 (pbk. : alk. paper)
1. Physical therapy for children. I. Title.
   [DNLM: 1. Physical Therapy Modalities. 2. Adolescent. 3. Child. 4. Congenital
   Abnormalities–rehabilitation. 5. Infant. 6. Nervous System Diseases–rehabilitation.
   7. Wounds and Injuries–rehabilitation. WB 460 O82p 2009]
   RJ53.P5O84 2009
   615.8'20832–dc22
                                               2008029619

Vice President and Publisher: Linda Duncan
Senior Editor: Kathy Falk
Senior Developmental Editor: Melissa Kuster Deutsch
Publishing Services Manager: Catherine Jackson
Senior Project Manager: Gena Magouirk-Singh
Design Direction: Maggie Reid

Printed in the United States of America

Last digit is the print number: 9 8 7 6 5 4 3 2

CONTRIBUTORS

Stacy L. Bauer, PT, PCS
Physical Therapist
Chicago, Illinois

Michelle Bulanda, PT, DPT, MS, PCS
Clinical Assistant Professor
Department of Physical Therapy
College of Applied Health Sciences
University of Illinois at Chicago
Chicago, Illinois

David Diers, EdD, MHS, PT, SCS, ATC
Associate Professor
Department of Physical Therapy
Governors State University
University Park, Illinois

Colleen E. Harper, PT
Manager
Rehabilitation Department
La Rabida Children's Hospital
Chicago, Illinois

Ann W. Jackson, PT, DPT, MPH
Owner and Principal Therapist
AJ's Therapuetic Services, Inc.
Flossmoor, Illinois;
Program Developer and Researcher
Department of Developmental and
    Rehabilitative Services
La Rabida Children's Hospital
Chicago, Illinois

Joanne Kelly, RN, BSN
Staff Nurse
Department of Orthopaedics
Northwestern Medical Faculty Foundation
Chicago, Illinois

Cheryl A. Mercado, OTR/L
Independent Provider/Sole Proprietor
Early Intervention Specialist
Chicago, Illinois

Christina Odeh, PT, MHS
Program Director
Physical Therapy Assistant Program
Herzing College
Winter Park, Florida

Margaret O'Shea, OTR/L
Occupational Therapist
Aurora, Illinois

Colleen Sullivan, PT, MS
Physical Therapist
Chicago, Illinois

Treat people as they are,
And they remain that way.
Treat them as though they are already what they can be,
And you help them become what they are capable of becoming.
Goethe

ACKNOWLEDGMENTS

This book is the product of many brilliant clinicians sharing their expertise and lessons, and I thank them for their teachings. Each of us has learned lessons from our textbooks and research, but we agree that the children and their families have taught us more important lessons than books ever will.

I personally want to express my complete gratitude and love to my husband Marty and my children Amanda Rose and Christopher Scott. They have supported me while I conceptualized and completed this project.

Deep thanks is given to my colleagues and students at Governors State University, my friends, and my extended family who have offered suggestions, camaraderie, and lots of hot tea … without these special people this project would never have been completed.

I would also like to thank the editorial staff at Elsevier. Without their guidance, attention to detail, and vision, this text would still be a pile of words stuck in my computer.

Finally, to the reader, may you be inspired to make a difference, complete a project or course of study, and help the world be a better place.

Roberta Kuchler O'Shea

PREFACE

Pediatrics for the Physical Therapist Assistant presents many pediatrics-related topics relevant to the physical therapist assistant (PTA) student or novice. The book is the compilation of several experts working diligently to present common topics regarding physical therapy for children and adolescents. Many chapters include case histories presented in the *Guide to Physical Therapy*/Nagi model with additional references to the cases using the WHO model.

WHO WILL BENEFIT FROM THIS BOOK?

This book is especially designed for the PTA student or novice clinician interested in pediatrics. It has a wide variety of topic chapters that span the broad spectrum of pediatrics.

WHY IS THIS BOOK IMPORTANT TO THE PROFESSION?

Pediatrics for the Physical Therapy Assistant is the only book on pediatrics specifically written for the PTA student. It covers topics commonly seen in pediatrics settings and encompasses several areas in pediatrics, from neurologic rehabilitation to sports injuries to congenital disorders.

CONCEPTUAL APPROACH

Where appropriate, case studies are included to assist in explaining the chapters. The case studies are presented in the *Guide to Physical Therapy* format as well as summarized in the WHO format. These practical examples help students build clinical reasoning skills when they connect theory to practice.

ORGANIZATION

- Part 1: Physical therapy practice issues including information regarding child development, assessment tools, general intervention principles and pedagogies, and a chapter on different models of teaming.
- Parts 2 and 3: Discussion of neurologic, musculoskeletal, and congenital disorders typically found in the pediatric healthcare arena. Many chapters include case studies to illustrate the chapter topics.
- Part 4: Special considerations chapters that describe topics that don't fit neatly into the other parts of the textbook.

DISTINCTIVE FEATURES OF THIS BOOK

- Case studies in the Nagi and WHO model formats
- "Clinical Signs" boxes
- "Intervention" boxes
- "Practice Pattern" boxes
- Templated structure: Each disorder is defined and its pathology and clinical signs explained; physical therapy assessment and intervention are described; a case study rounds out each chapter.

LEARNING AIDS (PEDAGOGICAL FEATURES)

- Key terms
- Clear chapter learning objectives
- Review questions and answers
- Important information presented in tables and figures

NOTE TO THE STUDENT

Frequently handouts are used to augment pediatrics curricula. However, this text allows the PTA student to maintain relevant information in a secure, durable format. The easy-to-read-and-understand style allows the student to learn pediatrics material easily. The topics cover a wide range of pediatrics topics and issues.

ANCILLARIES

The Evolve website has the following student resources:

- Learning activities
- Crossword puzzles

CONTENTS

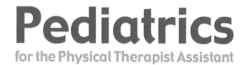

Pediatrics
for the Physical Therapist Assistant

Part ONE

Pediatric Physical Therapy Practice

Roberta Kuchler O'Shea, PT, PhD
Colleen E. Harper, PT

Chapter 1

Development

key terms

Blastocyte

Central nervous system (CNS)

Embryonic stage

Fetal stage

Germinal stage

Homunculus

Peripheral nervous system (PNS)

Primitive reflexes

Rigidity

Tone

Zygote

chapter outline

learning objectives

At the end of the chapter the reader will be able to do the following:

1. Trace the development of the neurologic system.

2. Identify the levels of the central nervous system (CNS).

3. Identify stages of development.

4. Recognize primitive reflexes and their impact on development.

5. Understand the issues of how tone can impact development.

6. Recognize the effects of poverty on child development.

A complete discussion of development should include a general understanding of how the brain, spinal cord, and nervous system develop. Disease or injury to the developing central nervous system or peripheral nervous system can result in disruption in development.

NERVOUS SYSTEM DEVELOPMENT

Nervous system development encompasses fascinating processes. The brain develops from a few dozen cells of the primitive ectoderm and weighs 800 grams at birth, approximately 1200 grams at age 6, and approximately 1400 grams at adulthood. By the sixth week of gestation the basic form of the human central nervous system is completed. Peak myelination of the nerves occurs during the third trimester of pregnancy, and development continues as life experiences contribute to functional maturity.[1]

The neural tube in the fetus develops into the brain and spinal cord, or the **central nervous system (CNS).** The rostral end becomes the brain, and the remainder of the tube closes to become the spinal cord. A condition called *spina bifida* results when the posterior tube does not properly close.

The spinal nerves, or the **peripheral nervous system (PNS),** can be described as *afferent, efferent, general,* or *special.* Afferent fibers carry sensory messages, efferent fibers carry motor messages, and general fibers innervate the skin, muscles, bones, and viscera. Special fibers innervate sensory organs in the head, such as taste buds, olfactory epithelium, retina, and cochlear and vestibular apparatus.[1]

Afferent fibers begin in the dorsal root ganglia and exit the spinal cord. Messages coming into the CNS regarding sensory information travel along these pathways. Conversely, efferent fibers originate in the ventral horn of the spinal cord and carry motor messages to the appropriate targets.[2]

NERVOUS SYSTEM FUNCTION

The human nervous system comprises three systems: CNS, PNS, and visceromotor nervous system. We will discuss the CNS and PNS in this section.

CENTRAL NERVOUS SYSTEM

The CNS consists of the brain and spinal cord. It begins in utero as the neural tube, and in a short time it folds on itself and differentiates into sections as previously discussed. At the basic level the nervous system is composed of neurons and glial cells. Neurons synapse with each other, allowing incoming sensory information and outgoing motor responses to pass between the periphery and the CNS. The CNS may be referred to as *gray matter* and *white matter.* This nomenclature indicates which structures are myelinated and which are not. Myelinated structures are considered to be white matter, whereas nonmyelinated structures are considered to be gray matter.

The CNS consists of the spinal cord, brainstem, and two cerebral hemispheres (Figure 1-1). The spinal cord has five levels: cervical, thoracic, lumbar, sacral, and coccygeal. Descending pathways (efferent) originate in the motor cortex and travel to the periphery carrying messages that control voluntary movement. Descending pathways will influence neuronal activity in the spinal cord gray matter. Specific parts of the motor cortex control specific areas of the body. As evident in the **homunculus** (Figure 1-2), the lower extremities are controlled in an area close to the central sulcus and midline, whereas upper extremities are controlled more laterally in the motor cortex. Ascending pathways (afferent) carry sensory information from the periphery to the cortex. There are several pathways that carry different sensations from the limbs to the cortex.

Similarly, the lobes of the cerebral hemispheres are diversified to control different functions. The

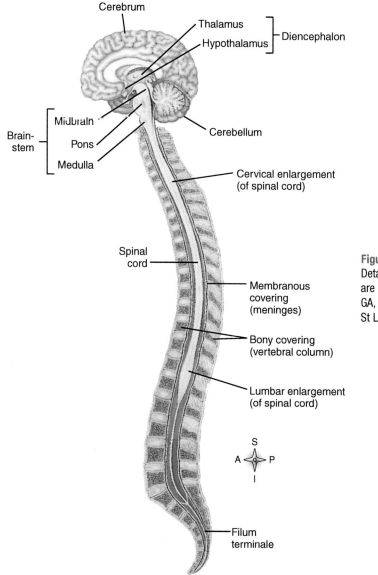

Cerebrum

Thalamus

Hypothalamus

Diencephalon

Midbrain

Brain-
stem

Pons

Medulla

Cerebellum

Cervical enlargement
(of spinal cord)

Spinal
cord

Membranous
covering
(meninges)

Bony covering
(vertebral column)

Lumbar enlargement
(of spinal cord)

S

A   P

I

Filum
terminale

Figure 1-1 The central nervous system. Details of both the brain and the spinal cord are easily seen in this figure. (From Thibodeau GA, Patton KT: *Anatomy & physiology,* ed 6, St Louis, 2007, Mosby.)

frontal lobe controls cognition and impulse control and contains the motor cortex; the occipital lobe controls visual stimuli; and the temporal lobe controls the language centers, including receptive and expressive language skills. The parietal lobe receives messages from all sensory neurons except those involved with vision and hearing.[3]

The brainstem consists of the medulla oblongata, pons, cerebellum, midbrain, and thalamus. The medulla contains ascending and descending pathways and some nuclei of

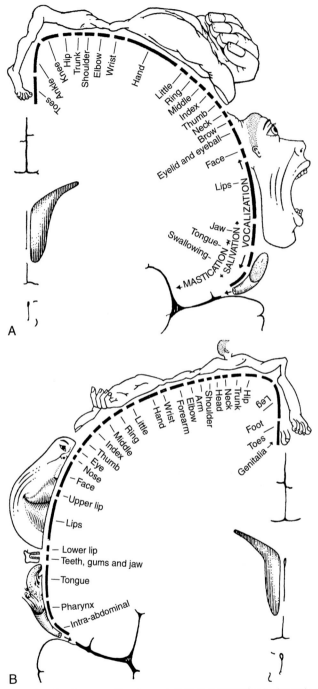

Figure 1-2 **A,** The motor homunculus showing proportional somatotopic representation in the main motor area. **B,** The sensory homunculus showing proportional somatotopic representation in the somesthetic cortex. (From Standring S: *Gray's anatomy: the anatomical basis of clinical practice,* ed 39, London, 2005, Churchill Livingstone.)

the cranial nerves. It is also an important relay center for the regulation of respiration, heart rate, and various visceral functions. Embryologically the pons and the cerebellum originate from the same part of the neural tube. The pons contains nuclei of several cranial nerves and acts as the relay station between the cortex, cerebellum, and descending motor fibers. The cerebellum controls coordination and helps the body produce smooth, purposeful movements. The midbrain houses the descending pathways and nuclei for several cranial nerves; midbrain centers are concerned with vision and auditory pathways, pain transmission, and motor function. The thalamus is surrounded almost completely by the cerebral hemispheres. Except for smell, all sensory information reaching the cortex passes through the thalamus. The thalamus conveys information regarding muscle tension and limb position sense to the cortex. This information allows for smooth, coordinated movements to take place. The relatively smaller hypothalamus influences sexual behavior, feeding, hormone output of the pituitary gland, and body temperature regulation.

There are two cerebral hemispheres. Each hemisphere has three subdivisions: the cortex, subcortical white matter, and the basal ganglia. The cortex covers the entire surface of each hemisphere. It is divided into sulci (the indentations in the brain surface) and gyri (the raised areas of the brain surface). The sulci and gyri formations of the brain allow an incredible amount of information to be stored; if the brain had a smooth surface, it would be limited in the amount of information it could process and store. The subcortical white matter is made up of myelinated axons carrying information to and from the cortex. The most organized portion of this white matter is known as the *internal capsule*. The basal ganglia contain a prominent group of cell bodies involved with motor function. Basal ganglia damage is implicated in disease processes such as Parkinson disease.

PERIPHERAL NERVOUS SYSTEM

The PNS is made up of the nerves and nerve pathways that allow signals to travel between the cortex, the spinal cord, and the peripheral muscles of the body (Figure 1-3). The PNS has sensory fibers and motor fibers that innervate glands and skeletal, cardiac, and

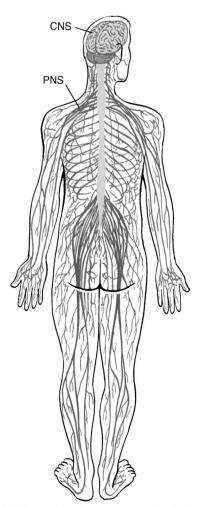

Figure 1-3 The peripheral nervous system is attached to the central nervous system, but its nerve fibers are distributed throughout the body. (From Nolte J: *The human brain: an introduction to its functional anatomy,* ed 5, St Louis, 2002, Mosby. Redrawn from Krstić RV: *General histology of the mammal,* Berlin, 1985, Springer-Verlag.)

smooth muscle. It can regenerate after an injury, whereas the CNS cannot. It is vital to human development that the nervous system form new pathways in the event of injury or damage. This ability to adapt is known as *plasticity*.

TYPICAL PHYSICAL DEVELOPMENT

Human physical development has been well documented and researched. This chapter will provide an overview of typical motor development in infants, toddlers, and children. Motor development can be influenced by individual social, emotional, and cognitive factors, as well as environmental and cultural factors. These influences are beyond the scope of this text and will not be discussed, but several chapters in addition to this one address atypical development secondary to risk factors and physical disabilities.

Typical physical development is based on an uncomplicated pregnancy lasting for a gestational period of approximately 40 weeks. During gestation the fetus undergoes significant changes. These changes continue after the child is born, some occurring well into adolescence and young adulthood.

At conception, fertilization occurs when the sperm and the ovum combine to form a new cell called a **zygote**. The zygote duplicates itself multiple times by cell division to eventually form a fetus. This duplication process is known as *mitosis* and also includes the duplication of all the genes and chromosomes. If there is a disruption in the duplication process—for instance, if there are too many or not enough chromosomes or the chromosomes are improperly located—typical development is compromised.

Each cell in the human body contains approximately 60,000 to 100,000 genes. Genes carry developmental instructions to form a human from a zygote. The genes are located in specific locations on the chromosomes. Each human cell, except the sex cells, should contain 23 pairs of chromosomes, totaling 46 chromosomes in all. The sex cells contain 23 single chromosomes, and when they combine at fertilization, the zygote has 46 chromosomes.

PRENATAL

There are three major stages in prenatal (before birth) development: germinal, embryonic, and fetal. The **germinal stage** occurs from fertilization until roughly 2 weeks gestational age. During this stage the zygote implants into the uterine wall and divides. As the cell divides it is no longer a zygote, but instead is referred to as a **blastocyte**. The blastocyte cells will begin to differentiate into several areas. A thickened area will evolve into two layers, the ectoderm and endoderm. The ectoderm will eventually become the outer layer of skin, nails, teeth, sensory organs, and nervous system, including the brain and spinal cord. The endoderm will transform into the digestive system, liver, pancreas, salivary glands, and respiratory system. In due time, a middle layer, the mesoderm, will differentiate and become the inner layer of skin, muscles, skeleton, and excretory and circulatory systems. Other areas of the blastocyte will evolve into protective components for the fetus, specifically the placenta, umbilical cord, and amniotic sac.

The **embryonic stage** occurs during weeks 2 to 8 of gestation. During this time there is continued rapid growth and development of the major body systems, including the respiratory, digestive, and nervous systems. This stage is considered a high-risk time, because the developing embryo can sustain significant damage from a host of factors. Most severely defective embryos will not survive past this stage.

The **fetal stage** constitutes the period between 8 weeks postconception and birth. During this stage, rapid growth continues, and organs and body systems become more refined (Table 1-1). Fingernails, toenails, and eyelashes develop. The fetus actively moves within the uterus, and these movements can

TABLE **1-1** Motor Development of the Fetus

	10-15 WEEKS	17-18 WEEKS	20 WEEKS
Upper extremity	Isolated extremity movements; hands to face; thumb sucking		Wide arcs of arm movement
Locomotion	Full body rotation around the umbilicus; climbing on the uterine wall	Vigorous extensor thrusts against uterine wall repositions fetus	Period of greatest mobility; creeping/crawling movement
Atypical behaviors	Fetal akinesia	Symmetric, stereotypic movements lacking dissociation	

From Long T, Toscano K: *Handbook of pediatric physical therapy*, ed 2, Philadelphia, 2002, Lippincott Williams & Wilkins.

be tracked by ultrasound. Motor patterns arise spontaneously and are not reflexive.[4] Male fetuses tend to be more active than females.[5] Other aspects of fetal development, including heart rate and cardiac activity and sleep/wake states, can also be monitored. Beginning at approximately 26 weeks gestation, fetuses also begin to respond to familiar voices, sounds (mother's heart beat), and external environmental stimuli (vibration). The fetus's brain is highly vascularized during the period between 28 and 32 weeks gestation.[2] If a child experiences aggressive movements (such as birth or being transferred via ambulance to a NICU) during this time, there is great potential for injury to the motor cortex.

POSTNATAL

Following birth the stages of human development continue. They include infant and toddler (0 to 3 years); early (3 to 6 years) and middle (6 to 12 years) childhood; adolescence (12 to 20 years); and young (20 to 40 years), middle (40 to 65 years), and late (older than 65 years) adulthood. Similar to prenatal development, childhood motor development is affected by several factors, including social-emotional and cognitive development, as well as the environment and culture.

Motor development in neonates and infants typically occurs in three directions: cephalocaudal, proximal-distal, and flexion into extension. The infant's movement must also be observed in several positions, including prone, supine, sitting, suspended prone, and standing. At birth the neonate is dominated by primitive reflexes and a flexion posture, but should be able to breathe and suck independently. Over the next few months, head and neck control and visual and auditory acuity are acquired. The baby will bat at objects, kick (randomly at first), and begin to prop up on forearms and later hands as the shoulder and hip/pelvis musculature become stronger. The baby learns to roll as he differentiates the upper half of his body from the lower half.

Reflexes

During the first year of life, children learn to roll, sit, crawl, and move into and out of those positions safely. Although primitive reflexes dominate the baby's movement as a young infant, as the child matures and develops control, the once obligatory reflexes become inhibited, and volitional control is available. Many of the postural reflexes, such as Landau, will assist the child in developing upright antigravity control. One may see a resurgence of reflexes when the child/adult is involved in high-stress situations. For example, *clonus* is the rapid beating of the foot in response to a quick stretch of the gastrocnemius tendon. If this reflex fails to be integrated, ambulation proves difficult. Picture a group of young adults experiencing a high ropes course for the first time. At 40 feet in the air, while standing on a 2-inch-diameter rope, the reoccurrence of clonus may occur in the novice climber. Uncontrolled foot tapping during an important exam, or even during an intense job interview, may also be observed. These uncontrolled foot-tapping behaviors, although very inhibited in normal situations, may be an indication of clonus.

Primitive reflexes are dominant when a child is born and oftentimes reappear in the presence of an upper motor neuron lesion. Reflexes are important to the infant as he learns to move against gravity and develops postural control. In infancy, as development proceeds, primitive reflexes become integrated as motor skills, and postural/balance reactions emerge.

The following reflexes will be described in more detail: suck/swallow, rooting, galant, flexor withdrawal, Landau, plantar and palmar grasp, and asymmetric tonic neck reflex (ATNR).

Suck/Swallow Reflex

Most babies are born with a strong suck/swallow reflex. This reflex allows the child to obtain and maintain oral nutrition. It usually integrates at 2 to 5 months. In response to a stimulus in the mouth, the baby begins to suck and swallow and learns how to nurse and control flow from a bottle. Some infants born with medical risks, especially prematurity, may lack the suck/swallow reflex. Early therapeutic intervention works to rectify the deficit and help the baby develop strong suck/swallow skills.

Rooting Reflex

The rooting reflex is related to the suck/swallow reflex and is integrated at three months. Stroking either side of its mouth will cause the baby to turn toward the ipsilateral (same) side. This reflex allows babies to locate their food source. When they feel the breast or bottle brush up against their cheek, they automatically turn toward the source. If it is a food source, the baby may find a nipple in his mouth, the suck/swallow reflex follows, and the baby is eating. If the rooting reflex is not appropriately integrated, the child may be obligated to turn the head toward whatever stimuli touches the cheek area. In a severe circumstance, if the child has a dominant rooting reflex, the child's wheelchair head rest/neck rest or even a strong breeze could elicit the rooting response, and the child may turn toward the stimulus even when it is not appropriate to do so.

Galant Reflex

The galant reflex occurs in response to stroking the paraspinals. The body's involuntary response is to bend to the stimulated side. This side bending helps a baby to develop rolling and controlled trunk movements. If not appropriately integrated bilaterally, the child may develop musculoskeletal deformities in response to repeated side-bending postures when stimulated by a back cushion or may be at risk for hip dislocation ipsilaterally.[3]

Flexor Withdrawal Reflex

Flexor withdrawal is a reflex that causes the baby to pull the lower extremity into flexion after sudden stimulus to the bottom of the foot. This reflex is helpful for safety reasons. For example, if you were walking along barefoot on a rug and stepped on a sharp tack, the flexor withdrawal reflex would cause you to pull your foot away immediately, thus keeping you safe. However, if you could not control this reflex, it stands to reason that every time you took a step, your lower extremities would go into an exaggerated lower extremity flexion movement pattern.

Landau Response

The Landau response is an extension response to being in the prone position. When prone the child plays in the "airplane position": extension of the hips, shoulders, and trunk. While prone the child will also move into and out of flexion and extension patterns. The Landau response helps the infant develop co-contraction of the proximal joints and coordination of movement between flexion and extension. The Landau response usually integrates by 6 months, as the child learns to push up into a 4-point position, requiring flexion of the hips and shoulders while maintaining trunk extension.

Grasp Reflexes

Plantar grasp is the curling of the toes in response to pressure at the ball of the foot; palmar grasp is the curling of the hand and fingers in response to pressure in the palm. This reflex makes it difficult to put on an infant's shoes. Dominant plantar reflexes may inhibit children from walking with a typical gait pattern.

The palmar grasp indirectly assists in bonding. Some infant-parent dyads have difficulty bonding for a myriad of reasons (such as social-emotional issues and medical frailty). The palmar grasp results in a child automatically grasping and not releasing an object put into the hand. While the baby is feeding, the mother or father can massage the baby's palm, and that hand will immediately assume the grasping position and maintain a hold on the parent's fingers for a bit. The best outcome will be that the parent feels the child is expressing love, and the upward cycle begins: parent plays with child, child inadvertently grasps parent, parent finds this cute and encourages the behavior. This behavior works well for an infant, but the obligatory grasp inhibits development if not integrated. Imagine the toddler or preschooler who cannot release an object. If this child grabs something hot and holds on, the child will be injured. Both the palmar and plantar grasps should be integrated by 9 months.

Asymmetric Tonic Neck Reflex

The asymmetric tonic neck reflex (ATNR) is often referred to as the *fencing reflex* and is normally seen in children 3 to 5 months old. As they turn to look to the left or right, the ipsilateral upper extremity goes into extension, and the contralateral upper extremity comes up into horizontal flexion. Similarly, the ipsilateral lower extremity extends, and the contralateral lower extremity flexes, hence the baby appears to be "fencing." This reflex is helpful when the child is developing hand-eye coordination and learning about cause and effect. For example, a noise on the left might attract a baby's attention. The child looks left, causing the left upper extremity to extend, and while extending, this arm inadvertently hits the child's overhead mobile and causes the toy to make a movement and noise; the child notices this new object (cause-and-effect knowledge develops). Although the ATNR is useful to the developing infant, a person with an inappropriately dominant ATNR will have difficulty completing midline, two-handed activities and difficulty mastering independent living skills such as self-feeding and dressing.

Motor Development

Typical motor milestones for infants are as follows: head control develops at 4 months, rolling begins between 6 and 8 months, sitting develops between 5 and 7 months, creeping usually appears at 9 to 10 months, the infant is competent in cruising furniture at 10 to 11 months, and ambulation skills are mastered between 12 and 15 months (Table 1-2). Some children will walk as early as 10 months or as late as 15 or 16 months. Children who have not begun ambulating by 16 months should be assessed by a developmental professional. Infants gain the status of toddlers after mastering ambulation. As the child becomes a toddler and masters upright mobility, developmental fine-tuning emerges.

As children learn to roll, they begin to differentiate segments of their bodies. The head and trunk and legs learn to move independently of one another. Similarly, children learn to differentiate between moving the left side of their body and the right side of their body. This allows for reciprocal movements between the arms and legs when crawling, walking, and bike riding.

TABLE **1-2** Motor Milestones for Infants

SKILL	TYPICAL ACQUISITION AGE
Head control	4 months
Rolling	6-8 months
Sitting	5-7 months
Creeping	9-10 months
Cruising	10-11 months
Ambulation	12-15 months
Steps and higher level skills	18 months

As the child grows and develops, typical gait parameters (step and stride length, base of support, cadence) change. These changes happen in response to overall changes occurring system-wide and include changes in the neuromuscular system, the musculoskeletal system, and the sensory system.[6] Children begin to ambulate with a wide base of support, upper extremities in a high- or low-guard position, and lower extremities in slight flexion. At this phase the child tends to posture with the upper extremities in high-guard or arms-in-the-air position, where the shoulders are horizontally flexed to approximately 90 degrees, the elbows are flexed to 90 degrees, the wrist and hands are extended, and the hands are at about the level of the child's ears. As balance develops, the toddler will assume a low-guard position of the upper extremities. In this posture the shoulders tend to be more in neutral, with the elbows in flexion and the hands/fingers in extension. Thus the child's arms are closer to waist level, but the child is prepared for a stumble or fall, using upper extremity extension as needed.

As the child gains confidence and experience in ambulating, the base of support narrows, the step length and stride length increase, and the child moves with a slower cadence. The overall gait cycle becomes smoother and more fluid. Near 17 months, or after a few months of mobility practice, the child will begin to demonstrate a more heel-toe gait pattern, lateral weight shift, and reciprocal arm swing. After 18 months a typically developing child begins to ascend and descend steps, kick and catch a ball, and try to jump, hop, and run well. The child masters the three latter skills at about 3 years of age. Between 6 and 10 years the child should have mastered the adult forms of running, hopping, jumping, and throwing.[7]

ATYPICAL DEVELOPMENT

Several factors will affect a child's development. There are hallmark methods to describe delays or differences in development, including increases and decreases in tone, delayed motor development, delayed cognitive and communicative development, and inappropriately dominant primitive reflexes. Some of the delays may be significant at birth but diminish over time. Other delays will influence the child's growth and development over the entire life span. Atypical development may be caused by upper motor neuron disease, lower motor neuron disease, muscle disease, or genetic malformation and toxin exposure.

Upper motor neuron diseases affect the upper motor neuron systems in the central nervous system: the cortex, cranial nerve nuclei in the brainstem, and spinal cord. Cerebral palsy and spinal cord injury are examples of upper motor neuron pathologies. Lower motor neurons include the PNS and cranial nerves. Erb's palsy is an example of a lower motor neuron disease. Muscle disease, such as muscular dystrophy, will also cause disruptions in development.

TONE

Tone is the normal tension found in muscles. It can be described as the slight resistance felt when a joint is moving in its total range of motion.[8] Atypical tone becomes an issue when it affects the child's ability to move and be independent. Tone is often a relative term when considering the total population, and the range of normal is quite variable. As clinicians become more experienced with the feeling of tone, they are able to discriminate when variances may cause developmental complications.

Atypical tone includes hypertonia, mixed or fluctuating tone, rigidity, and hypotonia. The Modified Ashworth Scale of spasticity (Table 1-3) can be used to quantitatively describe tone. The Modified Ashworth Scale represents a grading scale for degree of spasticity. The patient receives a grade of 0 for no tone; 1 for slight increase in tone, with minimal resistance during flexion and extension; 1+ for slight increase in tone, with minimal resistance in remainder of range of motion;

TABLE **1-3** Modified Ashworth Scale

GRADE	DESCRIPTION
0	No increase in muscle tone
1	Slight increase in muscle tone, manifested by a catch and release or by minimal resistance at the end of the ROM when the affected part(s) is moved in flexion or extension
1+	Slight increase in muscle tone, manifested by a catch, followed by minimal resistance throughout the remainder (less than half) of the ROM
2	More marked increase in muscle tone through most of the ROM, but affected parts move easily
3	Considerable increase in muscle tone; passive movement difficult
4	Affected part(s) rigid in flexion or extension

2 for marked increased tone, but the limb can be easily flexed; 3 for considerable increase in tone, making passive range of motion (PROM) difficult; and 4 for rigidity in flexion and extension.[3]

Increased tone is also known as *hypertonia*. Hypertonia is commonly seen in individuals with upper motor neuron disease and is described as an increase in stiffness in muscles of the limb or trunk; it may also be called *spasticity*. Resistance to movement increases in response to rapid movement of the joint or limb, as if the joint were "catching." Hypertonia can often be reduced using handling techniques and orthotics.

Athetoid tone involves writhing, uncontrolled movements. Athetoid tone is a result of damage to the extrapyramidal region near the basal ganglia, not damage in the motor cortex. Fluctuating tone indicates fluctuations between hypertonia and near-normal tone. Children with spastic cerebral palsy often have underlying athetoid movements of the extremities and may exhibit fluctuating tone. Orthotic intervention techniques to normalize tone will be described in later chapters in detail.

Rigidity is also a significant resistance to movement; however, the cause is typically from extrapyramidal syndromes (dystonias) and damage such as that from Parkinson disease or after an anoxic event. Rigidity differs from spasticity because it is present through the entire range of motion. It is described as "lead pipe" or "cogwheel rigidity." In the first type the individual's extreme tone does not break and feels as if you are bending a lead pipe. Cogwheel rigidity is described as intermittent breaks in increased tone throughout range of motion, so the limb moves in a cogwheel pattern.[8]

Hypotonia, on the other hand, is "floppiness" or lack of resistance to movement. Marked hypotonia is referred to as *flaccidity*. Hypotonia may be associated with lower motor neuron involvement and would be present in polio, spinal cord injury, or brachial plexus injuries. Additionally, some genetic diseases, such as Down syndrome, are often characterized by increased hypotonia.

OTHER DEVELOPMENTAL ISSUES

Other developmental issues will also affect typical development. If a child is born blind or with visual impairments, acquisition of gross motor movements will be delayed. As the child learns about the environment and begins to explore, motor skills rapidly improve. Typically by the time the child is a toddler, motor skills are age-appropriate.

Conversely, children with hearing impairments appear to develop typically as infants, but as they age it becomes apparent that they have cognitive and language delays. With intervention, many of these delays can be minimized. Children with peripheral nerve damage or missing limbs may also experience early motor delays. As children cognitively advance and learn how to adapt their movements using intact body segments or prosthetics or orthotics, motor skills and independent activities-of-daily-living skills develop. More often than not, by the time the children are nearing early childhood (ages 3 to 5), they have adapted their movement patterns and skills and are independently age-appropriate. Several developmental sequelae and relevant interventions are discussed in depth in the following chapters.

POVERTY

Poverty seriously affects health and human development, and it has a significant and detrimental effect on child development. An American child is more likely to live in poverty than a child in 17 other wealthy industrialized nations for which data exist, according to the cross-national Luxembourg Income Study.[9] In the United States a child living in poverty has an increased likelihood of acquiring asthma, diabetes, morbid obesity, high lead levels (almost 900,000 children under the age of 5 currently have elevated blood-lead levels), or depression or becoming a victim of violence.[9,10] Each of these pathologies has significant health implications, and some are discussed elsewhere in the text.

Living in poverty often results in suboptimal and infrequent healthcare, exacerbation of chronic conditions, and risky environments.[9,10] Interestingly, more children are affected by intermittent poverty than chronic poverty situations. Fifty percent of U.S. children live in

---

Box **1-1** Key Facts about American Children	
Every 10 seconds a high school student drops out.	1 in 3 is born to unmarried parents.
Every 13 seconds a public school student is corporally punished.	1 in 3 will be poor at some point in their childhood.
Every 19 seconds a child is arrested.	1 in 3 is behind a year or more in school.
Every 23 seconds a baby is born to an unmarried mother.	1 in 4 lives with only one parent family living arrangements.
Every 35 seconds a child is confirmed as abused or neglected.	1 in 5 is born to a mother who did not graduate from high school.
Every 37 seconds a baby is born to a mother who is not a high school graduate.	1 in 5 was born poor.
Every 40 seconds a baby is born into poverty.	1 in 5 children under 3 is poor now.
Every 51 seconds a baby is born without health insurance.	1 in 6 is poor now.
Every minute a baby is born to a teen mother.	1 in 6 is born to a mother who did not receive prenatal care in the first three months of pregnancy.
Every 2 minutes a baby is born at low birth weight.	1 in 7 children eligible for federal child care assistance through the Child Care and Development Block Grant receives it.
Every 4 minutes a baby is born to a mother who received late or no prenatal care.	1 in 7 never graduates from high school.
Every 4 minutes a child is arrested for drug abuse.	1 in 8 has no health insurance.
Every 8 minutes a child is arrested for violent crimes.	1 in 8 lives in a family receiving food stamps.
Every 19 minutes a baby dies before his first birthday.	1 in 8 has a worker in their family, but still is poor.
Every 43 minutes a child or teen dies in an accident.	1 in 9 is born to a teenage mother.
Every 3 hours a child or teen is killed by a firearm.	1 in 12 has a disability.
Every 5 hours a child or teen commits suicide.	1 in 13 was born with low birth weight.
Every 6 hours a child is killed by abuse or neglect.	1 in 13 will be arrested at least once before age 17.
Every 22 hours a mother dies in childbirth.	1 in 14 lives at less than half the poverty level.
3 in 5 preschoolers have their mothers in the labor force.	1 in 35 lives with grandparents (or other relative) but neither parent.
2 in 5 preschoolers eligible for Head Start do not participate.	1 in 28 is born to a mother who received late or no prenatal care.
1 in 2 never complete a single year of college.	1 in 60 sees their parents divorce in any year.
1 in 2 will live in a single-parent family at some point in childhood.	1 in 83 will be in state or federal prison before age 20.
	1 in 146 will die before their first birthday.
	1 in 1339 will be killed by guns before age 20.

From Children's Defense Fund (website): http://www.childrensdefense.org. Accessed June 8, 2004.

vulnerable economic conditions at least once in their lifetimes.[11] Poverty directly affects a society's health issues by increasing the number of premature births or infants with low birth weight resulting from inadequate maternal prenatal care. In 1999, 7.6% of babies were born at low birth weight (under 5 lb, 8 oz); 13.2% of babies born to black mothers were born at low birth weight, compared with 6.6% of babies born to white mothers.[9] Poverty limits the family's purchasing power to acquire adequate housing, food, and healthcare, all of which will negatively affect a child's health and development, and poverty restricts a family's available social capital in their neighborhoods and schools.[10] Interestingly, poverty causes the most harm to children because of its corrosive effects on parents (Box 1-1).[10]

Summary

Knowledge of typical and atypical child development is important because it forms a basis for physical therapy practice. Each child behaves differently, and recognizing the skills and abilities of each child enables the physical therapist assistant to manage successful interventions.

Chapter Discussion Questions
1. Identify three ways poverty may impact a child's development.
2. Conceptualize one community-based strategy to help address environmental deficit.
3. Identify the three components of the human nervous system.
4. Describe motor development progression and how that progression affects the developmental sequence.
5. What is the developmental impact on a child if the following are not integrated?
   a. Rooting reflex
   b. Asymmetric tonic neck reflex
   c. Galant reflex
6. Define hypotonia.
7. Choose a type of atypical tone and describe how this tonal influence can affect a 6-year-old child's ability to function in an inclusive classroom setting.
8. List the components of the central nervous system.
9. How does the central nervous system differ from the peripheral nervous system?
10. At what week of gestation is the basic central nervous system developed?

REFERENCES
1. Haines DE: *Fundamental neuroscience*, ed 2, New York, 2002, Churchill Livingstone.
2. Gilman S, Newman SW: *Essentials of clinical neuroanatomy and neurophysiology*, ed 10, Philadelphia, 2003, FA Davis.
3. Accardo PJ, Whitman BY: *Dictionary of developmental disabilities terminology*, ed 2, Baltimore, 2002, Paul H. Brookes.
4. Long T, Toscano K: *Handbook of pediatric physical therapy*, ed 2, Philadelphia, 2002, Lippincott Williams & Wilkins.
5. Papalia DE, Olds SW, Feldman RD: *Human development*, ed 9, New York, 2004, McGraw-Hill.
6. Bierman JC: Developing ambulation skills. In Connolly BH, Montgomery PC, editors: *Therapeutic exercise in developmental disabilities*, ed 3, Thorofare, NJ, 2005, Slack.
7. Cech D, Martin S: *Functional movement development across the life span*, ed 2, Philadelphia, 2002, Saunders.
8. Fuller G: *Neurological exam made easy*, ed 2, Edinburgh, 2002, Churchill Livingstone.
9. Children's Defense Fund (website): http://www.childrensdefense.org. Accessed June 8, 2004.
10. Smith CA: *The encyclopedia of parenting theory and research*, Westport, Conn, 1999, Greenwood.
11. Silverman WK, Ollendick TH: *Developmental issues in the clinical treatment of children*, Boston, 1999, Allyn & Bacon.

RESOURCES
National Institute of Child Health and Human Development
www.nichd.nih.gov

Society for Research and Child Development
University of Michigan
3131 S. State Street, #302
Ann Arbor, MI 48108-1623
734-998-6578
www.srcd.org

National Association for Child Development
549 25th Street
Ogden, Utah 84401-2422
800-621-8606
www.nacd.org

National Association for Black Children
1101 15th Street NW, #900
Washington, DC 20005
202-833-2220
www.nbcdi.org

Foundation for Child Development
145 E. 3rd Street, 44th floor
New York, NY 10016-6055
www.fcd-us.org

Children's Defense Fund
www.childrensdefense.org

Chapter 2

Roberta Kuchler O'Shea, PT, PhD
Michelle Bulanda, PT, DPT, MS, PCS

Assessments

key terms

Criterion-referenced assessment tools

Norm-referenced assessment tools

Qualitative assessment
Quantitative assessment

outline

Purpose
Qualitative Assessments
Quantitative Assessments

Standardized Assessment Tools
    Norm-Referenced Assessments
    Criterion-Referenced Assessments

learning objectives

At the end of the chapter the reader will be able to do the following:

1. Differentiate between norm- and criterion-referenced assessments.

2. Discuss psychometric properties of different assessments.

3. Determine the purpose and design of each assessment tool.

4. Appreciate that one assessment is not appropriate for all testing purposes and all children.

This chapter will introduce several assessment tools used in pediatric settings. Although the physical therapist assistant (PTA) does not evaluate children directly, it is helpful to be familiar with the types of assessments tools commonly used in pediatric physical therapy examination and diagnosis. Familiarity with this component of the record gives a PTA background knowledge essential to being able to read assessment reports and understand their content. Data describing motor development (Figure 2-1) are typically divided into three areas: gross motor skills, fine motor skills, and oral motor skills. Since physical therapy traditionally focuses on gross motor and fine motor development, only these two areas will be discussed in this chapter. Oral motor literature is outside the scope of this text.

PURPOSE

The purpose of assessment is to screen for delays or abnormalities, provide a diagnosis, evaluate outcomes and progress, develop goals, collect data, and determine a prognosis. When an assessment is used to develop a diagnosis, it is attempting to distinguish individual characteristics based on some feature of interest. Data can also be used to classify children for program placement. When making determinations or diagnosis decisions, it is best to use a standardized and norm-referenced assessment tool designed to be demographically representative of a given population as a whole. The reference group used in developing such tests is called a *norming sample.*

If an assessment tool is being used to evaluate outcomes and progress, the tool should document change over a period of time or evaluate the effectiveness of a program or intervention. The tool should be standardized and sensitive enough to measure change over time.

To develop goals and outcomes, the preferred assessment tool should measure individual competencies and needs, be standardized, and document validity of the intervention for program planning. Some definitions and

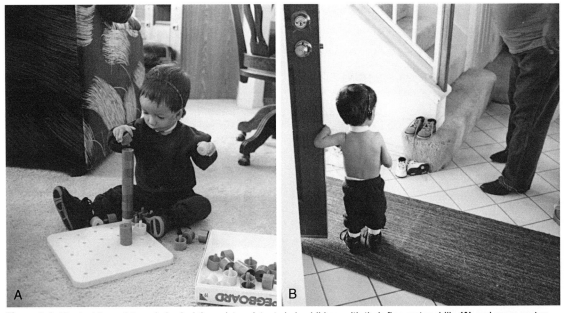

Figure 2-1 Physical therapists and physical therapist assistants help children with their fine motor skills **(A)** and gross motor skills **(B)**. (From Parham LD, Fazio LS: *Play in occupational therapy for children,* ed 2, St Louis, 2008, Mosby.)

descriptions you may find useful are as follows[1,2]:

- Age-equivalent score: the mean chronological age represented by a certain score. This score is useful when assessing and describing developmentally delayed children who cannot achieve a developmental index score. Parents and caregivers understand the age-equivalent scores more easily than other statistical data. However, these data are not necessarily statistically sound. It is better to use percentile or standard scores for data reporting.
- Percentile score: the percentage of children at the same age or grade level who should perform at a lower level. For example, if a boy is in the 60th percentile, he performed better than 60% of children in the norm group or reference group population. The average range of percentiles is between the 16th and 84th percentile.
- Percentage score: expresses the percent of items passed on a scale.
- Raw score: actual points earned on an assessment or number of items passed on a certain test. Several assessments require the child to achieve a basal (baseline) and a ceiling (cutoff) score. Each tool has particular criteria for establishing a child's basal and ceiling scores.
- Scaled score: provides an estimate of the child's ability level along a continuum of items. Scores range from 0 to 100; 0 is low capacity, and 100 is highly capable.
- Standard scores: describe deviations from the mean, or average, score for the group. Standard deviations are used to describe the divergence.
- Standard tests: tests that include a set of tasks or questions intended to assess a particular type of behavior when presented under standardized conditions.
- Reliability: determines if the tool is an accurate measure of what it claims to measure. Typically reliability is measured as the consistency of test item agreement between two or more observers or between two administrations of a test. Error in measurement can occur between two evaluators or because of errors in the test. The standard measure of error demonstrates the range of variability in which the true ability of an individual probably lies. Hence, it expresses test reliability for an individual independent of the variability found in a group.
- Validity: determines whether the assessment tool accomplishes its intended purpose. There are several types of validity. *Face validity* is the concept that the test strongly measures what it claims to measure. (Is the face value of the assessment valid and true?) *Content validity* requires that the assessment sample a reasonable range of target behaviors. (Is the content of the assessment measuring what it claims to measure?) *Concurrent validity* correlates the child's performance on an assessment to another valid assessment. (Will the child achieve the same age or developmental level on two different assessments given in the same time period?) *Construct validity* requires that the test explain the child's achievement within a theoretical framework. *Predictive validity* describes how well the assessment tool predicts the child's performance at a future date.[3]
- Responsiveness: the ability to detect minimally significant clinical change.

QUALITATIVE ASSESSMENTS

The primary purpose of **qualitative assessment** is to understand people's perspectives and their interpretation of behaviors and expressions.[4] There are several ways to assess a child and family, and using a combination of methods will provide a richer understanding of the child. Methods include an interview with the child, family, and caregivers; observation in settings familiar to the child (e.g., home, day care, and school); chart reviews of existing medical and educational records; and the standardized assessment tools.

When assessing a young child, it is imperative to discuss the child's progress or lack thereof with a person familiar to the child. The reporter may be able to provide necessary history and areas of concern. An older child may provide an understanding of his or her own motor concerns. In either case, identification of family/child priorities is vital to creating a successful plan of treatment. Existing medical or educational records provide the clinician with a window into the past; without having been there the clinician nevertheless gains insight into previous motor assessment performance. This insight can come from previously conducted standardized assessments and provider reports.[1]

QUANTITATIVE ASSESSMENTS

In **quantitative assessment,** researchers identify an inquiry area within a broad scope that requires investigation. The investigators' questions are narrow and have well-defined boundaries regarding who or what will be investigated. A specific experimental design is employed to answer the defined questions.[4]

STANDARDIZED ASSESSMENT TOOLS

Standardized assessments adhere to a formal administration and scoring protocol. These assessments can be categorized into two types: norm-referenced and criterion-referenced (Table 2-1). The differences between the two are significant and should be recognized prior to choosing an assessment tool.[1]

Norm-referenced assessment tools have been standardized on a demographically representative population and evaluate a child's performance based on comparisons with a normative typical-development sample (i.e., a representative group of the child's peers). Norming samples should mimic the racial and ethnic breakdown of the population being studied, typically the census in the United States. Normative assessments are valuable when diagnostic and qualifying information is needed to determine eligibility for services. Normative data allow standard scores, percentiles, and age-equivalent calculations to be made. Examples of norm-referenced assessments include the Bayley Scales of Infant Development, Third Edition (BSID-III); the Peabody Developmental Motor Scales, Second Edition (PDMS-2); the Test of Gross Motor Development, Second Edition (TGMD-2); and the Test of Infant Motor Performance (TIMP).

In contrast, **criterion-referenced assessment tools** are judgment-based and compare a child's performance to criteria that have been defined within the test.[5] They are often based on milestones of motor skills performed by typically developing children. Criterion-referenced assessments are more useful when developing a treatment plan or curriculum for a child. Examples of criterion-referenced assessments include the Gross Motor Function Measure (GMFM), the School Function Assessment (SFA), and the Hawaii Early Learning Profile (HELP).

NORM-REFERENCED ASSESSMENTS
Bayley Scales of Infant Development, Third Edition

The BSID-III[6] assesses the development of children from 1 to 42 months of age. It was standardized on a stratified random sample based on 2000 U.S. Census data. The BSID-III consists of five scales: cognitive, language, social-emotional, motor, and adaptive behavior.

The *cognitive scale* assesses sensory perceptual acuity and discrimination, object consistency, problem solving, early verbal communication, and early thinking abilities. The *motor scale* evaluates body control and fine and gross motor skills. Both scales yield standardized scores with a mean of 100 and a standard deviation of 15.

TABLE **2-1** Pediatric Physical Therapy Assessments

Assessment	Design	Authors/Date	Age Range	Measures
Alberta Infant Motor Scale (AIMS)	Norm-referenced	Piper, Darrah, 1994	Birth to 18 mo	Prone, supine, sit, and stand
Bayley Scales of Infant Development, Third Edition (BSID-III)	Norm-referenced	Bayley, 2005	1 to 42 mo	Cognitive, motor, language, social-emotional, and adaptive behavioral
Bruininks-Oseretsky Test of Motor Proficiency, Second Edition (BOT-2)	Norm-referenced	Bruininks, Bruininks, 2005	4 to 21 yr	Gross and fine motor skills
Gross Motor Function Measure (GMFM)	Criterion-referenced	Russell, Rosenbaum, Hardy and others, 1994		Motor function in: 1. lying and rolling 2. sitting 3. crawling and kneeling 4. standing 5. walking, running, and jumping
Hawaii Early Learning Profile	Criterion-referenced	Parks, 1997	Birth to 6 yr	1. cognition 2. gross motor 3. fine motor 4. social 5. self-help
Home Observation Measurement of the Environment (HOME)	Norm-referenced	Caldwell, Bradley, 1984	Birth to 10 yr	Quantity and quality of stimulation in the home environment
Peabody Developmental Motor Scales, Second Edition (PDMS-2)	Norm-referenced	Folio, Fewell, 2002	Birth to 6 yr	Gross and fine motor skills
Pediatric Evaluation of Disability Inventory (PEDI)	Criterion-referenced	Haley, Coster, Ludlow and others, 1992	6 mo to 7.5 yr	Self-care ability Social function
School Function Assessment (SFA)	Criterion-referenced	Coster, Deeney, Haltiwangar and others, 1998	Kindergarten to 6th grade	Participation Task support Activity performance Physical tasks Cognitive and behavioral tasks
Test of Gross Motor Development, Second Edition (TGMD-2)	Norm-referenced	Ulrich, 2000	3 to 10 yr	Locomotor and object control skills
Test of Infant Motor Performance (TIMP)	Norm-referenced	Campbell, Kolobe, Osten and others, 1995	Infants 32 wk gestation to 4 mo postterm	Functional motor performance

The BSID-III norming sample does not include children with diagnosed disabilities. For them the examiner has two scoring options. Examiners may either adapt the test items and not determine a standardized score or administer the test as directed and risk the child scoring significantly lower than the norm.

The BSID-III demonstrates concurrent validity with other reputable assessments, including the Motor Developmental Index with the McCarthy Scales of Children's Ability, the General Cognitive Index, and the Wechsler Preschool and Primary Scale of Intelligence, Third Edition.

Peabody Developmental Motor Scales, Second Edition

The PDMS-2[7] uses a stratified sample relative to the U.S. Census criteria. The PDMS-2 is designed to assess the gross and fine motor skills of children from birth through 6 years of age. Items are scored on a three-point scale. Age equivalents, motor quotients, percentile rankings, and standard scores can be calculated for each child.

The PDMS-2 gross motor scale assesses skills in four areas: reflexes, stationary, locomotion, and object manipulation. The fine motor scale assesses skills in two areas: grasping and visual-motor integration. Not all test items must be administered to achieve a basal and ceiling level.

The PDMS-2 has shown empirical reliability and validity. Updated features of the PDMS-2 include a software scoring and report system available as an additional option. Strengths include recently updated norms, revision of test items, optional awarding of partial credit on items, and an illustrated administrator's manual. Among its weaknesses are incomplete descriptions of scoring on some items, leading to subjective scoring, and increased administration time when assessing children with delays, because more time is needed to establish a basal score.

Test of Gross Motor Development, Second Edition

The TGMD-2[2,8] is appropriate for children 3 to 10 years of age. This norm-referenced scale identifies children who may be eligible for special services because of significantly delayed gross motor skills.

The TGMD-2 consists of two scales with six subtests. The locomotor scale includes run, gallop, hop, leap, horizontal jump, and slide. The object control scale includes striking a stationary ball, stationary dribble, kick, catch, overhand throw, and underhand roll. This assessment can be easily administered in less than 30 minutes. Scoring options include standard scores, percentile scores, age equivalents, and a gross motor quotient.

Test of Infant Motor Performance

The TIMP is a comprehensive motor test designed to assess functional motor performance of infants between 32 weeks gestational age and 16 weeks postterm. Initial reports on the TIMP suggest that it yields reliable measurements that are valid for discriminating optimal motor performance from poor motor performance in infants born preterm and very young infants.[9] Scoring on the TIMP has been reported to be sensitive to changes related to maturation and medical complications.

The TIMP consists of 59 items divided into 2 sections: elicited and observed. The elicited section items assess the infant's motor responses to placement in various positions and to visual or auditory stimulation.[10] The observed section items are used to rate spontaneous movement exhibited by the infant. The items on the TIMP have been shown to have ecological validity (i.e., the elicited section items are similar to demands placed on infants in everyday caregiving situations). Moderate concurrent validity with the Alberta Infant Motor Scale was demonstrated for infants at 3, 6, 9, and 12 months of age.[11,12]

Alberta Infant Motor Scale

The purpose of the Alberta Infant Motor Scale (AIMS)[13] is to provide an observational tool to be administered by a healthcare provider. It is a norm-referenced test using a representative infant population sample of Alberta, Canada, compiled between 1990 and 1992. There are four subscales accounting for 58 items: prone, supine, sit, and stand. Each item has descriptors for weightbearing, posture, and antigravity movements. The manual must be used to accurately score the items. Scores are presented exclusively as percentiles.

The strengths of this test are ease and speed of administering the assessment, its observational format, and its emphasis on quality of movement. Limitations are that therapists must subjectively convert percentile scores and that there are a limited number of items for birth to 4 months of age.

Bruininks-Oseretsky Test of Motor Proficiency, Second Edition (BOT-2)

The Bruininks-Oseretsky Test of Motor Proficiency, Second Edition (BOT-2)[14] assesses motor skills and discrimination in children with serious motor dysfunctions. It is a norm-referenced assessment tool with age ranges of 4 to 21 years. There are 8 subtests and a short- and long-scoring form. The long form takes approximately 60 minutes to administer.

The strengths of the BOT-2 are that it covers a wide age range and assesses unique aspects of motor development, including speed, agility, balance, strength, bilateral coordination, and upper-limb coordination. The tasks are child-friendly and include photos to accompany the simple instructions. Norms are based on U.S. Census data.

Home Observation Measurement of the Environment

The Home Observation Measurement of the Environment (HOME)[15] measures the quantity and quality of stimulation in the home environment, thus assessing the home environment from the child's vantage point. It can be used with children from birth to 10 years. The items assess types of toys available, family routines, discipline and interaction, learning materials, language stimulation, physical environment, academic stimulation, modeling, variety, and acceptance. The HOME can be administered via interview or observation and usually takes 45 minutes to complete.

The strengths of the HOME are that it is a systematic data-collection system for the home environment, it is easy to administer, it covers a wide age range, and it is used extensively in

research. Unfortunately the scoring criteria can be rather ambiguous.

The Pediatric Evaluation of Disability Inventory

The PEDI[16] is a norm-referenced tool that assesses functional skills of children aged 6 months to 7.5 years, although some selected scales can be used for children older than 7.5 years. The PEDI allows therapists to measure performance over time. Children with motor delays can be assessed using the PEDI, provided their skills do not exceed those of a typical 7.5-year-old. The PEDI measures capability and performance of functional activities in three content areas: self-care, ability, and social function. Additionally, the PEDI records the amount of caregiver assistance the child needs to complete a skill and any equipment/object modifications that may be necessary. Scores may be obtained from interviews with parents or primary caregivers or from observation of the child.

The strengths of the PEDI are that it is designed for use with children with disabilities, it can be administered easily, decisions regarding goals and further referrals can be determined from test results, and there is a score range (standard error of measurement) and caregiver-assistance scale. Its limitations are that no composite score can be calculated and the test was normed on a relatively small regional sample.

CRITERION-REFERENCED ASSESSMENTS
Gross Motor Function Measure

The GMFM[17] allows a therapist to measure a change in motor function over time in a child with cerebral palsy. It is a criterion-referenced assessment that focuses on how much (the quantity) of an activity the child can accomplish rather than how well (the quality) the child performs the movement. Eighty-eight items assess activities of motor function over five areas. These areas include lying and rolling; sitting; crawling and kneeling; standing; and walking, running, and jumping. All items found on this assessment can be accomplished by a typically developing 5-year-old child.

The strengths of the GMFM are that it covers a wide age range, various dimensions can be scored, and there is a goal score. Limitations are that each item must be administered and only items administered and performed during the testing session can be scored.

School Function Assessment

The purpose of the SFA[2,18] is to assess a child's function and guide program planning for students with disabilities within their educational abilities. This is a criterion-referenced assessment for children in kindergarten through 6th grade. It tests skills in the following areas: participation, task support, activity performance, physical tasks, and cognitive and behavioral tasks.

The strengths of the SFA are that its content is specific to children with physical or sensory impairments and clinical judgment is based on typical performance. Its limitations are that it requires collaboration and coordination among team members to obtain valid information, and it is time-consuming to administer.

Hawaii Early Learning Profile

The HELP[19] is a comprehensive and developmentally sequenced, curriculum-based assessment tool that include six domains: cognitive, language, gross motor, fine motor, social, and self-help. The HELP promotes a cross-disciplinary, integrated approach that focuses on the whole child and includes the importance of supportive environments and interactions, building on strengths, and providing activities for working on specific needs within a curriculum for children from birth to 6 years of age.

Summary

The assessment tools described in this chapter can be used to complete initial evaluations of the child and to collect data. These measurements can be used to benchmark progress as time goes on and change the plan of care as needed. They can also be used as ongoing assessment strategies in reevaluating a child's abilities and needs across the spectrum of growth and development. In this way, the assessment tools allow the therapist to measure developmental progress.

Chapter Discussion Questions

1. Why is reliability important in regard to assessment tools?
2. Should a raw score be used to compare a group of children over time? Why or why not?
3. List at least three purposes of assessment. Describe a setting or environment and why you would use assessment measures in this setting.
4. When and why would you report age-equivalent scores?
5. Why is test validity an important construct?
6. Describe at least two types of test validity. What would be the consequence of violating each of these constructs?
7. Identify one benefit of using qualitative assessment.
8. Compare and contrast criterion-referenced assessments and norm-referenced assessments.
9. Identify and describe one criterion-referenced assessment tool and one norm-referenced assessment tool.
10. Describe a scenario in which you would use quantitative assessment and a scenario in which you would use qualitative assessment.

REFERENCES

1. Brenneman S: Assessment and testing of infant and child development. In Tecklin JS: *Pediatric physical therapy*, ed 3, Philadelphia, 1999, Lippincott Williams & Wilkins.
2. Long T, Toscano K: *Handbook of pediatric physical therapy*, ed 2, Philadelphia, 2002, Lippincott Williams & Wilkins.

3. Accardo PJ, Whitman BY: *Dictionary of developmental disabilities terminology*, Baltimore, 1996, Paul H Brookes.

4. DePoy E, Gitlin LN: *Introduction to research*, St Louis, 1994, Mosby.

5. Guralnick M: *Interdisciplinary clinical assessment of young children with developmental disabilities*, Baltimore, 2000, Brookes.

6. Bayley N: *Bayley scales of infant development manual*, ed 3, San Antonio, 2005, Psychological Corporation.

7. Folio MR, Fewell RR: *Peabody developmental motor scales*, ed 2, Austin, 2002, PRO-ED.

8. Ulrich DA: Test of gross motor development-second edition (TGMD-2), Austin, 2000, PRO-ED.

9. Campbell SK: Test-retest reliability of the test of infant motor performance, *Pediatr Phys Ther* 11:60, 1999.

10. Campbell SK, Kolobe THA, Osten ET, and others: Construct validity of the test of infant motor performance, *Phys Ther* 75:585, 1995.

11. Campbell SK, Kolobe THA: Concurrent validity of the test of infant motor performance with the Alberta infant motor scale, *Pediatr Phys Ther* 12:1, 2000.

12. Campbell SK, Kolobe THA, Wright BD, and others: Validity of the test of infant motor performance for prediction of 6-, 9- and 12-month scores on the Alberta infant motor scale, *Dev Med Child Neurol* 44(4):263, 2002.

13. Piper MC, Darrah J: *Motor assessment of the developing infant*, Philadelphia, 1994, Saunders.

14. Bruininks RH, Bruininks BD: *Bruininks-Oseretsky test of infant motor proficiency*, Second Edition, Circle Pines, Minn, 2005, American Guidance Center.

15. Caldwell B, Bradley R: *Home observation for measurement of the environment (HOME)-Revised Edition*, Little Rock, 1984, University of Arkansas.

16. Haley SM, Coster WJ, Ludlow LH, and others: *Pediatric evaluation of disability inventory (PEDI): development, standardization, and administration manual*, Boston, 1992, New England Medical Center Hospitals and PEDI Research Group.

17. Russell D, Rosenbaum P, Hardy S, and others: Gross motor function measure: methodological and practical issues, *Phys Ther* 74(7):630, 1994.

18. Coster W, Deeney T, Haltiwangar J, and others: *School function assessment*, San Antonio, 1998, Therapy Skill Builders.

19. Parks S: *Hawaii early learning profile (HELP)*, Palo Alto, Calif, 1997, Vort.

RESOURCES

University of New Mexico Center for Developmental Disability

2300 Menaul Blvd NE
Albuquerque, NM 87107
www.newassessment.org
This site provides an overview of early childhood assessment tools.

Chapter 3

Roberta Kuchler O'Shea, PT, PhD

Overview of Physical Therapy Interventions

learning objectives

At the end of the chapter the reader will be able to do the following:

1. Identify the differences between intervention philosophies.

2. Recognize which interventions would be most appropriate for a given situation.

3. Understand why one intervention may not be appropriate for all situations and all children.

Physical therapy interventions vary, depending on many scenarios. There are standards in the profession that the physical therapist assistant (PTA) will encounter. This chapter is designed to help you become familiar with some of the more common pediatric physical therapy interventions and environments you may encounter. Interestingly, research has not proven one intervention better or worse than another when used appropriately. This may be because so many factors influence effectiveness. Master clinicians use a wide variety of techniques and interventions that can be modified based on variables including but not limited to the child's pathology, family structure, living situation, age, and past history. The following discussion is by no means an all-inclusive discussion of PT interventions; it should be used as an overview and guide.

TERMINOLOGY

Recently there has been a call to describe individuals with disabilities in terms of *enablement* models instead of *disablement* models. In the past, the **Nagi model of disablement** (Figure 3-1) has been widely used to describe patients and the effect of their injuries or pathologies on their livelihood. The new movement has adopted the **World Health Organization model of enablement**: International Classification of Functioning, Disability, and Health (ICF) (Figure 3-2).[1] This model describes how the patient's injury or pathology impacts his or her activities and participation in society. The components of the framework are body structure and function, activity limitations and participation restrictions, and environmental factors. Although the cases in this text follow the Guide to Physical Therapy

Practice format, the ICF framework has been included following each case to demonstrate for the reader how each case can be analyzed from an enablement model. Treatment goals and interventions are then formulated from the enablement perspective, with the patient and/or family actively participating in the formulation of goals.

GOALS OF INTERVENTION

Regardless of the age of the child, goals of intervention must be established before treatment begins. Goals should be functional and realistic. A goal becomes meaningful only when it is relevant to the child's lifestyle. For instance, a child and therapist should not be working on increasing active range of motion merely for the sake of increased range. What will the child be able to do differently or more efficiently with increased range of motion? Will the child's gait pattern improve? Will the distance of ambulation increase? Thus the goal of improving knee extension by 10 degrees is no longer acceptable in pediatric practice. Why does the child need this increased range of motion? The goal should reflect what the child will be accomplishing with improved range of motion. A more appropriate goal would be that the child will ambulate a certain distance in order to play with peers or ambulate to class.

Another example regards head control. Many a goal has been written stating the child will independently hold the head up for a certain amount of time. If the goal is limited to maintaining an upright head position, it can be accomplished with standard head rest/support equipment. The goal is met simply and without extended therapy. It is doubtful that this is the

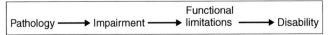

Figure 3-1 Schematic representation of the four components of health status and the process of disablement in the model developed by Nagi.

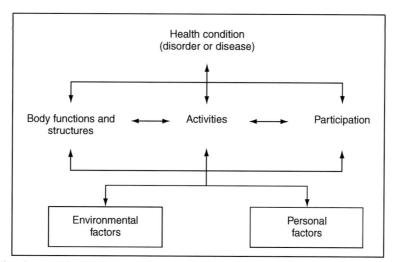

Figure 3-2 Interactions between the components of the International Classification of Function. (From World Health Organization: *International Classification of Functioning, Disability, and Health (ICF)*, Geneva, 2001, WHO.)

actual goal of a child or parent. The actual goal would be that the child can hold the head up to participate in an activity/program, communicate with family or peers, or navigate through an environment. A more meaningful statement of the goal might be that the child will be able to maintain an upright head posture in order to drive a power chair safely or participate in dinner.

Goals are meant to be met, modified, or changed. Reassessment of the goals should occur somewhat frequently. The goals will either be met or require revision. Revision or elimination of the goal should occur when it becomes evident that the goal will not be met. Many times it becomes apparent that what at one time appeared to be a relevant functional goal is no longer so. When this occurs, the goal should be revised to make it more applicable.

INTERVENTION PLAN

After goals have been established, an intervention plan can be devised. The intervention plan will reflect the child's current needs and capabilities. Interventions should be based on what is appropriate for both the child and the family. It is best to first think about intervention based on the age of the child and the pathology. If the injury is acute in nature (flare-up in arthritis, soft tissue shortening secondary to immobilization, torticollis, or an injury/surgery that requires gait training with an assistive device), then service delivery will look very different from therapy given for a chronic pathology (cerebral palsy, traumatic brain injury, Down syndrome, developmental delay).

For American children in the age range of birth to 3 years, pediatric physical therapy intervention may take place within Early Intervention, Part C, protocols. (Early intervention [EI] is discussed in more depth in Chapter 4.) Services delivered in this way must be family-centered. Historically EI services were child-centered and mostly focused on the specific needs of the child. Family-centered service broadens the scope of the interventions and focuses therapy on the family and the child's position in the family. Therapists assume more of a coaching role, working with the child through the family.

Intervention should also be embedded in routines that already occur in the home or within the child's day. Thus lots of time and energy will be focused on teaching the family members how to handle, position, and interact with the child to get optimal performance from the child over the span of the day. Therapy goals are worked on throughout the entire day, not just at therapy-designated time. If a child needs to increase strength, then appropriate activities will be designed so that the child works on strength while participating in his or her regularly scheduled activities. Leg strength can be improved with squat-to-stand activities. If a container/toy is placed on a low table surface, and all of the pieces are on the floor, the child must repeatedly perform squat-to-stand activities to put all the pieces into the container. Likewise, if therapy is focusing on improved fine motor skills, pulling diaper wipes from a container will work on grasp-and-release movements. These are activities embedded in typically occurring routines. If the child needs to improve a gait pattern, the parent will be taught stretching activities that can occur at every diaper change, for instance. Ambulation can be built into going to check for mail at the box or cruising around the bedroom or kitchen. (A child will be more inclined to cruise if furniture is placed close together to provide ready support.)

Often the therapist must invest a great deal of effort in slowing down the caregiver to permit time for the child to practice movements/activities. Instead of letting the parent completely dress the child to speed up the process, the therapist should encourage the parent to allow the child to complete some of the activity—pulling the shirt over the head, putting the foot into the shoe, using pull-to-sit activities instead of always being scooped up. Thus the child receives more meaningful practice opportunities and in the long run learns new skills in the context of where they need to be applied.

As the child enters school age, the focus of therapy may switch from a family-centered to an education-centered approach. Therapies delivered within an educational environment must focus on improving school performance. Therapy services outside the educational system may continue to be more child/family centered. For example, a 6-year-old child with diplegic cerebral palsy attends school. The child lives on the second floor of a two-story walkup building. There are no elevators in this building. The child has difficulty ambulating up the many steep steps to his apartment. His school is in a single-story building without steps. If the family wanted this child to improve his safety on the steps at the apartment, providing practice opportunities would be outside the mandates of the school therapist, since there are no steps in the school building. Thus the goal is not educationally relevant. However, the astute therapist will think about the child's participation in school activities outside of the building, such as ascending and descending the school bus steps or the playground equipment. In this way therapy could focus on stair climbing, which is important to the child's ability to be independent and safe both at home and within his educational environment. Additionally, the family may choose to engage the services of a community-based therapist to work on noneducation-based goals.

After the therapist, family, and child (if appropriate) have developed goals, the therapist should decide what intervention technique(s) may be most efficient and effective at helping the child meet the goals. There are several types of interventions and differing philosophies. In this chapter several of the interventions will be discussed. By no means is this an all-inclusive list or a ranking of the "best" interventions. This chapter is designed to give the reader an overview of what is currently practiced, most commonly, in the United States. It should be used as a guide to build on as the therapist accumulates experience and breadth and depth of knowledge.

TYPES OF INTERVENTIONS

Common interventions include the following (Table 3-1):
- Neurodevelopmental treatment (Bobath)
- Proprioceptive neuromuscular facilitation (Kabat, Knott, Voss)
- Conductive education (Peto)
- Strengthening and stability
- Therapeutic taping
- Sensory integration (Ayers)

The basis for all treatments must embrace in some form the dynamic systems model of motor control and motor learning. This model explains that all components of a child's world must be considered and will be influenced by all systems working in concert or conflict with each other. Fay Horak wrote that humans accomplish tasks using interacting systems that work together in an integrated fashion with shifting dominance.[2] There are several physiologic systems, as well as environmental and cultural systems, to consider before determining the optimal intervention. If any component of any of these systems is not on target and not working in concert with the other systems, dysfunction will occur. It is up to the treating therapist to collect all the clues and decipher which component is not up to par, then determine if intervention focus should correct the malfunctioning component or assist the child and family to adapt and learn new strategies in order to function as independently and optimally as possible.

The physiologic systems include the *commanding system*, the *regulating and comparing*

TABLE **3-1** Comparison of Common Interventions

INTERVENTION	PHILOSOPHY	APPROPRIATE USE
Neurodevelopmental treatment (NDT)	Uses motor control to effect postural control and interactions between many neurologic and physiologic systems. Enhances the individual's capacity to function.	Children with cerebral palsy and motor disorders
Proprioceptive neuromuscular facilitation (PNF)	Strengthens muscle groups within diagonal and rotational movement patterns, based on developmental sequence and the sequential mastery of motor milestones.	Children with muscle imbalances
Conductive education (CE)	Views child as a whole child, using learning concepts, motor control/motor learning, and the group model to improve function. Learning movements and functional skills requires practice, intention, group motivation, and breaking down skills into task series. Uses specialized equipment to enhance child's orthofunction (ability to be functional and independent).	Children with CP, spina bifida, and other motor disorders
Strengthening and stability	Improved function through improved strength, bone density, joint structures, muscle function, and management of obesity.	Children with weakness and muscle imbalances
Therapeutic taping	Uses rigid or flexible taping to support and influence muscle groups.	Children with muscle weakness, joint instability, joint malalignment, and postural asymmetries
Sensory integration (SI)	Provides controlled sensory input to help children with sensory processing.	Children with sensory processing dysfunction; children exhibiting dysfunction in ability to take in and process sensory information, organize behaviors and movements, or formulate/plan/ and execute motor plans.

system, the *sensorimotor system* and the *musculoskeletal system*. In order to operate functionally, a person's commanding system must integrate and act on stimulation from the sensory system, the cognitive system, and the emotional system. The body also must be able to regulate and compare actions in order to modify and learn new skills. The comparing and regulating system includes the predictive central set, accurate knowledge of results, and adequate knowledge of performance. The body must be able to activate an intrinsic error-detection system. An adequately functioning sensorimotor system includes postural orientation made up of a working visual system, a working somatosensory system, and a working vestibular/proprioceptive system; the ability to adapt to the environment; sensory and processing skills; and motor coordination. The typical musculoskeletal system includes postural alignment, appropriate tone, intact primary sensory function, adequate range of motion, appropriate strength, lack of pain, and sufficient coordination.

If a child cannot utilize his vestibular/proprioceptive systems efficiently, significant delays in balance and coordination may result. The treating therapist must keep this in mind. A child who appears to fall frequently may do so in response to decreased muscle tone or decreased muscle strength. However, this clumsy child may be just as likely to have delayed balance and vestibular responses that prevent successful efforts to catch himself as he begins to fall; or she may never see the horizon as straight and the ground as being still. A child with vestibular/processing issues will not benefit significantly from a strengthening program, but will benefit greatly from a program that emphasizes linear swinging and vestibular training.

In addition to the physiologic systems, each child is influenced by environmental and cultural systems. Environmental systems include the child's primary living habitat, school or day care facility, neighborhood, and resources to function in these environments. Cultural systems include the family's traditions and beliefs, the extended families' traditions and beliefs (which may differ somewhat from the immediate family's), and known or perceived expectations of the child from society at large.

In order for an intervention plan to be successful, all the described systems that have an effect on a child must be continually assessed and monitored. Although a child may have a primary pathology or functional limitation, various influences from other systems may negatively affect the child and impact the primary impairment.

In the following sections several common interventions are described. Most require additional training and experience on the part of the therapist. Each intervention has unique principles, but the interventions also have overlapping themes. It is up to the therapist to determine, in light of the whole child and what is causing the relevant dysfunction, which interventions to use and when. Often several different interventions can be employed to provide the child and family with optimal experiences. The master clinician is able to adapt and modify interventions to meet the child and family's ever-changing needs.

NEURODEVELOPMENTAL TREATMENT

Neurodevelopmental treatment (NDT) originally was theorized by Berta and Carl Bobath. Since its inception in the late 1940s, the approach underwent a major shift of focus in the 1990s. Originally the approach focused on patterns of movement. Dysfunction of the movement patterns was thought to be caused by a loss of control from damaged higher centers in the brain. These lesions unleashed abnormal reflex activity. In the 1990s a shift from an orthopedic model to a biomechanical and systems model occurred. Current NDT theory embraces knowledge of motor control and looks at the effects of postural control as a result of interactions between many neurologic and physiologic systems.

The overall goal of management and treatment, according to NDT theory and tenets, is to enhance the individual's capacity to function. Intervention involves a hands-on approach when working with individuals with central nervous system insults that create difficulties in controlling movements, with NDT embracing several general treatment principles[3]:

- A child with cerebral palsy must be treated as a whole child with a whole personality.
- A good evaluation or assessment of the child must be completed.
- From the time of initial assessment, treatment programs should be customized to meet the needs of the individual child.
- The child's responses to treatment should be reassessed often.
- Realistic and reachable treatment goals are essential.
- Key points of control are used in treatment. Key points of control are parts of the body, typically proximally, where the therapist can apply light pressure to influence movement through the rest of the body.
- Teamwork is essential and must include the family.

In summary, pediatric NDT is primarily used to treat children with cerebral palsy and other movement disorders. However, aspects of the theory are applicable to many different clinical scenarios.

PROPRIOCEPTIVE NEUROMUSCULAR FACILITATION

Proprioceptive neuromuscular facilitation (PNF) was developed in the early 1950s by Dr. Herman Kabat and Maggie Knott. The goal of PNF was to strengthen muscles within functional movement patterns rather than straight-plane or anatomic-plane motions. These movement patterns are known as *diagonals*. Physical therapist Dorothy Voss added many clinically relevant techniques to the PNF patterns. The theoretical basis for PNF rests within the hierarchical model of development. Hence PNF theory is based on the developmental sequence and the sequential mastery of motor milestones.

Diagonal movement patterns are vitally important, because they represent mass movements characteristic of normal motor activity. The spiral and diagonal components are directly related to the spiral and rotary characteristics of skeletal muscle. Diagonal patterns can efficiently and effectively address specific problems of musculoskeletal weakness, and PNF is based on the principle that human beings respond in accordance with the demand placed upon the neuromusculoskeletal system. Two diagonals of motion exist for each major part of the body, and each diagonal is made up of two patterns that are antagonistic to each other. Each pattern has a component of flexion or extension. Each diagonal involves movement toward and across the midline or movement across and away from the midline and includes rotation with a flexion or extension pattern. When assessing the patient, PNF treatment protocols will look first at the patient's functional abilities. The identified stronger areas (agonist) will be used within the treatment session to assist the weaker areas (antagonist). Treatment movement patterns must be specific and directed toward a goal. Additionally, activity that will best develop coordination, strength, and endurance is necessary. Stronger body parts assist in strengthening weaker body parts though cooperation of muscle groups to achieve optimal function. For this reason PNF places great emphasis on using maximal resistance tolerated throughout the entire range of motion; by resisting stronger muscles, weaker muscles will receive overflow/reinforcement to help them become stronger and more coordinated. To initiate a movement, PNF technique may call for a stretch of the synergist. This provides the increased proprioceptive stimulation necessary to create a chain of muscle activity from a completely lengthened state to a completely shortened state, where the shortened muscle is the agonist.

In summary the PNF techniques work optimally in individuals with muscle imbalances secondary to spasticity, flaccidity, weakness, or pain. As a patient improves, coordination and balance activities can be added. Treatments tend to be intensive, using the patient's existing capabilities and skills without increasing pain or fatigue. The overall emphasis is on improving the person's function.[4]

CONDUCTIVE EDUCATION

Conductive education was theorized by Andres Peto in 1948 in Budapest, Hungary. It is an integrated system that allows a child with motor dysfunction to learn to move within functional skills. Peto believed that children with motor disorders could learn to move by utilizing their brain's plasticity. He believed that learning movement required practice as well as rhythmic intention, so he based his technique on the educational principles of group learning and motivation.[5]

Conductive education is based on four primary principles: a conductor, the group setting, rhythmic intention, and a specific task series for each functional skill. A conductor or a therapist trained in conductive education leads a session. The children attend in a group setting, with a typical ratio of 3 children to 1 adult. Skills are broken down into a series of tasks by the conductor. Children receive individual assistance as needed in order to complete the task at hand. The group of children practices each task until mastered, and then individual tasks are built into mastering skills. Rhythmic intention is the cadence set to time a movement or series of movements. Rhythmic intention allows children to replay the cadence and perform newly learned movements on their own. The cadence helps the child initiate a movement, sequence a movement, and complete the movement. Conductive education focuses on the functional skills a child needs to be optimally independent. This notion is also known as *orthofunction*. Motor learning and motor control principles come into play, and intensive amounts of practice time are part of conductive education programs.

Conductive education programs use specifically designed equipment that assists the child to perform a movement. Slatted plinths and benches allow the child to grasp between the slats for stability. Additionally, horizontal or vertical posts can be attached to table tops to provide anchors for children to use to stabilize themselves against gravity. Ladder-back standers and ladder-back chairs also provide graspable uprights to use while practicing ambulation. Conductive education programs in the United States are typically 3 to 4 hours per session, with sessions occurring 3 to 5 times per week. Given that generous amount of treatment time, there is wonderful opportunity to practice and use feedback and feed-forward mechanisms to master a task and eventually master the skill.

In the United States the trend is to develop transdisciplinary or interdisciplinary teams to provide conductive education programs, using conductors and therapists working together. Some programs also use a hybrid system that allows the child to simultaneously attend their educational program (school) and a conductive education program.

Conductors, who until recently could only receive training in Europe or Hungary, can now earn a teaching certificate with an emphasis on conductive education pedagogy in the United States, and therapists in the United States can receive additional training in the pedagogy of conductive education and be certified as well.

In summary, conductive education is an intensive motor training program that uses motor learning and motor control principles, along with educational learning principles, to teach children with movement disorders to move to their highest potential. This leads to the child being as functional as possible. Conductive education is not appropriate for all children. However, many of the principles and tenets of conductive education can be used successfully with children who may not be eligible for an entire conductive education program.

STRENGTHENING AND STABILITY

Current theories in rehabilitation support the fundamental notion that children with motor impairments must work on strengthening and stability. As seen in the previous discussion on theoretical interventions, there are several methods to accomplish strength training in children with pathologies. Diane Damiano has studied and written about the importance of strengthening for children with spasticity.[6] Appropriate weightbearing through the long bones helps to maintain bone density and joint structure. Exercise and strengthening are mandatory for a child with movement disorders to prevent overuse of the strong muscles, atrophy and wasting of weaker muscles, and obesity for children who cannot move as efficiently as their typically developing peers.[7-9] In each of the following chapters dealing with a specific pathology, strengthening techniques specific to that pathology are addressed. In this chapter different tools to help a child become stronger and more motorically efficient are discussed. These techniques may be used in addition to any of the other therapeutic techniques when working with a child and/or the child's family.

THERAPEUTIC TAPING

Therapeutic taping is used to provide support or input to a muscle group. Flexible taping is also known as *Kinesio taping*, while rigid taping is known as *Leukotaping* or *strapping*.

Kinesio taping helps to support weakened muscles or prevent muscle overuse. Kinesio tape is flexible and has elastic properties. To strengthen a weakened muscle, the tape is applied from origin to insertion. To prevent cramping or overcontraction of a muscle, tape should be applied from insertion to origin.[10,11]

Leukotaping (named after Leuko sports tape) is rigid strapping used to support a joint in normal alignment. Muscle facilitation for appropriate firing can be achieved by laying the tape parallel to the muscle fibers. Similarly muscles can be inhibited by laying the tape perpendicular to the muscle fibers.[12] Over time it has been demonstrated that bony remodeling can occur with appropriate and consistent rigid taping.

TheraTogs is an orthotic product designed to capture the benefits achieved with taping without directly adhering to the skin. The client wears a vest and shorts made of a neoprene-type material. With additional arm and leg cuffs, flexible or rigid straps can be added to the suit to facilitate or inhibit movements. TheraTogs are easy to don and doff, should be worn directly next to the skin, and easily fit under typical street clothes and diapers. The TheraTogs provide consistent input, essentially where a therapist would provide manual input for the child, in the absence of handling the child.

SENSORY INTEGRATION

Sensory integration therapy assists the child by using controlled sensory input to help children with sensory processing difficulties.[13] It is a theory of brain-behavior relationships.[11] The theory has three major components: normal sensory function, sensory integration dysfunction, and a programmatic guide for using sensory integration techniques. Ayers felt that learning is dependent on the person's ability to take in and process sensory information from the environment and self-movements, then organize behavior and movements in response to these inputs.[11] If an individual has difficulty integrating and processing, the result will be deficits in planning and executing movements and in motor learning. To remedy this dysfunction in motor learning, intervention within a meaningful context must occur to improve the ability of the central nervous system to process and integrate sensory inputs.[14]

In summary, sensory integration treatment encapsulates three areas: the theory, the evaluation, and the treatment. Each is vital in treating the child. A clinician can receive additional training in sensory integration theory and treatments.

Summary

Therapists have a plethora of intervention techniques available to them. It is the responsibility of the therapist to use appropriate interventions that promote improved patient function and independence. Interventions should also be consistent with plan-of-care goals identified for each child.

Chapter Discussion Questions

1. How can a child practice standing and weight shifting while in the family's kitchen/food preparation area?
2. Design two physical therapy–related treatment activities that focus on either dressing or feeding.
3. Describe the benefit of including typically developing peers within a treatment session.
4. Think of three community-based programs/resources that could be utilized by children/families to augment services.
5. What are the underlying foundational beliefs of NDT?
6. What are the underlying foundational beliefs of PNF?
7. What are the underlying foundational beliefs of conductive education?
8. How do strengthening and stability influence the ability of a child with CP to move independently?
9. How are TheraTogs and taping similar?

REFERENCES

1. World Health Organization: *International Classification of Functioning, Disability and Health (ICF)* (website): www.who.int/classification/icf. Accessed August 14, 2005.
2. Horak F: Assumptions of underlying motor control for neurological rehabilitation. In Shumway-Cook A, Woollacott MH, editors: *Motor control: theory and practical applications*, ed 2, Philadelphia, 2001, Lippincott Williams & Wilkins.
3. Bly L: *NDT theoretical assumptions*, Laguna Beach, Calif, 1997, NDT Instructors Group.
4. Voss DE, Ionta MK, Myers BJ: *Proprioceptive neuromuscular facilitation*, ed 3, Philadelphia, 1985, Harper & Row.
5. O'Connor J, Yu E, Guohui L: *Moving ahead: a training manual for children with motor disorders*, New York, 1998, Springer-Verlag.
6. Dodd KJ, Damiano DL: A systematic review of the effectiveness of strength-training programs for people with cerebral palsy, *Arch Phys Med Rehabil* 83(8):1157, 2002.
7. Chad KE, Bailey DA, McKay HA, and others: The effects of a weightbearing physical activity program on bone mineral content and estimated volumetric density in children with spastic cerebral palsy, *J Pediatr* 135(1):115, 1999.
8. Slemenda CW, Miller JZ, Hui SL, and others: Role of physical activity in the development of skeletal mass in children, *J Bone Miner Res* 6(11):1227, 1991.
9. Stuberg WA: Considerations related to weightbearing prognosis in children with developmental disabilities, *Phys Ther* 72:35, 1992.
10. Kase K, Hashimoto T, Okane T: *Kinesio taping perfect manual*, Albuquerque, 1996, Kinesio Taping Association.
11. Kase K, Wallis J, Kase T: *Clinical therapeutic applications of the kinesio taping method*, Albuquerque, 2003, Kinesio Taping Association.
12. Alexander CM, Stynes S, Thomas A, and others: Does tape facilitate or inhibit lower fibers of the trapezius? *Man Ther* 8(1):37, 2003.
13. Fisher AG, Murray EA: Introduction to sensory integration theory. In Fisher AG, Murray EA, Bundy AC, editors: *Sensory integration: theory and practice*, Philadelphia, 1991, FA Davis.
14. Long T, Toscano K: *Handbook of pediatric physical therapy*, ed 2, Philadelphia, 2002, Lippincott Williams & Wilkins.

RESOURCES

Neurodevelopmental Treatment Association (NDTA)

1540 S. Coast Highway, Suite 203
Laguna Beach, CA 92651
800-869-9295
www.ndta.org

Conductive Education Information

www.conductive-ed.org.uk

InterAmerican Conductive Education Association (IACEA)

PO Box 3169
Toms River, NJ 08756-3169
800-824-2232
www.iacea.org

Certificate in the Principles of Conductive Education

Governors State University
PT Program
1 University Parkway
University Park, IL 60466
www.govst.edu/cecert

Kinesio Taping Association

3939 San Pedro Dr. NE
Bldg C, Suite 6
Albuquerque, NM 87110
888-320-8273
www.kinesiotaping.com

Sensory Processing Disorder (SPD)

1901 W. Littleton Blvd
Littleton, CO 80120
303-794-1182
www.spdnetwork.org

Sensory Integration International

PO Box 5339
Torrance, CA 90510-5339
310-787-8805
www.sensoryint.com

4

Roberta Kuchler O'Shea, PT, PhD

Pediatric Therapy Teams

key terms

Individualized Educational Plan (IEP)

Individualized Family Service Plan (IFSP)

Interdisciplinary

Multidisciplinary

Transdisciplinary

outline

Pediatric Physical Therapy Environments
  Medical Model
  Outpatient Clinical Model
  School Model
  Early Intervention Model

Models of Service Delivery/Team Interaction
  Multidisciplinary Model
  Interdisciplinary Model
  Transdisciplinary Model

learning objectives

At the end of the chapter the reader will be able to do the following:

1. Identify categories of various environments of therapeutic intervention.

2. Compare and contrast the various models of intervention.

3. Identify the strengths and weakness of each intervention model.

PEDIATRIC PHYSICAL THERAPY ENVIRONMENTS

Rehabilitation and therapy teams are made up of several variations of members. General categories of team models include the traditional inpatient and outpatient medical model, the outpatient clinic model, and the school model, including (Part B) the early intervention model. Each of the models is unique in its nuances and requires different roles and responsibilities of the team members (Figure 4-1). Additionally, service delivery can be described in terms of multidisciplinary, interdisciplinary, or trans-disciplinary models.

MEDICAL MODEL

Medical rehabilitation teams typically refers to services delivered to a child during an inpatient stay at a hospital; this includes intensive care and acute care units. Medical rehabilitation teams can also function in outpatient clinic models, which include outpatient services at a hospital or freestanding clinic. Most pediatric clinics and hospitals treat children until they reach adulthood.

The *Guide to Physical Therapy Practice* recommends that specific coordination, communication, documentation, and patient/client-related instruction be provided as part of physical therapy intervention for all patients. Coordinated services can be provided between therapists working within a variety of settings. A benefit of hospital-based services is the availability of medical providers, specialists, and other healthcare providers. Depending on the system, a child can be followed by the same rehabilitation team regardless of inpatient or outpatient status. Typically medical rehabilitation teams (Figure 4-2) consist of physical therapists (PTs), occupational therapists (OTs), speech/language therapists, recreational therapists or child life specialists, social workers, psychologists, physicians, nutritionists, respiratory therapists, and nurses. Assistive technology, prosthetics, and orthotics specialists often consult with teams as well.

OUTPATIENT CLINICAL MODEL

Outpatient clinics may have PT, OT, speech/language, and social work as primary components of the team. Other specialists may consult with the team as needed. These specialties may include orthotics, prosthetics, nutrition, mental health practitioners, respiratory therapists, and assistive technology providers. Additionally, many PTs have freestanding clinics and practice as the sole practitioner.

Support staff and related services teams typically include PT, OT, and speech/language

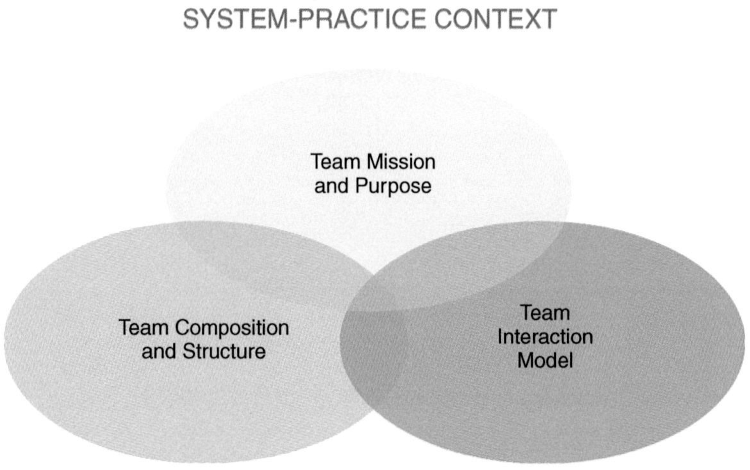

SYSTEM-PRACTICE CONTEXT

Figure 4-1 Model of team dynamics. (From Case-Smith J: *Play in occupational therapy for children*, ed 5, St Louis, 2005, Mosby.)

Team Mission and Purpose

Team Composition and Structure

Team Interaction Model

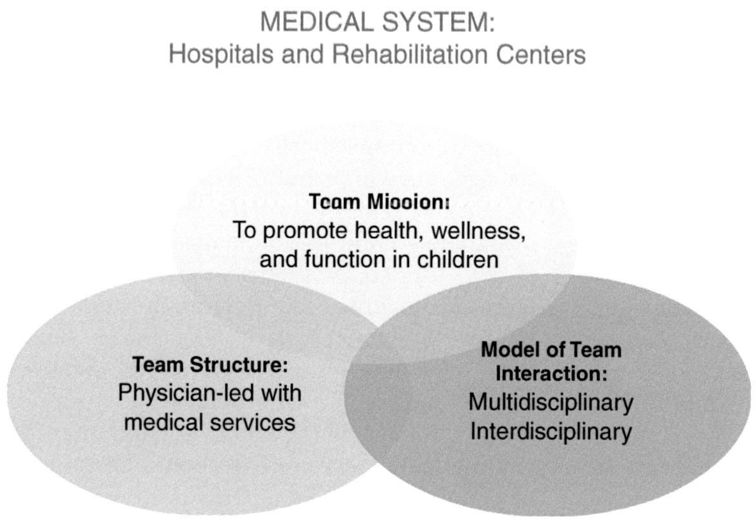

MEDICAL SYSTEM:
Hospitals and Rehabilitation Centers

Team Mission:
To promote health, wellness,
and function in children

Team Structure:
Physician-led with
medical services

**Model of Team
Interaction:**
Multidisciplinary
Interdisciplinary

Figure 4-2 Example of team
dynamics in the medical system.
(From Case-Smith J: *Play in occupational therapy for children*, ed 5,
St Louis, 2005, Mosby.)

therapists, vision specialists, hearing specialists, nurses, and workers in school systems. Ideally the team of therapists is transdisciplinary, where role release occurs and all therapists work on all the goals.

SCHOOL MODEL

Physical therapists in a school setting are only mandated to work on goals that will enhance the child's educational experience (Figure 4-3).

This aspect of the PT's role is often misunderstood by non–school-related therapists and parents and may lead to conflicts among the child's therapy providers, so coordination and communication across settings is vital. Each child receiving school services will have an **Individualized Educational Plan (IEP).** The IEP outlines all the services the child should be receiving during the school year, the amount of time services are to be delivered, and educationally

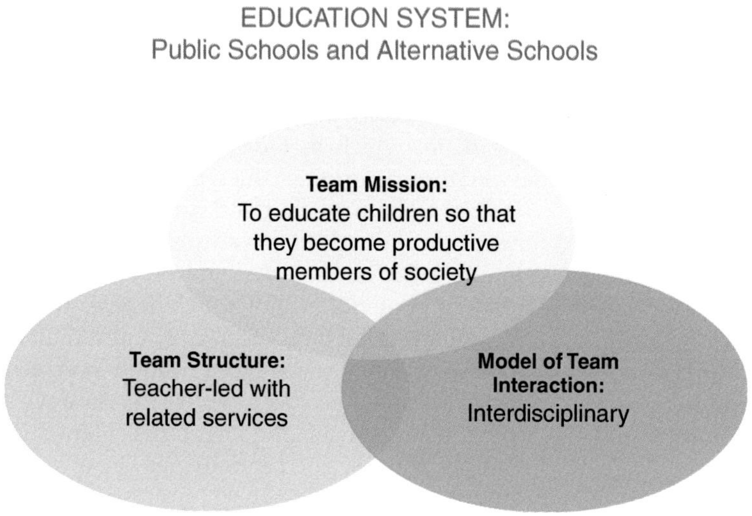

EDUCATION SYSTEM:
Public Schools and Alternative Schools

Team Mission:
To educate children so that
they become productive
members of society

Team Structure:
Teacher-led with
related services

**Model of Team
Interaction:**
Interdisciplinary

Figure 4-3 Example of team dynamics in the educational system. (From Case-Smith J: *Play in occupational therapy for children*, ed 5, St Louis, 2005, Mosby.)

relevant goals for the year. The IEP contains contributions from all relevant team members, including the child (if an appropriate age) and the child's caregivers. School therapists work closely with the school's other therapeutic service professionals in regular education, special education, and adaptive physical education. Let us revisit the example from the previous chapter: If a child living on the second floor of a two-story building attends school in a single-level building and does not encounter steps during the school day, a school therapist need not work with the child to practice going up and down steps. This skill would not be educationally relevant for this particular child. With good communication between team members, innovative treatment plans can be established. For example, in this case, the therapist might be able to work on steps going up and down the slide or onto and off of the school bus that would allow the therapist to work on steps as part of the school program and indirectly impact home functioning.

Federal legislation helped to mandate services for children with disabilities within the school setting. In particular, PL 94-142 (Education for All Handicapped Children Act of 1975) was designed to ensure that all children with disabilities receive a free and appropriate education and individualized educational programming. This law also guaranteed that children would be appropriately tested for special education services, that an IEP would be developed to meet the unique needs of each child with a disability, and that services would be delivered in the least restrictive environment for the student. In 1990 PL 94-142 was reauthorized and changed a bit. The change brought a new name to the law, now referred to as the Individuals with Disabilities Education Act (IDEA; PL 101-476). The new wording of the law used "people first" language and expanded available services to children with autism and traumatic brain injury and created research and technology centers.[1]

EARLY INTERVENTION MODEL

Early intervention (EI) services are mandated by guidelines set forth in Part C of IDEA. Early intervention specifically refers to children in the age range of birth to 3 years. Each state establishes eligibility criteria. Medical criteria designate a child as automatically eligible for Part C–funded programs in cases of certain medical diagnoses that potentially could lead to developmental delays (e.g., birth weight lower than 1000 grams, Down syndrome).

If a child is showing delays but does not meet automatic eligibility, the child may be eligible for EI services based on a percentage of developmental delay. This percentage varies from state to state, some states requiring the child to demonstrate at least a 30% delay, others ranging between a 25% and 50% delay. Therapists should contact their state's Part C representatives to determine state-specific criteria. Additionally, a therapist may create eligibility using clinical judgment. For instance, a child who weighed 1500 grams at birth may be showing some warning signs of atypical development, but not at a high enough rate of delay. The evaluating therapist could state developmental concerns in a clear clinical judgment statement and request service.

After eligibility is established, an **Individualized Family Service Plan (IFSP)** is created. The IFSP meeting establishes outcomes and related strategies based on the caregiver's priorities, concerns, and professional assessments. The team, which includes the family and all evaluators, determines the type and amount of services to be provided and how best to meet the needs of the child in a natural environment (Figure 4-4). The *natural environment* has been a point of contention and grand debate. It has been determined that a natural environment is not necessarily a place but a routine in which the child can be involved with typically developing peers on an ongoing basis. Hence EI services should not be delivered in a clinic

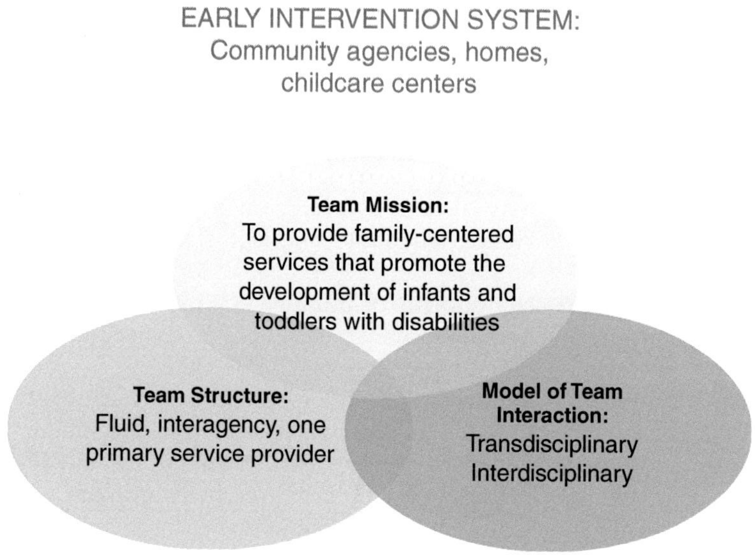

EARLY INTERVENTION SYSTEM:
Community agencies, homes,
childcare centers

Team Mission:
To provide family-centered
services that promote the
development of infants and
toddlers with disabilities

Team Structure:
Fluid, interagency, one
primary service provider

**Model of Team
Interaction:**
Transdisciplinary
Interdisciplinary

Figure 4-4 Example of team dynamics in early intervention systems. (From Case-Smith J: *Play in occupational therapy for children*, ed 5, St Louis, 2005, Mosby.)

room with the caregiver sitting in another room. Commonly EI services are delivered at the child's home, in the babysitter/day care setting, or in a center-based program. Center-based programs should include children with varying degrees of abilities and typically developing children who are not at risk for developmental delay.

Another important focus of EI services is how the family unit is coping with a child who has special needs. The family is an integral part of the team and vital to the child's potential improvement. Family education should include embedding therapy activities into family routines—having the child practice standing while helping to wash dishes, for instance, or incorporating range of motion (ROM) and activities to decrease tone into diaper changing or dressing activities.

MODELS OF SERVICE DELIVERY/TEAM INTERACTION

Therapy can be delivered in one of three program delivery models: multidisciplinary, interdisciplinary, and transdisciplinary. Each of

the models embraces a unique philosophy and set of expectations of team members.

MULTIDISCIPLINARY MODEL

In the **multidisciplinary** model, the team members recognize the importance of each member. However, the child receives services from one to several providers working in isolation while treating the child. Each discipline assesses the child individually without input from the other team members. The child and family are potentially exposed to several therapy services with unrelated goals and routines. Multidisciplinary team recommendations may conflict with each other and lead to confusion for the caregivers.[2] The providers and family may not consider themselves to be working as a team.

INTERDISCIPLINARY MODEL

The **interdisciplinary** team members share responsibility for service delivery. Child assessments occur separately by discipline; however, results are shared between providers. Goals are discipline-specific but are shared with other team members to form a single plan of intervention. The family may not consider themselves central to the interdisciplinary team. Team members implement their own specific portion of the plan. Collaboration between service providers occurs regularly, and some potential co-treatment opportunities between disciplines may exist. Hospital systems generally conform to the interdisciplinary model. Small interdisciplinary teams may also be established within the overall interdisciplinary model.

TRANSDISCIPLINARY MODEL

The most integrated of service delivery models is the **transdisciplinary** team model. The team members commit to work and learn across disciplinary boundaries. Families are integral parts of the team, and goals are based on the family's priorities and concerns in concert with the service provider's concerns. Assessments characteristically occur arena-style, in which the child is assessed by all team members simultaneously.

All disciplines work on all goals, and treatment interventions typically include strategies from all disciplines. For instance, the PT may be working on language goals while working on standing activities. In this case as the child participates in standing activities, the PT may also be encouraging verbalizations and communication development. In another example the child working on sit-to-stand activities may also be working on dressing activities. Hence, when the child is in standing position, he shifts his weight, raises a leg, and practices components of pulling on a pair of pants. Or perhaps when the child is in standing position, he practices buttoning skills.

Early intervention protocols and school settings encourage the use of transdisciplinary delivery services. Ideally, the family and one primary service provider carry out the program with input from other team members.

Transdisciplinary teams require a high level of training and experience to work effectively. Further, team members must be able to work together successfully. Box 4-1 lists a five-step process for problem solving that encourages all members to contribute and ensures that all solutions are considered.

Box 4-1   Steps in Team Problem Solving

STEP 1: DEFINE THE PROBLEM OR ISSUE
- The problem is defined clearly and objectively.
- The team develops a comprehensive description of the problem, including individual and environmental factors that influence the issue.
- Team members make a commitment to solving the problem.

STEP 2: GATHER INFORMATION ABOUT THE PROBLEM
- Team members work to thoroughly understand the problem.
- Barriers and supports/resources are identified.

STEP 3: GENERATE AND CONSIDER ALTERNATIVE STRATEGIES
- Alternative strategies are formulated.
- Creative and divergent thinking is helpful.
- Team members identify as many strategies as possible to reduce barriers and increase supports.

STEP 4: DECIDE ON AND IMPLEMENT A STRATEGY
- Each alternative is discussed, with team members identifying the resources needed and assessing the probability of success.
- Consensus decision making is used.
- Once a decision has been made, a plan is developed for achieving the solution.
- The plan identifies specific action, the team members responsible, and a timeline for implementation.

STEP 5: EVALUATE THE SUCCESS OF THE PLAN
- The team determines whether the strategies were correctly implemented. If they were, the outcome of each strategy is evaluated.
- If the outcome does not meet the goals, the barriers are analyzed, new approaches are generated, an alternative strategy is selected, and a new plan is developed.

Data from Johnson DW, Johnson FP: *Joining together: group theory and group skills*, ed 4, Englewood Cliffs, NJ, 1994, Prentice-Hall; and Rainforth B, York-Barr J: *Collaborative teams for students with severe disabilities: integrating therapy and education services*, ed 2, Baltimore, 1997, Brookes.

Chapter Discussion Questions

1. Why is the caregiver/family the primary member of the therapeutic team?
2. Identify two ways that interdisciplinary teams differ from transdisciplinary teams.
3. Justify why transdisciplinary teams can be more effective or efficient than multidisciplinary teams.
4. Identify mandated limitations for school-based therapists.
5. How does the concept of the Individualized Family Service Plan (IFSP) differ from the Individualized Educational Plan (IEP)?
6. Describe the benefit of including typically developing peers within a treatment session.
7. Think of three community-based programs/resources that could be utilized by children/families to augment services.
8. Identify the strengths and weaknesses of multidisciplinary, interdisciplinary, and transdisciplinary teams.

REFERENCES

1. Accardo PJ, Whitman BY: *Dictionary of developmental disabilities terminology*, Baltimore, 1996, Paul H Brookes.
2. Johnson LJ, Gallagher RJ, LaMontagne MJ, and others: *Meeting EI challenges: issues from birth to three*, ed 2, Baltimore, 1994, Paul H Brookes.

RESOURCES

American Physical Therapy Association (APTA)
www.apta.org

Pediatric Section of the APTA
www.pediatricapta.org

Neurology Section of the APTA
www.neuropt.org

Individuals with Disabilities Education Act homepage
www.ed.gov/policy/speced/guid/idea/idea2004.html

Office of Special Education Programs (OSEP) homepage
www.ed.gov/about/offices/list/osers/osep/index.html

Part TWO

Neurologic and Muscular Disorders

Chapter 5

Christina Odeh, PT, MHS

Cerebral Palsy

Guide Pattern 5C: Impaired Motor Function and Sensory Integrity Associated with Non-Progressive Disorders of the Central Nervous System—Congenital Origin or Acquired in Infancy or Childhood

key terms

Cerebral palsy

Diplegia

Gross Motor Functional
  Classification

Hemiparesis

Hypertonia

Hypotonia

Spasticity

Spastic quadriplegia

Tetraparesis

Triplegia

outline

learning objectives

At the end of the chapter the reader will be able to do the following:

1. Understand the etiology and causes of cerebral palsy.

2. Identify the various types of cerebral palsy and their characteristics.

3. Understand the various sensory, medical, and cognitive problems associated with cerebral palsy.

4. Understand the role of evaluation and ongoing assessment in the treatment of a child with cerebral palsy.

5. Identify appropriate treatment strategies for the entire age span of a child with cerebral palsy.

6. Understand the roles of other healthcare professionals in the management of a child with cerebral palsy.

7. Be familiar with the various assistive technologies that may be used for intervention.

DEFINITION

Cerebral palsy (CP) is a permanent, non-progressive neurologic disorder of motor function. In other words, *cerebral palsy* is a broad term used to describe a group of chronic conditions impairing control of posture and movement. Motor disturbances appear in the first few years of life and generally do not worsen until later in life. Cerebral palsy is a result of faulty development, injury, or damage to motor areas in the brain, disrupting the brain's ability to control movement and posture. Early signs of CP usually appear before 3 years of age. Some characteristic signs may be spasticity, muscle weakness, ataxia, rigidity, or atypical movement patterns. Infants with CP are frequently slow to reach developmental motor milestones.

Cerebral palsy affects joint motion, muscle strength, balance, and coordination (Figure 5-1). These problems are first noted in early childhood and continue into adult life. The muscles of speech, swallowing, and breathing may be involved. Intellectual disabilities (mental retardation) and seizures can also occur, but these problems are not always present. There are about 500,000 persons who have CP in the United States, and a 2002 estimate of the cost of care for these individuals was $8.2 billion.[1-3]

PATHOLOGY

Cerebral palsy is a medical condition caused by a permanent brain insult during pregnancy (prenatal), delivery (perinatal), or shortly after

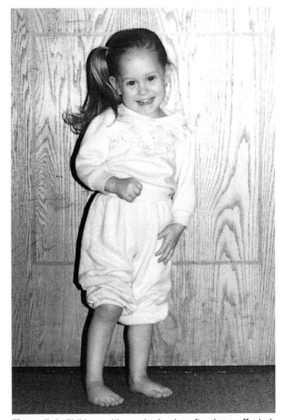

Figure 5-1 Children with cerebral palsy often have affected joint motion, muscle strength, balance, and coordination. (From Zitelli BJ, Davis HW: *Atlas of pediatric physical diagnosis*, ed 5, Philadelphia, 2007, Mosby.)

birth (postnatal). Premature birth is associated with an increased risk of CP. Brain damage may be traced to several factors, depending on the type of CP, its onset, and the health history of mother and child. Prior to the 1980s, it was believed that most cases were caused by birth trauma. However, it is now clear that only a small fraction of cases are due to birth trauma.[4,5] Cerebral palsy is either congenital (present at birth) or acquired after birth within the first few years of life. In many cases the actual cause may be unknown.[6]

Congenital cerebral palsy results from brain damage during pregnancy or around the time of birth. Very low birth weight infants and premature infants are at increased risk for CP. Improved neonatal intensive care has resulted in increased survival rates for these at-risk infants.[7] Children born of multiple pregnancy (twins, triplets, or more) are also at increased risk for congenital CP. Congenital CP can be caused by a variety of conditions:

- Infection during pregnancy: a number of infections can affect both mother and child (e.g., rubella, cytomegalovirus, and toxoplasmosis). These infections can cause damage to the nervous system of the developing fetus.
- Jaundice: severe, untreated jaundice (known as *neonatal hyperbilirubinemia*) can result in brain damage and athetoid CP.
- Rh incompatibility: a blood condition that causes the mother's immune cells to attack the fetus, resulting in jaundice, which in turn may result in athetoid CP. Because Rh disease can be prevented with immunization of the mother at appropriate times, this is an uncommon risk factor or cause of CP in the United States.
- Oxygen shortage: if the oxygen supply to the brain is severely low during pregnancy or at the time of birth, the infant may suffer a type of brain damage called *hypoxic-ischemic encephalopathy*.
- Stroke: women who suffer from coagulation disorders may be at increased risk for stroke in the fetus. Premature infants have immature brain tissue that is susceptible to cerebrovascular injury as well.
- Toxicity: drug or alcohol use during pregnancy can result in brain damage.

- Bleeding: prolonged bleeding in the infant's brain shortly after birth can cause brain damage.
- Kidney and urinary tract infections: these infections in the mother can lead to brain damage in the fetus.

Acquired cerebral palsy results from brain damage in the first few months or years of life and can be caused by conditions such as brain infections (e.g., encephalitis or meningitis) or head trauma or injury (e.g., falls, automobile accidents, or child abuse). Several causes of congenital and acquired CP are preventable or treatable: Rh incompatibility, rubella (German measles), jaundice, and head injury. Although CP cannot be cured, early diagnosis and treatment can improve a child's chances of becoming independent.

While the cause of CP is often linked to maternal or child health history or accidents that result in brain damage, it has been estimated that 17% to 60% of all cases of CP have no known perinatal or neonatal complications.[3] Undocumented antenatal events may cause brain damage or increase the infant's vulnerability to future events. The prevalence of CP has remained relatively constant; however, its incidence in the preterm population has increased with the improved survival rate of very-low-birth-weight infants. Children with CP display a wide range of capabilities and level of involvement.

Cerebral palsy has been classified several ways, according to the quality of muscle tone or movement, pattern of motor impairment, and severity.[8] *Muscle tone* is the amount of resistance to movement in a muscle. Muscle tone keeps the body in a certain posture or position (e.g., sitting upright). Typical changes in muscle tone allow movement. For example, to bring your hand to your face, the tone in your biceps muscle at the front of your arm must increase, while the tone in the triceps muscle at the back of your arm must decrease. The tone in different muscle groups must be balanced for you to move smoothly. Cerebral palsy has been classified into types of muscle tone or movement: spastic (hypertonic), hypotonic, ataxic, and athetoid (dyskinetic). The Modified Ashworth Scale (Table 5-1) provides a standard method of describing tone.

Spastic cerebral palsy is the most common form under this classification. In most cases the involved muscles of the body are stiff and tight and do not allow normal movement. There is increased resistance to passive stretch, which may be velocity dependent (**spasticity**), and in many cases there is also the presence of abnormal neurologic reflexes, such as clonus, hypersensitivity to sensory stimuli, and hyperactive deep tendon reflexes. Hypertonia can be so severe that joint movement is difficult or impossible; this leads to abnormal posturing and joint deformities. Frequently a child with **spastic quadriplegia**, for example, may have increased tone and spasticity in the arms and legs but decreased underlying tone of the trunk and head/neck.

When children exhibit decreased tone throughout their body, they may be classified as having *hypotonic cerebral palsy*. Typically they will present with poorly defined muscles, decreased responses to deep tendon reflexes, and hypermobile joints. They also typically have decreased ability to generate enough force for a sustained muscle contraction. This diagnosis may be made in infancy or when the child is a toddler. As children grow, abnormal movement patterns that would place them in a different classification, such as athetoid CP, may develop.

A child with *athetoid cerebral palsy* typically shows signs of fluctuating tone, muscles that stiffen on their own to cause abnormal postures of the arms or legs, and/or writhing movements. Children with *ataxic cerebral palsy* have poor balance and coordination, and the gait pattern typically requires a wide base of support.

The second type of classification of CP indicates the pattern of motor involvement. Some children have weakness and poor motor control of one arm and one leg on the same side of the body. This is called **hemiparesis**. Many have problems in all four extremities, or **tetraparesis**. Another category, **diplegia,** describes involvement primarily in the legs, with little or no involvement in the arms. Less frequently there may be a diagnosis of **triplegia,** in which one arm and hand are virtually uninvolved, whereas all other limbs are. These two classification schemes can be combined for a more descriptive diagnosis such as spastic quadriplegia.

The third type of classification is a **Gross Motor Functional Classification** system (Table 5-2), which categorizes children by degree of severity or functional capability. This system provides a qualitative, objective measure of prognosis for gross motor skills. A child can be classified at one of five levels, depending on the child's skill level, not age.[9]

LEVEL I

Infants in this category can move in and out of sitting, floor sit independently, and manipulate objects with their hands before 18 months. This same child is able to independently ambulate before 2 years of age without an assistive device. By 4 years of age, the child can get up from the floor into standing without assistance.

TABLE **5-1** Modified Ashworth Scale

GRADE	DESCRIPTION
0	No increase in muscle tone
1	Slight increase in muscle tone, manifested by a catch and release or by minimal resistance at the end of the ROM when the affected part(s) is moved in flexion or extension
1+	Slight increase in muscle tone, manifested by a catch, followed by minimal resistance throughout the remainder (less than half) of the ROM
2	More marked increase in muscle tone through most of the ROM, but affected parts move easily
3	Considerable increase in muscle tone; passive movement difficult
4	Affected part(s) rigid in flexion or extension

TABLE **5-2** Gross Motor Functional Classification System

	INFANCY	CHILDHOOD	ADOLESCENCE
Level 1	Independent head control, moves in and out of sitting independently	Independent ambulation, rises from floor independently, manages steps independently	Independent ambulation, runs and jumps, reduced speed, balance, and agility
Level 2	Uses upper extremity (UE) support to maintain sitting	Continues to use UE for support in sitting, independently rises from floor, reciprocal crawling, ambulates with assistive technology	
Level 3	Maintains floor sitting when low back is supported, can roll and creep forward on stomach	"W" sits, may require adult assistance to assume sitting, creeps on stomach or crawls on hands and knees, may pull to stand on a stable surface and cruise short distances, walks short distances indoors using an assistive mobility device, sits independently	Community ambulators with an assistive device, climbs steps using a railing, uses wheeled mobility for longer distances
Level 4		Ambulates short distances, wheeled mobility in community	Uses wheeled mobility
Level 5	Limited voluntary control		Extensive use of adaptive equipment

By age 6 the child can climb stairs. By age 12 a child performing at this level is able to ambulate without assistance on all surfaces and can successfully complete more advanced gross motor skills. The Level I child can run and jump with reduced speed, balance, and coordination.

LEVEL II

An infant who is classified as functioning at Level II is able to maintain floor sitting, but needs to use their hands to maintain balance. This child is "commando" or belly crawling, pulling to stand by using furniture, and beginning to cruise before age 2. By age 4 the child continues to require one or two hands to balance in floor sitting, so the hands are not free to manipulate objects bilaterally in space. Transitions in and out of sitting are accomplished independently; the child can pull to stand on a stable surface (Figure 5-2). Crawling is accomplished with a reciprocal pattern, and ambulation can be accomplished with an assistive device. At 6 years the child can sit on the floor independently with both hands free, can get up from the floor using a stable surface, and

ambulate short distances without an assistive device. These children usually require an assistive device when walking outdoors and in the community until about age 12. They can climb stairs using the railing, but cannot run or jump. By age 12, uneven surfaces, inclines, and crowds are still difficult for these children to negotiate. For most conditions, they are able to ambulate without an assistive device.

LEVEL III

Infants are able to maintain floor sitting when their lower back is supported. These children are able to roll and creep forward on their stomachs. Between the ages of 2 and 4, these children often "W" sit (sitting between flexed and internally rotated hips and knees) and may require adult assistance to assume an optimal sitting position. These children creep on their stomachs or crawl on hands and knees (often without reciprocal leg movements). They may pull to stand on a stable surface and cruise short distances. They may walk short distances indoors using an assistive mobility device, but need assistance for steering and

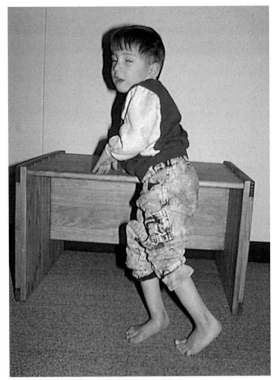

Figure 5-2 Some children with cerebral palsy are able to pull themselves into a standing position by using a stable surface, such as a piece of furniture, as leverage. (From Zitelli BJ, Davis HW: *Atlas of pediatric physical diagnosis*, ed 5, Philadelphia, 2007, Mosby.)

standing. They are able to roll and creep, but do not use reciprocal leg movements. By their sixth birthday, these children can sit independently in a chair, but require truncal stabilization to maximize hand function. Transfers require minimal adult assistance. Ambulation is accomplished using assistive devices for short distances, but adult supervision is required, and difficulty persists in negotiating turns and uneven surfaces. These children use wheeled mobility systems in the community and may achieve independence using a powered mobility system. By age 12 these children may accomplish higher levels of function but may still rely on wheeled mobility systems.

LEVEL V

Before their second birthdays, children functioning at this level have limited voluntary control of movement. They are unable to hold up their head or trunk against gravity and require adult assistance to roll. By age 12 these children cannot sit, stand, or walk. Adaptive equipment and assistive technology are used extensively to attempt to compensate for the child's motor deficits. Some children are able to use power mobility systems.

CLINICAL SIGNS

Children with CP sustain damage in the areas of the brain that control movement and muscle tone. While this brain lesion does not change over time, the clinical manifestations may change as the child grows. Many of these children have normal intelligence, even though they have difficulty with motor control and movement. The condition causes different types of motor disability in each child. Depending on the severity of the problem, a child with CP may simply be a little clumsy or awkward, or he may be unable to walk. In some children, the muscle tone generally is increased (spasticity or **hypertonia**), whereas others are abnormally limp (**hypotonia**). Speech may be

turning. By age 6 these children sit independently in a chair, transfer using a stable object, walk with an assistive device, and climb stairs with assistance. By age 12 they can independently ambulate the community with the help of an assistive device, climb steps using a railing, and use a wheelchair for longer distances.

LEVEL IV

Infants and toddlers in this category have head control, but truncal support is needed for sitting. These children can usually roll independently by age 2. By age 4 they can sit when placed, but they need both hands on the floor to maintain balance. These children need adaptive devices to accomplish sitting and affected as well. Typically, children with hypertonia in the extremities may have hypotonia in the trunk and neck region. Hypertonia can lead to joint contractures and postural malalignment.

Cerebral Palsy Clinical Signs

- Difficulty with motor control and movement
- Difficulty maintaining normal posture
- Affected tone
- Affected speech

Signs of CP typically include involuntary movements, difficulty with fine motor tasks (e.g., writing or using scissors), and difficulty with gross motor skills such as maintaining balance, sitting, crawling, or walking. The symptoms differ from person to person and may change over time. Because there are many different types of CP and the severity of the disability can vary tremendously, there is a wide range of signs and symptoms to consider when making the diagnosis. The primary clue that a child might have CP is a delay in achieving developmental motor milestones such as learning to roll over, sit, crawl, smile, or walk. Some specific warning signs are given in Table 5-3.

DIAGNOSIS OF CEREBRAL PALSY

Doctors typically diagnose CP by testing motor skills and reflexes, looking into medical history, and employing a variety of specialized tests, such as magnetic resonance imaging (MRI). If parents have any concerns about their child's development, they are encouraged to talk to their pediatrician at routine wellness visits. However, because children's rates of development vary widely, it is sometimes difficult to make a definite diagnosis of mild CP in the first year or two of life. Often the child may be labeled as *developmentally delayed* and referred for early intervention services. A consultation from a developmental

TABLE 5-3 Common Warning Signs of Cerebral Palsy

AGE OF INFANT	SIGNS
Over 2 months	Head lags with pull to sit
	Muscles or joint movement feels stiff
	Generally feels floppy, hypotonic, or joints are hypermobile
	Extensor tendencies: the child seems to overextend the back and neck, constantly acts as if he or she is pushing away from you when held in a cradled position
	Legs may get stiff and they cross or "scissor" when the child is picked up
Over 6 months	Continues to have the asymmetric tonic neck reflex
	Reaches out with only one hand while keeping the other fisted
Over 10 months	Crawls in a lopsided manner, pushing off with one hand and leg while dragging the opposite hand and leg
	Scoots around on buttocks or hops on knees, but does not crawl on all fours

pediatrician or pediatric neurologist may be recommended to assist in the diagnosis. A CT scan or MRI of the head may also be recommended to determine whether a brain abnormality exists. Even when a firm diagnosis is made during these early years, it often is difficult to predict how severe the disability will be in the future. However, usually by 4 years of age, there is enough information to predict accurately how a child will function in years to come.

SECONDARY CONDITIONS

The disabilities associated with CP can vary greatly in severity. For example, one child with mild CP may have no obvious impairment other than a slight lack of coordination, while another with a severe form may be unable to walk, talk, see, or feed himself. Some children with CP are also affected by other medical disorders, including seizures or mental impairment. However, CP does not always cause profound impairment. This section will outline some common associated problems with CP.

MENTAL RETARDATION

An estimated 30% of children with CP have problems with intellectual functioning (thinking, problem solving). Many are classified as *mentally retarded*, while others have average abilities with some learning disorders.

SEIZURES

One out of every three individuals with CP has or will develop seizures. Some children start having seizures years after the brain is damaged. There are many different types of seizures that may occur, and these are discussed in another chapter. Fortunately, in most cases these seizures can usually be controlled with anticonvulsant medications.

VISION IMPAIRMENTS

The coordination of the eye muscles is often affected by the brain damage causing CP. More than three out of four children with CP have *strabismus*, a problem with one eye turning in or out, with or without nearsightedness. If this problem is not corrected early, the vision in the affected eye will get worse and eventually will be lost permanently. Approximately 20% to 40% of children with CP develop visual perceptual problems. This makes it extremely important to encourage families to have their child's eyes checked.

ORTHOPEDIC ISSUES

In most cases a decrease in a child's joint range of motion is detected first; the decrease may be functional or fixed. This decrease in range of motion at the joint is most often caused by unequal tone, spasticity, or muscle tension. A functional shortening is generally caused by increased tone and passive resistance to stretch or irritability of the child (which can be an active resistance to the stretch); it may be positionally dependent. A fixed-muscle shortening is referred to as a *contracture*. An orthopedic surgeon should be consulted if a contracture is noticed. If untreated, contractures may lead to other orthopedic deformities, such as hip subluxation or dislocation, scoliosis, foot equinus, equinovarus, and moderate to severe functional limitations of the upper and lower extremities. Of those children with hemiparesis, many will develop a shortening of the involved leg and arm. The difference between the legs is rarely more than two inches, but an orthopedic surgeon should be consulted if shortening is noticed. Depending on the degree of difference between the legs, a heel or sole lift may be prescribed to fit into the shoe on the shorter side. This is done to prevent a tilt of the pelvis, which can lead to scoliosis when standing or walking. Orthotics, splinting, casting, or medication may be used to improve joint mobility and stability. Sometimes surgery is required to correct serious orthopedic deformities.

DENTAL PROBLEMS

Many children with CP have more than the average number of cavities. One reason may be that it is difficult for them to brush their teeth. However, they also have enamel defects more frequently than normal children, making their teeth more susceptible to decay.

HEARING LOSS

Some children with CP have a complete or partial hearing loss. This most often happens when the CP is a result of severe jaundice at birth. If an infant does not blink in response to loud noises by 1 month, turn the head or otherwise respond to sound by 3 to 4 months, or say words by 12 months, referral for a hearing screen or assessment is recommended.

ORAL MOTOR DYSFUNCTION

Cerebral palsy is a neuromuscular disorder that affects the body's ability to generate enough force for a muscle contraction or maintain the proper tone necessary for good oral motor control. Often children with spastic quadriplegia, athetosis, ataxia, or CP that affects the whole body will have difficulty with tongue control, swallowing, eating, creating sounds, babbling, and talking. However, the extent of a child's oral motor dysfunction may not be predicted by their physical disability. A child may be severely impaired physically with spastic quadriplegia, yet still able to talk and communicate effectively; or a child or adolescent with CP may be able to ambulate functionally, but be unable to talk or communicate effectively.

PROBLEMS WITH SPATIAL AWARENESS

Over half the children with hemiparesis cannot sense the position of their arm or hand on the affected side. For example, when the involved hand is relaxed, the child cannot tell whether the fingers are pointing up or down without looking at them. When this problem is present, the child rarely will attempt to use the involved hand, even if the motor disability is minimal.

MANAGEMENT

There is no standard therapy that works for all patients. Medications can be used to control seizures and muscle spasms, and custom orthotics can compensate for muscle imbalance. Surgery, mechanical aids to help overcome impairments, counseling for emotional and psychologic needs, and physical, occupational, speech, and behavioral therapy may be employed.

MEDICAL MANAGEMENT

Because of the vast array of potential associated disorders, a multidisciplinary approach is necessary in the management of CP. A child with CP may be seen by a pediatrician, neurologist, orthopedic surgeon, physiatrist, optometrist or developmental optometrist, physical therapist, occupational therapist, speech and language pathologist, developmental therapist, audiologist, dietician, or other specialists to address their individual needs.

PHARMACEUTICAL INTERVENTION

Pharmaceuticals are used for a number of associated conditions, such as spasticity,[10] management of seizure disorders, or reflux. Treatment for the reduction of hypertonia or spasticity may include drugs such as baclofen, diazepam, and dantrolene. All of these drugs can be taken by mouth, but baclofen may also be delivered directly into the cerebrospinal canal through an intrathecal baclofen pump. Intrathecal administration is the preferred route because it does not produce the systemic side effects (drowsiness, dizziness, weakness, confusion, upset stomach) that occur with oral baclofen. Also, because oral baclofen does not cross the blood-brain barrier effectively, maintaining optimum levels of the drug requires larger doses, whereas much smaller intrathecal doses can produce the desired therapeutic effect. The intrathecal baclofen pump is surgically implanted under the subcutaneous fat of the abdomen and administers a constant flow of medication into the cerebrospinal fluid to reduce spasticity. The pump is rarely implanted in children under the age of 4, since small children lack the body mass to support a pump. Before implanting the pump in anyone, doctors typically administer a trial dose of baclofen to see how well a patient's muscles relax.

Injections of botulinum toxin are a treatment for chronic hypertonia in CP, spasticity, and other disorders.[11] Often pediatric physiatrists perform the Botox injections with or without the use of an electromyogram (EMG), depending on the location and size of the muscle to be injected. If the child has significantly impaired range of motion, he may be sent to a physical therapy team to receive serial casting 2 to 3 weeks after the injections to maximize the functional benefits of the Botox injection. Alternatively, some physicians may inject phenol into the nerve innervating the spastic muscle. The phenol strips the myelin from the nerve sheath and thus reduces the input to the muscle, reducing the muscle tone. Rehabilitative treatment may involve range of motion, active stretching, functional training, and strengthening programs.

Seizure disorders are also treated with pharmaceutical intervention. Children with generalized tonic-clonic seizures are usually first treated with phenobarbital, phenytoin (Dilantin), carbamazepine (Tegretol), or sodium valproate (Depakene or Depakote). Absence seizures are usually best treated with either sodium valproate (Depakene or Depakote) or ethosuximide (Zarontin). Initial treatment for partial seizures is often started with carbamazepine (Tegretol), phenytoin (Dilantin), or sodium valproate (Depakene or Depakote).

While many children have their seizures managed with a single medicine (monotherapy), some require more than one medication (polytherapy) for effective control. If seizures are poorly controlled, the dosage of a single medication is usually increased until either the seizures are controlled or the child is having too many side effects. At that point, either the medicine will be changed or an additional medicine will be started. Newer medications that can be used to treat seizures include lamotrigine (Lamictal) and gabapentin (Neurontin).

SURGICAL INTERVENTION

Surgical intervention may be used to manage various associated medical complications an individual with CP might experience. The most common use of surgical intervention is to correct or prevent orthopedic deformities, such as contractures, hip dislocation, hip subluxation, or scoliosis. Some children may undergo any of those surgeries or a tendon transfer to improve functional capabilities. Much less frequently children may have surgery for neurologic intervention; for example, a shunt placement and revisions if hydrocephalus is present in infancy or selective dorsal rhizotomy for spasticity management. Some children with CP have oral motor dysfunction, which impairs safe and effective chewing or swallowing. These children may benefit from a G-tube or J-tube to augment or replace their nutritional intake.

PHYSICAL THERAPY MANAGEMENT

The five elements of client management are examination, evaluation, diagnosis, prognosis, and intervention. The physical therapist is responsible for the completion of the first four elements prior to intervention by a physical therapist assistant. The *examination* should contain the following components: a history, a systems review, and selection and administration of specific appropriate tests and measures. The history should include any significant occurrences during prenatal and labor/delivery care, current health status, developmental milestones achieved, social history, and identification of patient/family expectations and desired outcomes. This history assists in guiding the physical therapist through a relevant systems review, which should include the physiologic status of the musculoskeletal, neuromuscular, cardiopulmonary, and integumentary systems and the child's overall affect, general cognition, primary language, ability to communicate, and ability to follow directions.

The history and systems review are analyzed to develop a hypothesis about the child's potential problems, impairments, and functional limitations so the appropriate tests and measures can be selected. There are a number of different styles of assessments that may be performed. A multidisciplinary assessment is a form of developmental assessment in which a group of professionals with different kinds of training and experience works with a child and family, directly or indirectly. Frequently a team of therapists (physical, occupational, speech, developmental) may perform a multidisciplinary assessment on a young child with CP. This type of assessment can be helpful, because professionals with different kinds of training are skilled in observing and interpreting different aspects of a child's development and behavior.

There are standardized assessment tools appropriate to examination of a child with CP during various stages of development. The Motor Assessment of Infants (MAI), Test of

Infant Motor Performance (TIMP), Alberta Infant Motor Scale (AIMS), Gross Motor Function Measure (GMFM), and Pediatric Evaluation of Disability Inventory (PEDI) may be used. An assessment of range of motion, reflexes, tone, strength, balance, and any atypical movement patterns should also be reported in the examination.

The next element of patient management is the *evaluation*, a dynamic process in which the physical therapist makes clinical judgments based on the information gathered during the examination. The results of the tests and measures are generally utilized to confirm the potential impairments, functional limitations, and disabilities of the child with a developmental delay. These potential impairments may be decreased or increased tone, decreased strength, diminished or poor balance, diminished bilateral coordination, decreased arousal and attention, and clumsiness during play. Delayed motor skills, delayed oral motor development, impaired locomotion, and poor sensory integration are potential functional limitations. Actual impairments and functional limitations will depend on the type and severity of CP and help to establish the physical therapy *diagnosis*.

Once the impairments and functional limitations are identified, the *prognosis* is determined. The prognosis will include the predicted optimal level of functional improvement, recommendation for amount of service, and establishment of a plan of care. The prognosis will depend on the severity of the CP, impairments, and functional limitations. The recommended amount of therapy and the establishment of a plan of care are the critical elements to establish prior to the start of intervention by a physical therapist or a physical therapist assistant.

INTERVENTION

Intervention is defined as the purposeful and skilled interaction with the patient/client, including coordination, communication, documentation, patient/client-related instruction, and procedural interventions. The PT intervention will address the identified impairments or functional limitations of the child. Clinical intervention should be a team effort and should never lose sight of the whole child. Physical therapy may focus on reducing tone, increasing range of motion, increasing strength, improving functional motor skills and mobility, and caregiver education regarding interventions, including positioning and handling issues. It is vital to the success of therapy that both the child, if appropriate, and the caregiver be fully educated in the interventions occurring in PT. If the family does not understand how to perform the interventions, carryover outside of therapy sessions will be diminished. Furthermore, great effort should be taken to embed therapy into the family's naturally occurring routines. For example, range of motion and stretching activities could occur in conjunction with diaper changing or dressing activities. If a child is working on transitional movements (sit-to-stand, standing, and squatting) the child's home environment should be set up to encourage these activities. Toys can be moved up onto a low table top or cabinet instead of left on the floor. The child can stand at the sink and help with rinsing the dishes or preparing food. Additionally, therapy might also focus on limiting or minimizing the child's disability within the community. This would involve identifying barriers in the home or community and recommending modifications that will make the environment more accessible.

Cerebral Palsy Interventions

- Address impairments and functional limitations
- Reduce tone
- Increase range of motion
- Increase strength
- Improve functional motor skills and mobility
- Educate caregivers
- Identify barriers and recommend modifications to make environment more accessible

PROGNOSIS

At this time, cerebral palsy cannot be cured, but many individuals with CP can enjoy normal lives if their neurologic problems are properly managed. Hypertonia is sometimes painful and can lead to functional limitation, disability, or, in severe cases, reduced quality of life. Although its symptoms may change over time, CP by definition is not progressive, so if a patient shows increased impairment, the problem may be something other than CP.

RESEARCH

Research suggests that CP may result from incorrect cell development early in pregnancy. For example, a group of researchers has recently observed that more than one third of children with CP also have missing enamel on certain teeth. Scientists are also examining other events—bleeding in the brain, seizures, and breathing and circulation problems—that threaten the brain of a newborn baby. Some investigators are conducting studies to learn whether certain drugs can help prevent neonatal stroke, and others are examining the causes of low birth weight. Scientists are exploring how brain insults (like brain damage from a shortage of oxygen or blood flow, bleeding in the brain, and seizures) can cause the abnormal release of brain chemicals and trigger brain disease.

The National Institute of Neurological Disorders and Stroke (NINDS)[12] supports research on brain and spinal cord disorders that can cause hypertonia. The goals of this research are to learn more about how the nervous system adapts after injury or disease and to find ways to prevent and treat these disorders.

Text continued on page 64

CASE OF A CHILD WITH CEREBRAL PALSY

EXAMINATION

History

Amy was born prematurely on January 25, 1997, at 28 weeks gestation. She was hospitalized for a total of 3 months. After her first month of life, a computerized tomography (CT) scan of her brain was performed. Enlarged ventricles were reported, and hydrocephalus was diagnosed. She received a ventriculoperitoneal (VP) shunt for treatment of the hydrocephalus and recovered well. Amy underwent additional tests and procedures for diagnosis and treatment. She was placed on seizure medication after an electroencephalogram (EEG) detected abnormal/seizure activity. She was discharged home at the end of the 3-month hospital stay and referred to the Easter Seals early intervention program.

Amy's diagnoses were spastic quadriplegic cerebral palsy, cortical blindness, and a seizure disorder. When she was a year old, she had bilateral tympanostomy tubes placed in her ears to relieve the symptoms of chronic ear infections. When she was 4, she was evaluated for VP shunt malfunction. A CT scan at the time indicated that her ventricles had shrunk or collapsed. Her neurosurgeon stated that the shunt was overcompensating, but the shunt was not removed.

Based on her initial outpatient evaluation at an Easter Seals clinic in 1997, Amy received physical therapy, speech, and occupational early-intervention services until she was 3 years old. She received the following equipment while at the clinic: Panda stroller (stroller base with adaptive seating), TherAdapt supine stander, Rifton table and chair, and bilateral solid ankle foot orthotics (AFOs).

She was transitioned out of Easter Seals and began services at an outpatient clinic when she was 3. At that time Amy's family had grown from one child to four. She had a younger sister who was born 18 months after Amy and a twin brother and sister who were born in early 2000. Amy's father was in law school until 2001 and initially attended all her therapy sessions. After he took the bar exam and began to work, he was unable to attend the sessions but visited occasionally.

CASE OF A CHILD WITH CEREBRAL PALSY—cont'd

Amy's mother worked full-time, but she attended therapy sessions whenever she had days off. Amy's extended family was extremely helpful in assisting whenever needed. One aunt in particular eventually became Amy's primary caregiver.

Tests and Measures

Amy was reassessed at the new clinic to develop fresh goals and a treatment plan. Assessment consisted of range of motion (ROM), tone and strength assessment, tolerance, and response to handling and various developmental positions, using clinical observations and professional judgment. The outcome measure used to document functional performance was the WeeFIM System, and the evaluator was certified to administer the test. Amy was dependent for all items in the mobility, self-care, and communication domains, with the exception of exhibiting maximal assistance in comprehension and social interaction. She assisted with rolling supine to side-lying or prone by bringing her nonweightbearing arm around to the front of her body, but she could not independently perform any transitions or mobility skills. Joint passive range of motion (PROM) was within normal limits, except for moderately decreased PROM of bilateral hamstrings and decreased PROM of bilateral adductors. Amy displayed poor head and trunk control. She kept her head turned to the right 75% of the time. She also had decreased left neck rotation and lateral flexion ROM. Amy did not actively bear weight in her upper or lower extremities and had spasticity of bilateral upper and lower extremities and underlying hypotonia, particularly in the trunk. She tolerated handling well and enjoyed being talked to by the therapist. According to the Gross Motor Function Classification (GMFC) Scale, Amy's functioning is categorized as level V—severely limited in self-mobility, even when using assistive technology.

EVALUATION

Weekly physical therapy was recommended. Amy also began to receive weekly occupational and speech therapy in the same outpatient clinic. She seemed frail and lethargic at times. Her seizure medications were adjusted; she was weaned off Dilantin and phenobarbital and placed on Topamax. Within 3 to 4 weeks, she appeared much more alert and interactive during therapy sessions. Her parents and caregivers were concerned with how thin she was, despite the amount of food she consumed. Amy underwent G-tube surgery to help increase the number of calories she ingested and improve her nutritional status. She was placed on a continuous drip of PediaSure while she slept. Increased care was required with feedings at night, as well as the care and cleaning of the surgical site, which would not heal. This placed an additional strain on the family dynamics. Amy spent at least 50% of her time with her maternal aunt and uncle.

Diagnosis

Amy's diagnosis falls into the Guide to PT Pattern 5A: Impaired ROM, strength, self-care abilities, mobility with need for assistive technology, and impaired motor function and neuromotor development.

Prognosis

Given the extent and severity of Amy's impairments and functional limitations, she will likely require extensive assistance to meet her daily needs. Ongoing weekly physical, occupational, and speech therapies were recommended.

DIRECT INTERVENTION

Coordination/Communication

At this time the family had been battling with the school system to provide appropriate care and education for Amy. Two school therapists and a teacher insisted that she was functioning at a "brainstem" level and refused to provide the services the parents thought were appropriate. Amy reportedly spent the majority of her time in school sitting/lying in a beanbag chair because she had outgrown the Rifton chair. Amy's parents refused to sign the IEP at the end of the 2000-2001 school year and requested independent evaluations to assess her cognitive, visual, and communicative capabilities.

Amy was referred to a pediatric physiatrist and a pediatric orthopedic surgeon regarding spasticity management and contractures. She also needed prescriptions for adaptive equipment. Various options to manage spasticity were discussed, but ultimately orthopedic surgery was recommended to lengthen the hamstrings and hip adductors to address her lower extremity contractures. Amy's parents decided they wanted a second opinion and

Continued

CASE OF A CHILD WITH CEREBRAL PALSY—cont'd

asked her therapist and other parents for recommendations. The same recommendations came from several parents and other physical therapists at the center: consultation with a well-regarded local orthopedic surgeon. The parents were concerned that Amy had also begun to develop a scoliosis, so the physical therapist agreed to attend the consultation with the family for support. After the initial consultation and an MRI were performed, several surgical interventions were recommended. They included bilateral hamstring, adductor, and hip flexor tenotomies, right varus derotation osteotomy, and pelvic osteotomy. These interventions would address the contractures, femoral anteversion, acetabular dysplasia, and hip subluxation with migration of 70% on the right. The physician concluded that with the migration index of her left hip at 40%, the contractures of her left lower extremity, the abnormal forces of spasticity, and her abnormal movement patterns, Amy most likely would eventually need the varus derotation osteotomy. He recommended she have both hips done at the same time.

The decision to consent to the surgery was difficult for the family. They really did not want to subject Amy to such an extensive procedure. However, the surgeon felt strongly that since he was going to perform the surgery, he might as well do it all now. Based on his extensive research and experience, the osteotomies were inevitable. Finally they agreed and scheduled the surgery. The day before the surgery, Amy's parents got a call from the physician's office. Due to irregularities in her preoperative blood tests, Amy's surgery was postponed until her blood coagulation levels normalized. After months of blood work and testing, they found out that the initial report was a lab error, and the surgery could go forward. In the interim (during the summer), Amy's aunt began hippotherapy and aquatics for Amy while she continued all other therapies.

Therapeutic Exercise

Amy's PROM was good, with the exception of her hamstrings, until she turned 4. She began to grow and "bulk up" after insertion of the G-tube. By March 2001 she had outgrown her stander and chair at home and had maxed out the adjustability of the Panda stroller. Increased tightness and deformities began to develop. Significant tightness was noted in her neck and bilateral upper and lower extremities. Specifically, the popliteal angle was 40 to 50 degrees bilaterally. She began to develop a "windswept" posture of her pelvis and lower extremities and would not actively bear weight on her lower extremities, nor would she take steps in her gait trainer.

Assistive Devices

Physical and occupational therapy was increased to twice weekly. Amy began responding very well to a light box that was introduced in therapy, and she was beginning to functionally use her vision. As a team, we also began to work on appropriate positioning and use of her left upper extremity for communication devices and switch activation. Amy's aunt became very involved in this whole process, purchasing any necessary tools or equipment that was not approved by insurance (e.g., gait trainer, light box, switches) and working with her on almost a daily basis. Amy began to identify pictures, letters, and concepts (big/small) with varying accuracy from 30% to 70%. With physical fatigue, Amy became less accurate.

PRESURGICAL GOALS

Short-term goals for Amy prior to surgery were:
1. Amy will long sit on the floor while maintaining head in midline for 20 seconds; maximal support at her trunk and knees in no more than 30 degrees of flexion.
2. Amy will activate quads in supported standing for 2 out of 5 trials.
3. Amy will sit on a bench for 60 seconds with upper extremities supported on a table and support only at her pelvis.
4. Amy will roll from supine to prone with moderate assist through her pelvis for 2 out of 5 trials, initiating the movement by lifting her right or left arm.

NEW EPISODE: PLAN OF CARE

Amy underwent extensive bilateral orthopedic surgery just prior to her fifth birthday. She was immobilized with a hip spica cast for 6 weeks. This was a very difficult time for Amy's parents. The hospital was about 1½ hours away from

CASE OF A CHILD WITH CEREBRAL PALSY—cont'd

their home, and Amy experienced some minor complications postoperatively. The parents alternated who stayed overnight at the hospital with her. She was hospitalized for a week. Amy's parents did not own a van and were unsure of how they were going to transport her from the hospital to home, so prior to surgery the physician's office assisted with the preparation for postoperative transport and care. Her parents opted to keep Amy home from school for the 6 weeks she was in a cast. They attempted to rent a handicap-accessible van without success and became concerned she would have be transported lying on the back seat of the car secured by pillows and seat belts. Fortunately Amy's aunt sold her car and bought a van that could be used to transport the child to and from the hospital and therapy. Amy's parents were able to rent a reclining wheelchair for her.

REEVALUATION

Two days after surgery, in physical therapy, Amy began weightbearing exercises as tolerated while in the hip spica cast. The therapists instructed her parents on care and hygiene related to the cast. One week after discharge, Amy resumed outpatient physical and occupational therapy twice a week for trunk strengthening and improving hand/arm use and head control. She also received speech therapy once a week. When the spica cast was removed, the orthopedic surgeon ordered PT 5 times per week for 4 weeks, with a decrease to 4 times per week for 4 weeks, then 3 times per week for 4 weeks. Amy's goals also changed postoperatively.

Once the intensive postoperative rehabilitation was completed, therapy continued twice weekly. Amy's aunt reported that Amy had begun to wake up several times during the night crying and had muscle spasms. Massage helped alleviate the spasms and calmed Amy. She began to see a massage therapist weekly and receive increased water/fluids through her G-tube, but after 6 weeks she was still having muscle spasms every night. Amy's aunt purchased Usanimals, a multivitamin from Usana Health Sciences. Within 2 days, the spasms had stopped completely and Amy now, more than a year later, takes a multivitamin daily and sleeps well through the night without muscle spasms. The most dramatic improvement postoperatively was Amy's ability to sit with her legs extended.

DIRECT INTERVENTION

Orthotics

While wearing the TLSO brace, which had been modified into a sitting brace, Amy was able to sit with her arms on a support surface while activating a switch and keep her head up in midline for short periods. She began to accept weight on her lower extremities, with active pushing approximately 30% of the time. With prepping and use of her TLSO, Amy has actually demonstrated full weightbearing with hands held for up to 5 seconds.

GOALS

After surgery Amy was reassessed, and her goals were revised as follows:
1. Once placed, Amy will long sit utilizing a TLSO with supervision for 20 seconds while activating a switch toy with her left upper extremity.
2. Amy will stand with bilateral knee immobilizers, AFOs, and a TLSO with upper extremities on a support surface and minimal cues to maintain midline for 10 seconds.
3. Amy will ambulate in her Pony gait trainer for 20 feet with assist to turn or avoid obstacles.
4. Amy will roll to left and right side-lying independently.
5. Amy will perform sit to stand from a bench with maximal assistance at her trunk for 4 out of 5 trials.

OUTCOMES

Amy responded very well to her orthopedic surgery. In an attempt to determine whether the surgical intervention and therapy had research-based evidence, an article published by O'Donnell and Roxborough[13] gave descriptions of the best sources of research evidence. According to these authors, the best sources of evidence are systems in which the latest professional evidence is integrated from an electronic health record with the client's current circumstances. In Amy's case a website, www.evidence.org, was searched without success in locating any information on children with CP.

Continued

CASE OF A CHILD WITH CEREBRAL PALSY—cont'd

The second best source reported was review articles. According to the review articles by Gormley,[14] the evidence supports the use of orthotics to minimize the potential abnormal positioning of the foot and contractures. The author also discussed the use of orthopedic surgery for correction of contractures and torsional deformities of the long bones (i.e., femur). Logan[15] discussed that diet and biomechanics are essential parts of the treatment of children with CP. G-tube surgery, orthotic use, and orthopedic intervention were all a part of Amy's care.

Logan[15] also discussed the need for therapists to have training in a variety of treatment options available and to approach treatment of the child as a whole. In Amy's therapy sessions, the clinic staff had attempted various treatment approaches. Over the course of the 3 years they treated Amy, they used neurodevelopmental treatment (NDT), Feldenkrais, massage, myofascial release, cranial sacral treatment, sensory integration and stimulation, and functional training approaches. The clinic's occupational therapist took classes on vision, and the speech therapists attempted several different modes of communication: simple sign language, vocalizations, eye gaze, switch activation, and assistive technology. Specific therapeutic treatment approaches are all lacking in true research-based evidence. There are no stringent research articles regarding the effects of myofascial release, cranial sacral therapy, Feldenkrais, or sensory integration on the functional improvements of a child with CP. There have been a few research studies regarding the positive outcomes of children with spastic quadriplegic CP with NDT[16,17] and

horseback riding,[18] but they lack quality research design, adequate sample size, and control groups.

On the other hand, outcomes of the specific surgical interventions (e.g., varus derotation osteotomy and pelvic osteotomy) in children with CP have been reported in several journals.[19-22] Surgical intervention for contractures, subluxed hips, and torsional deformities in a child with CP is well accepted in the medical community.[19-23] There is no research-based evidence regarding the combined surgical interventions as performed on Amy. She did, however, demonstrate a positive outcome overall, and the only surgical intervention that may be necessary in the next two decades is surgical fusion if her scoliosis continues to progress despite bracing.

ANALYSIS OF CASE USING THE ICF MODEL (POSTSURGICALLY):

Body functions: Lower extremity deformities requiring surgery bilaterally, hip spica cast, pain, decreased trunk strength, decreased head and neck control, decreased volitional hand/arm use, decreased communication skills, decreased range of motion.

Activity limitations: Decreased lower extremity weightbearing, decreased ability to play and interact with peers, limited independence, decreased sitting tolerance, difficulty with mobility.

Participation restrictions: Could not attend school, difficulty participating in family routines, difficulty in accessing environmental stimuli and playing with toys.

Environmental factors: Difficulty in finding transportation, limited resources, changes in nutritional vitamins, toys needed to be modified.

Chapter Discussion Questions

1. What are the hallmark signs of cerebral palsy? When do these signs begin to diminish?
2. Describe four possible causes for the occurrence of CP and the classifications of CP.
3. Provide details of the Gross Motor Function Classification System at each of its levels. How can CP be described by the medical community?

REFERENCES

1. Batshaw ML: *Children with disabilities*, ed 5, Baltimore, 2002, Paul H Brookes.
2. Campbell SK: *Physical therapy for children*, ed 3, Philadelphia, 2006, Saunders.
3. Davis DW: Review of cerebral palsy, Part I: description, incidence, and etiology, *Neonatal Netw* 16(3):7, 1997.
4. Accardo PL, Whitman BY, Behr SK: *Dictionary of developmental disabilities terminology*, ed 2, Baltimore, 2002, Paul H Brookes.

5. Korman LA, Smith BP, Shilt JS: Cerebral palsy, *Lancet* 363:1619, 2004.
6. Shelov SP, Hannemann RE: *Caring for baby and young child: birth to age 5*, New York, 1999, Bantam.
7. O'Shea TM, Preisser JS, Klinepeter KL, and others: Trends in mortality and cerebral palsy in a geographically based cohort of very low birth weight neonates born between 1982-1994, *Pediatrics* 101:642, 1998.
8. Palisano R, Rosenbaum P, Walter S, and others: Gross motor function classification system for cerebral palsy, *Dev Med Child Neurol* 9:214, 1997.
9. Rosenbaum PL, Walter SD, Hanna SE, and others: Prognosis for gross motor function in cerebral palsy, *JAMA* 288:1357, 2002.
10. KoKo C, Ward A: Management of spasticity, *Br J Hosp Med* 58:400, 1997.
11. Korman LA, Smith BP, Balkrishnan R: Spasticity associated with cerebral palsy in children: guidelines for the use of botulinum A toxin, *Paediatr Drugs* 5:11, 2003.
12. National Institute of Neurological Disorder and Stroke: *Cerebral palsy information page* (website): http://www.ninds.nih.gov/disorders/cerebral_palsy/cerebral_palsy.htm. Accessed July 10, 2004.
13. O'Donnell ME, Roxborough L: Evidence-based practice in pediatric rehabilitation, *Phys Med Rehabil Clin N Am* 13(4):991, 2002.
14. Gormley ME Jr: Treatment of neuromuscular and musculoskeletal problems in cerebral palsy, *Pediatr Rehabil* 4(1):5, 2001.
15. Logan LR: Facts and myths about therapeutic interventions in cerebral palsy: integrated goal development, *Phys Med Rehabil Clin N Am* 13(4):979, 2002.
16. Bar-Haim S, Harries N, Belokopytov M, and others: Comparison of efficacy of Adeli suit and neurodevelopmental treatments in children with cerebral palsy, *Dev Med Child Neurol* 48(5):325, 2006.
17. Kluzik J, Fetters L, Coryell J: Quantification of control: a preliminary study of effects of neurodevelopmental treatment on reaching in children with spastic cerebral palsy, *Phys Ther* 70(2):65, 1990.
18. Sterba JA, Rogers BT, France AP, and others: Horseback riding in children with cerebral palsy: effect on gross motor function, *Dev Med Child Neurol* 44(5):301, 2002.
19. Gamble JG, Rinsky LA, Bleck EE: Established hip dislocations in children with cerebral palsy, *Clin Orthop Relat Res* Apr(253):90, 1990.
20. Noonan KJ, Walker TL, Kayes KJ, and others: Varus derotation osteotomy for the treatment of hip subluxation and dislocation in cerebral palsy: statistical analysis in 73 hips, *J Pediatr Orthop B* 10(4):279, 2001.
21. Poul J, Pesl M, Pokorna M: [Bone surgery for unstable hips in patients with cerebral palsy], *Acta Chir Orthop Traumatol Cech* 71(6):360, 2004.
22. Roye DP Jr, Chorney GS, Deutsch LE, and others: Femoral varus and acetabular osteotomies in cerebral palsy, *Orthopedics* 13(11):1239, 1990.
23. Abel MF, Blanco JS, Pavlovich L, and others: Asymmetric hip deformity and subluxation in cerebral palsy: an analysis of surgical treatment, *J Pediatr Orthop* 19(4):479, 1999.

RESOURCES

National Institute of Neurological Disorder and Stroke
www.ninds.nih.gov

American Academy of Cerebral Palsy and Developmental Medicine
www.aacpdm.org

National Disability Sports Alliance
25 W. Independence Way
Kingston, RI 02881
401-792-7130
www.ndsaonline.org

United Cerebral Palsy
1600 L Street NW #700
Washington, DC 20036
800-872-5827
www.ucp.org

Easter Seals
230 W. Monroe Street #1800
Chicago, IL 60606-4802
800-221-6827
www.easter-seals.org

March of Dimes Birth Defects Foundation
1275 Mamaroneck Ave
White Plains, NY 10605
888-663-4637
www.marchofdimes.com

Children's Hemiplegic and Stroke Association
4101 West Green Oaks Blvd
PMB #146
Arlington, TX 76016
817-492-4325
www.hemikids.org

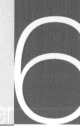

Chapter 6

Stacy L. Bauer, PT, PCS

Pediatric Traumatic Brain Injury

Guide Pattern 5C: Impaired Motor Function and Sensory Integrity Associated with Nonprogressive Disorders of the Central Nervous System—Congenital Origin or Acquired in Infancy or Childhood

key terms

Acceleration-dependent injury

Contrecoup injury

Coup injury

Glasgow Coma Scale (GCS)

Heterotopic ossification (HO)

Rancho Los Amigos Levels of Cognitive Functioning

Rotational injury

Translational injury

Traumatic brain injury (TBI)

outline

Definition
Pathology
Clinical Signs

Intervention
 Physical Therapy Assessment
 Physical Therapy Intervention

learning objectives

At the end of the chapter the reader will be able to do the following:

1. Identify causes of traumatic brain injury.

2. Characterize the brain injury by severity.

3. Describe the importance of the Glasgow Coma Scale and the Rancho Los Amigos Levels of Cognitive Functioning.

4. Identify treatment plan components.

Traumatic brain injury in infants and children (Figure 6-1) is a fairly common occurrence, although the mechanisms of injury are quite varied. In this chapter, mechanisms, incidence, demographics, and management and treatment of brain injuries are outlined. The effects of a traumatic brain injury can be quite devastating not only to the infant or child, but also to the family, including siblings, parents, and/or caregivers. Depending on the severity of the traumatic brain injury, the lifelong implications for a particular infant or child can be mild, moderate, or severe, in some cases requiring full-time nursing care. Understanding all the potential mechanisms and outcomes is vital to the successful rehabilitation of these infants and children and to the education of their families.

DEFINITION

According to the *Guide to Physical Therapist Practice*, Second Edition,[1] traumatic brain injury is found in the Neuromuscular Preferred Practice Pattern C and has an ICD-9 code of 854.01.

Traumatic brain injury (TBI) is classified as a traumatically induced physiologic disruption of brain functioning, resulting in partial or total impairments of one or more areas of functioning.[2] The areas of functioning potentially affected include, but are not limited to, the following: cognition; memory; attention; reasoning; abstract thinking; judgment; problem solving; information processing; speech and language; psychosocial behavior; sensory, perceptual, and motor abilities; and physical functioning.

PATHOLOGY

In the United States, traumatic brain injury is the leading cause of death and injury-related disabilities among children and young adults. According to national statistics, more than 1 million children per year are injured.[2] Based upon the Glasgow Coma Scale (GCS), which will be discussed at length later in this chapter, 5% of all children who present with traumatic brain injury are pronounced dead on arrival to an emergency room, 6% are classified as having a severe brain injury (<8 on the GCS), 8% are

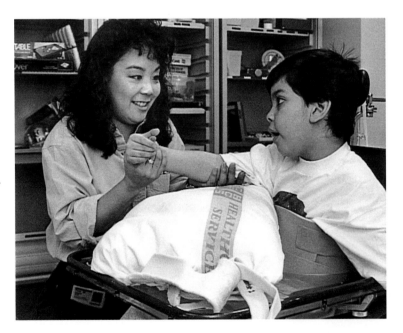

Figure 6-1 Although traumatic brain injury is a fairly common occurrence in children, injuries can be varied. (From Case-Smith J: *Occupational therapy for children*, ed 5, St Louis, 2005, Mosby.)

classified as having a moderate brain injury (9-12 on the GCS), and 82% are classified as having a mild brain injury (13-15 on the GCS).[3] Every year in the United States, more than 30,000 children exhibit a permanent disability following brain injury. Brain injury is also more common in boys compared to girls and is often attributed to the more daring nature of boys' behavior compared to that of girls, especially in the teenage years.[4]

There are many mechanisms of TBI to infants and children, but within these different mechanisms, the severities of the injuries are also quite varied. The potential mechanisms of injury include motor vehicle accidents (MVA), either with the infant or child restrained or unrestrained or MVA-versus-pedestrian collisions; sports injuries; anoxia; seizure disorders or epilepsy; shaken baby syndrome (SBS); cerebrovascular accidents (CVA); tumors/neoplasms; infections; penetrating injuries; near-drowning injuries; neurotoxic events; and hydrocephalus. Traumatic brain injury does not include brain dysfunctions caused by congenital or degenerative disorders or birth trauma. Falls and abuse-related brain injuries are the most common mechanisms of injuries in infants from birth to 2 years of age.

Shaken baby syndrome has increased in prevalence in the past few years in the United States as a mechanism of injury, and SBS is a leading cause of morbidity and mortality in infants.[5] Not only does SBS cause diffuse brain damage due to the shaking of the infant, it also results in bruising of cerebral tissue when it strikes the rigid, rough inner skull surface. The cerebrum is suspended within the cerebral cavity in cerebrospinal fluid (CSF). When an infant is shaken, the brain bounces back and forth within the skull, and the consequence is brain tissue injury or destruction. Violent shaking can also produce rotational "shearing" forces; these cause additional brain injury and often visual deficits secondary to retinal bleeding and/or detachment. Blood vessels that supply the brain can also be torn, causing intracranial bleeding. Shaken baby syndrome is discussed in more detail in Chapter 7.

With preschool-aged children, falls and injuries associated with MVA are quite common. Often children in this age group are not properly restrained while riding in a vehicle, or they are not closely supervised while playing outdoors and are struck when they run out into the street to retrieve a ball or toy. In the school-aged population (ages 5-11) MVA and MVA-versus-pedestrian collisions, falls, and sports and recreation injuries are the most common causes of morbidity and mortality.[6] Sports and recreation-based activities are also implicated in the most common injuries to children in the early adolescent and adolescent age groups and contribute to the high number of mild brain injuries reported each year in the United States.

CLINICAL SIGNS

The short- and long-term effects of these injuries to the brain are highly dependent upon their location within the brain, the age of the infant or child, and the length of time elapsed since the injury. Traumatic brain injuries involve both primary and secondary injuries.

Primary injuries are related to the forces that occur at the time of the initial impact; they can be grouped with respect to the role played by acceleration factors.[6] An **acceleration-dependent injury** is related to the effects that occur when a force is applied to a movable head. It may be either translational or rotational in nature.[6] A **translational injury** causes lateral movement of both the skull and the brain in response to a force applied to the side of the skull. As the skull is impacted, it rapidly decelerates, but the brain inside does not. Rather, it continues to move until it is stopped by the skull on the side opposite the impact. A **coup injury** occurs at the point of impact, and when the brain strikes the skull opposite the area of direct impact (secondary to the initial force/injury), a **contrecoup injury** occurs.[7]

Both coup and contrecoup injuries can cause significant brain damage. A **rotational injury** occurs when the brain remains stationary on a moving, rotating skull. As a result the forces on the brain are rotational in nature. Rotational injuries are related to shearing trauma, which also has been associated with diffuse axonal injuries.[8]

Secondary injuries occur because of processes induced in response to the initial trauma. These secondary injuries account for a significant amount of the overall damage that occurs with TBI. Examples of secondary injuries include scalp injuries, skull fractures, cerebral edema, epidural hematomas, acute subdural hematomas, subarachnoid hemorrhages, increased intracranial pressure, organ damage, and fractures.[2] Medical management of secondary injuries tries to minimize the damage caused by the primary injuries, mostly with surgical intervention, pharmacologic management, and mechanical ventilation. The main goal of all of these interventions is to sustain life and prevent further injury.

Traumatic brain injuries are classified as mild, moderate, or severe (Box 6-1), typically based on a standardized classification system utilized by emergency medical personnel at the onset of the injury. The **Glasgow Coma Scale (GCS)**, an observational scale utilized in emergency rooms and intensive care units following TBI, rates the injury on a newly injured infant or child.[3] This scale is used to project a future prognosis for the child's possible outcome. The items rated include eye opening, motor response, and verbal response (Table 6-1). Based upon a total from all three categories, scores of 3 to 8 are defined as a severe injury, 8 or 9 to 12 as a moderate injury, and 13 to 15 as a mild injury. A modified GCS for infants was created to accommodate for their preverbal status. This is not widely used to date.

Mild TBI is the most common type of brain injury and describes the initial insult relative to its neurologic severity. Concussions and whiplash injuries are often consistent with a diagnosis of a mild brain injury, but often in the sports medicine literature, they are not described as such. Mild brain injuries are currently increasing in number for both boys and girls because of increases in recreational and contact sports activities for children in the United States.[9] Certain activities and sports place children, especially preteens and teens, at risk. Common examples are boxing, soccer, football, bike riding, skiing, baseball, inline skating and skateboarding, and horseback riding. The use of helmets with many recreational and sporting activities has increased in recent years. Helmets are a simple, low-cost strategy that may prevent mild brain injuries, but mandating their use is not always greeted with enthusiasm by the general public.

| Box **6-1** | TBI Classifications |

MILD TBI

Early-appearing signs and symptoms: headaches, nausea and vomiting, blurred vision, tinnitus, dizziness, stiff neck, fatigue, and light and noise sensitivity

Late-appearing signs and symptoms: slowed or impaired information processing, disorganization, reduced frustration tolerance, rapid mood changes and increased irritability, difficulties retrieving previous information, increased sensitivity to noise, and reports of being overloaded or overwhelmed

MODERATE TBI

Loss of consciousness and/or posttraumatic amnesia of greater than 30 minutes but less than 24 hours and/or the presence of a skull fracture

SEVERE TBI

Loss of consciousness or posttraumatic amnesia lasting greater than 24 hours, a Glasgow Coma Scale of less than 8, extensive physical impairments with possible respiratory compromise, and a slowed overall recovery

TABLE **6-1** Glasgow Coma Scale

	EYE OPENING	MOTOR RESPONSE	VERBAL RESPONSE
6	N/A	Obeys commands	N/A
5	N/A	Localizes	Is oriented
4	Spontaneous	Withdraws	Confused conversation
3	To speech	Abnormal flexion	Inappropriate words
2	To pain	Extensor response	Incomprehensible sounds
1	None	None	None

Data from Teasdale G, Jennett B: Assessment of coma and impaired consciousness. A practical scale, *Lancet* 2:81-84, 1974.

Mild TBI is defined by: any period of a loss of consciousness, any loss of memory for events immediately before or after the accident, any alteration in mental status at the time of the accident, any focal neurologic deficit that may or may not be transient in nature but does not exceed a loss of consciousness of approximately 30 minutes or less, an initial GCS score of 13-15 after 30 minutes, and/or posttraumatic amnesia of no more than 24 hours.[10] Common symptoms of mild traumatic brain injury are divided into "early" and "late" symptoms.

Common "early" symptoms, described as those symptoms present at the time of the injury, are headaches, nausea and vomiting, blurred vision, tinnitus (ringing in the ear), dizziness, stiff neck, fatigue, and light and noise sensitivity. These symptoms can have an adverse impact on a child's academic performance and interpersonal skills. Because children with mild brain injuries do not typically have associated physical injuries, their behaviors in school or at home may be misconstrued as attention problems, increased negative behaviors, poor motivation, or a "negative" attitude.

"Late" symptoms are those that may appear days after the child sustains the mild brain injury. These can become apparent when the child is in a more challenging, cognitively demanding school and psychosocial environment.[9] These symptoms include slowed or impaired information processing, disorganization, reduced frustration tolerance, rapid mood changes and increased irritability, difficulties retrieving previous information, increased sensitivity to noise, and reports of being "overloaded" or "overwhelmed."

Moderate brain injury is characterized by: a loss of consciousness and/or posttraumatic amnesia of greater than 30 minutes but less than 24 hours and/or the presence of a skull fracture. As stated earlier, it is typically differentiated by a GCS score of 8 or 9 to 12. A severe brain injury is characterized by: a loss of consciousness or posttraumatic amnesia lasting greater than 24 hours, a GCS of less than 8, extensive physical impairments with possible respiratory compromise, and a slowed overall recovery.[2] These extensive physical impairments are often the result of brainstem or more diffuse cortical damage.[11]

With both moderate and severe brain injuries, common impairments are noted in the physical, cognitive, sensory, speech and language, personality, and behavioral domains. Neurologic, musculoskeletal, and sensory impairments vary depending on the location of the injury, severity of the injury, and age of the child. Disturbances typically involve limitations in independence with mobility, impaired strength, limited range of motion, impaired motor planning and coordination, vision deficits (including visual field deficits), decreased perceptual abilities, hearing impairment or loss, impaired sensation (including decreased kinesthetic awareness and proprioception), impaired balance (both static and dynamic), decreased safety awareness, and increased impulsivity. There is also the possibility of seizure activity.

The development of **heterotopic ossification (HO)** is a common risk for children who experience brain injury. In HO there is pathologic bone formation around a joint in the pericapsular space.[11] This often causes pain, decreased range of motion, and swelling of the joint. The etiology of HO is unclear, but appears to be caused by increased muscle tone around a joint.[1] Approximately 3% to 20% of children who sustain a brain injury will develop HO.[12] If suspected or diagnosed, HO should be treated aggressively by physical therapists, including the use of splinting if required.

Speech and language problems often result from a moderate to severe brain injury, and these include difficulty with articulation, fluency of speech, echolalia, aphasia (both expressive and receptive), and word-finding difficulties. Feeding and swallowing issues also commonly occur and require comprehensive assessment by a speech-language pathologist.

Cognitive impairments for children with moderate and severe brain injuries are typically long-lasting and in some cases very devastating. As with physical impairments, cognitive impairments vary, but often include arousal problems, poor/diminished concentration and attention, long- and short-term memory deficits, limited insight into one's own deficits, organizational deficits, executive functioning deficits, problem-solving deficits, and impaired ability for new learning.[13] Early in the rehabilitative process, sustaining arousal is of primary focus. Arousal is controlled by the reticular activating system, and with moderate to severe brain injury, this system is often impaired, resulting in difficulty with sensory modulation of both internal and external environmental stimulants.

Social/emotional and behavioral changes are also prevalent; these include increased anxiety, emotional lability, low self-esteem, increased restlessness, increased agitation, increased mood swings, excessive emotional shifts, depression, lack of motivation, lowered frustration tolerance, lack of inhibition and increased impulsivity, difficulty with peer relationships, and poor or diminished social skills. Often these children experience a sense of grief and loss.

Traumatic Brain Injury Clinical Signs
Partial or total impairments of one or more of the following areas of functioning: • Cognition and reasoning • Memory and attention • Abstract thinking • Judgment • Problem solving • Information processing • Receptive and expressive language • Psychosocial behavior • Sensory and perceptual abilities • Motor function • Physical functioning

INTERVENTION

Once an infant or child is medically stable in the acute care setting, deciding what will be the most appropriate next step for that child's recovery and rehabilitation is paramount. Physical therapy, as well as occupational and speech therapy, is often ordered in the acute care setting.

One option for furthering the child's recovery is transitioning him or her to an inpatient rehabilitation program. This option offers the child the benefits of intensive, comprehensive therapies. Depending upon the nature and extent of the child's injuries, the length of stay for this course of treatment is quite variable.

For children who do not require the intensive nature of an inpatient rehabilitation program, other options include day rehab programs, outpatient therapies, or early intervention therapy for those under 3 years of age. Day rehab programs offer intensive daily therapies in a clinic environment, but allow children to be at home at night with their caregivers and family. For many children, less often for infants with brain injury, day rehab programs may be a natural progression from more intensive inpatient rehabilitation programs. Outpatient therapies are often appropriate for an infant or child with deficits in only one or two areas and allow for specifically focused services for those deficits (e.g., outpatient occupational and physical therapy for right hemiplegia without cognitive deficits). Early intervention services, either home- or center-based, can be implemented for infants from birth to 3 years of age. However, early intervention services focus primarily on the achievement of developmental milestones, rather than rehabilitation from a traumatic injury. Several day rehabilitation programs are now accepting infants under the age of 3 for a modified day rehabilitation program, such as 2 to 3 times per week for 1 to 2 hours a day. More traditional day rehab programming often involves daily therapy for 4 to 6 hours a day.

PHYSICAL THERAPY ASSESSMENT

The physical therapy examination is a comprehensive assessment and testing process that leads to a diagnostic classification and in some cases referral to another medical/healthcare professional. Components of the physical therapy examination include a thorough patient history; systems review and in-depth assessment of the child's cognition, including

orientation, Rancho Los Amigos Levels of Cognitive Functioning, attention, alertness, memory, agitation level, and safety awareness; range of motion; neuromuscular assessment, including muscle tone, reflexes, neurologic signs, and posturing; muscle strength assessment; endurance; balance; posture; pain assessment; skin and skull integrity; coordination; sensory functioning, including tactile, auditory, olfactory, vestibular, visual, proprioceptive, and stereognostic; and motor control, including initiation, sequencing, quality of movement, planning, grading, termination, compensatory patterns, and asymmetries.

The **Rancho Los Amigos Levels of Cognitive Functioning** (Table 6-2) is a multi-level scale of cognitive recovery developed by the professional staff of the Rancho Los Amigos Hospital in Downey, California.[3] This scale is used for assessment of recovery, communication between medical professionals and facilities, and to measure change and progress during the rehabilitation course. Anthropometric characteristics; assistive and adaptive devices; circulation; cranial and peripheral nerve integrity; environmental, home, and play barriers; gait and locomotion; neuromotor development

TABLE **6-2** The Rancho Los Amigos Levels of Cognitive Functioning

LEVELS OF RECOVERY	DESCRIPTION
Level I	No Response—to pain, touch, sound, or sight
Level II	Generalized Response—to pain
Level III	Localized Response—Blinks to strong light, turns toward/away from sound, responds to physical discomfort, inconsistent response to commands
Level IV	Confused-Agitated—Alert, very active, aggressive or bizarre behaviors, performs motor activities but behavior is non-purposeful, extremely short attention span
Level V	Confused-Non-Agitated—Gross attention to environment, highly distractible, requires continual redirection, difficulty learning new tasks, agitated by too much stimulation. May engage in social conversations but with inappropriate verbalizations
Level VI	Confused-Appropriate—Inconsistent orientation to time and place, retention span/recent memory is impaired, begins to recall past, consistently follows simple directions, and goal-directed behavior with assistance
Level VII	Automatic-Appropriate—Performs daily routine in highly familiar environment in a non-confused but automatic, robotlike manner; skills noticeably deteriorate in unfamiliar environments. Lacks realistic planning for own future
Level VIII	Purposeful-Appropriate

Data from Rancho Los Amigos National Rehabilitation Center, Downey, California.

and sensory integration; and orthotic, prosthetic, and supportive devices are also assessed during the examination.

PHYSICAL THERAPY INTERVENTION

Based upon this thorough examination, the physical therapist completes the evaluation, synthesizing the data and making clinical judgments. A physical therapy diagnosis is then determined, in which the primary dysfunctions are identified and become the focus of the direct interventions. Lastly, the plan of care is created, through which the functional and measurable goals and expected outcomes are established. It is of great importance to include in this process the goals of the family/caregivers and even the child, if able and appropriate, to ensure their full participation in the recovery process.

A variety of treatment approaches exists for infants and children with brain injuries. Each should have an individualized program created that will make the most of their potential for recovery. Treatment planning should include addressing the identified primary and secondary impairments, with the ultimate goal of maximizing independence in mobility, self-care, and reintegration of that infant or child into their family and community. Allowances must also be made for preinjury functional abilities, age, interests, and activities, especially in the case of school-aged children.

Primary impairments are atypical components of any individual system that contributes to abnormal tone and/or secondary impairments. These include insufficient force generation (i.e., strength), spasticity (velocity-dependent increased resistance to passive movement), abnormal extensibility/range of motion, and exaggerated or hyperactive reflexes. *Secondary impairments* are postures or movements observed during the performance of a task; these are compensatory, due to the lack of the normal or adequate component. They include malalignment issues, such as increased hip flexion, adduction and internal rotation with knee flexion, and ankle dorsiflexion during "crouch" gait patterns.[12]

Once the primary and secondary impairments are identified, this knowledge can allow the physical therapist to create (and the physical therapist assistant to execute) effective interventions for treatment. Based upon the Rancho Los Amigos Levels of Cognitive Functioning score, if appropriate, coma stimulation interventions can be initiated to promote increased arousal with modulation, increased attention and following of simple one-step commands, increased eye contact upon request, and activation of trunk and extremity musculature with purpose and intention of movement. These therapeutic interventions can be progressed in difficulty and demand on the infant or child, depending on the child's responses and ability to maintain an alert, modulated state while receiving auditory, visual, tactile, olfactory, and/or gustatory input. Providing a variety of sensory input, albeit one type of input at a time initially to avoid overstimulation, will assist in activating various centers within the brain, increasing arousal, and promoting the maximization of the neural plasticity potential of the damaged areas.[14] Environmental modifications can also be made to ensure an infant or child does not experience overstimulation, especially during the early stages of coma recovery (Rancho Level I-V). Limiting outside noises (television, radio, music), decreasing direct lighting, modulating auditory input from staff and family members, and providing therapy in a small, quiet, stimulation-controlled environment are all helpful approaches.

Restoration of trunk and extremity strength, static and dynamic sitting and standing balance, and reeducation of developmental motor skills appropriate for the infant or child's age are vital treatment strategies for infants and children with brain injury. The restoration of motor functioning should include eliciting improved motor control, planning and sequencing skills, and addressing any sensory impairments, such as decreased kinesthetic awareness and decreased proprioception. Sensory integration treatment can be implemented if appropriate, including use of swinging, swaddling, various textures for sensitization or desensitization, and garments (e.g., Benik vests, TheraTogs) or weighting of the trunk or extremities to increase kinesthetic awareness. Along with the use of compression garments to increase kinesthetic awareness, Kinesio taping and the use of wraps such as Fabrifoam are other available adjunctive treatment measures.

Treatment interventions should also address any truncal or extremity asymmetries caused by the brain injury or by limitations in strength, power or endurance. In the case of an infant or child with a hemiplegia, the resultant musculoskeletal deformities that can develop if not appropriately treated can be long-lasting and lead to more aggressive treatment requirements in the future (e.g., orthopedic surgery). As the child's functional and cognitive skills improve, providing more challenging cognitive tasks while performing more challenging motor tasks will test the ability to multi-task a variety of sensory inputs. The child will learn to process various, possibly conflicting, information while improving motor planning and sequencing and executive functioning skills.

When range of motion or flexibility concerns are present, a variety of treatment interventions can be implemented. The use of orthotics, splinting, knee immobilizers, or serial casting are available treatment interventions for range-of-motion impairments.[15] Aquatic therapy interventions can also be very effective for the treatment of children with brain injury. If any hemodynamic or temperature abnormalities are present, however, aquatic therapy is contraindicated. For infants and children with more severe impairments, increasing tolerance to handling, sensory input, upright anti-gravity movement activities, and maintaining and improving range of motion for basic hygiene and functional tasks are appropriate interventions.

Depending on the appropriateness for each individual child, adaptive equipment can be utilized to augment functional mobility; it may be a temporary measure or provide modified independence for the future. Adaptive equipment varies from walkers, crutches, canes, adaptive strollers, wheelchairs (both manual and powered mobility), standers, and gait trainers. The decision to utilize adaptive equipment should be based upon the individual child's needs and potential abilities for recovery, with the goal of restoring the greatest level of independence given functional mobility. In some instances a wheelchair may be used temporarily to transport a child to and from the therapy gym until the child can ambulate the requisite distance with or without assistance and possesses the required endurance.

In addition to physical and sensory issues, physical therapy treatment may also have to incorporate strategies for modifying inappropriate behavior and emotional responses. Adaptations for cognitive delays and memory loss may also be an integral part of physical therapy.[16] Special education programs are well equipped to assist the child with community reintegration and cognitive therapy. In order to minimize objectionable behaviors and assist with regaining memory, therapy schedules, routines, and expectations should be consistent. Rewards and consequences must be carefully and repeatedly explained and reinforced with the child. Clear, simple expectations explained in a cognitively appropriate manner will benefit children after TBI. Schedules, personal identification, and family members' names should be written out for the child who can read. Older children may benefit from a "helper book" that records all daily routines, important phone numbers, and lists of family, friends, and therapeutic/medical staff.[10] Some children may require picture charts and color organization to assist them in remembering important facts and routines. Regular periods of unrestricted physical activity will help the child release excessive energy and impulsivity. All adults should be behavioral role models so that the child can reinforce learned skills; positive reinforcement of acceptable behaviors is essential. Referral to a behavioral specialist may be required if behavioral disruptions persist.[16]

Involving family and caregivers in the recovery process is vital to the infant or child with a brain injury. Their ability to participate in the therapy sessions and to carry over the treatment interventions to the home environment, or during nontherapy times if hospitalized, will exponentially influence and benefit the child's therapy process. It is the therapist's responsibility to include the family/caregivers and empower them to again feel as though they are effective caregivers for their infant or child with a brain injury.

Traumatic Brain Injury Interventions

- Provide a variety of sensory input to assist in activating various centers within the brain
- Modify the environment to ensure the infant or child does not experience overstimulation
- Use orthotics, splints, knee immobilizers, and/or serial casting for range-of-motion limitations
- Augment functional mobility with adaptive devices
- Incorporate strategies for modifying inappropriate behavior and emotional responses
- Involve family and caregivers in the recovery process

Summary

Traumatic brain injuries in infants and children are highly common and occur through a variety of mechanisms. The potential outcomes following brain injury are highly dependent upon the severity and location of the actual injury. According to Kraus and colleagues, at discharge 3% of those with mild brain injury exhibited neurologic sequelae, 94% of those with moderate brain injury exhibited neurologic sequelae, and 100% of those with severe brain injury exhibited neurologic sequelae.[5] With effective early treatment, the functional abilities of these children can be highly improved. Treatment for TBI should focus on minimizing primary and secondary impairments, reintegrating the infant or child into the family unit as soon as possible, and providing the family/caregivers with effective methods for interacting with the child.

Text continued on page 79

CASE STUDY OF A CHILD WITH TRAUMATIC BRAIN INJURY

EXAMINATION

History

R.J. is a 6-year-old boy who fell from a third-story window while sitting on the ledge at home. The screen fell out of the window, and as a result he fell, striking the concrete sidewalk and sustaining a traumatic brain injury. Upon initial examination in the emergency room, R.J. was given a Glasgow Coma Scale score of 5. He was diagnosed with a left temporal subdural hematoma, a skull fracture, and a fractured left femur.

He was in the pediatric intensive care unit (PICU) for 2½ weeks following his injuries, during which time he was intubated for 3 days and then extubated without incident. R.J. underwent open reduction and internal fixation of his left femur fracture, a procedure completed by the orthopedic surgeon. He had his intracranial pressures (ICP) monitored while in the PICU, and he received placement of a nasogastric tube for nutrition because of concerns about his ability to effectively and safely swallow. Physical therapy services were initiated in the PICU following the removal of the intracranial pressure bolt 8 days after his traumatic brain injury. After 2½ weeks in the PICU, R.J. was transferred from the acute care pediatric hospital to a small rehabilitation program within a specialized pediatric hospital.

He did not have a cast in place, but he was not to bear weight on the left lower extremity, under the recommendation of the orthopedic surgeon. This nonweightbearing status was in place for 3 weeks, at which time he was seen for reevaluation by orthopedics, and his weightbearing status was changed to weightbearing as tolerated. R.J. had developed excellent callus formation of the left femur fracture during these 3 weeks.

R.J. lived at home with his mother and 4-year-old and 1-year-old sisters in a public housing

CASE STUDY OF A CHILD WITH TRAUMATIC BRAIN INJURY—cont'd

project on the south side of a large metropolitan area. According to his mother, R.J. was developing typically until this accident and was not yet attending preschool, although she was planning on enrolling him in the fall. At the time of the initial evaluation, R.J.'s mother was able to identify several of his current limitations and stated three goals for his treatment:

1. R.J. will eat by mouth with assistance.
2. R.J. will walk with or without assistance.
3. R.J. will tell me what he needs by talking.

Review of Systems

Upon initial examination of R.J., the following items were noted:

1. R.J. responded to pain by grimacing.
2. R.J. was able to open his eyes upon verbal request in 3 of 5 attempts, but he was unable to make eye contact with the therapist. When R.J.'s eyes were open, he maintained his visual gaze to the left.
3. R.J. demonstrated an increased heart rate and respiratory rate when the therapist provided verbal or tactile input. He also began to yawn and make munching movements with his mouth.
4. R.J. was able to move his left upper extremity independently, but in a random, inconsistently purposeful fashion.
5. R.J. was able to move his left foot and ankle independently and tolerated gentle range of motion of his left knee and hip (as was approved by orthopedics).
6. R.J. was unable to move his right upper and lower extremity, except for inconsistent movement of his right hand, which was noted only twice.
7. R.J. was unable to independently perform any functional gross motor skills.
8. R.J. was unable to control his secretions.
9. R.J. was unable to vocalize.

At the time of admission to the inpatient rehabilitation program, referrals for occupational and speech therapy were written. It was recommended that R.J. receive these therapies to address feeding/swallowing, cognition, developmental skills, and activities of daily living.

Tests and Measures

Impairments:

R.J. was noted to have a flaccid right upper and lower extremity, and his left upper extremity exhibited spontaneous movement, although not with consistent purpose. His left lower extremity exhibited movement at his foot and ankle, and he tolerated gentle range of motion of the left hip and knee joints. His muscle tone throughout his trunk was decreased significantly, as was tone in the right upper and lower extremities. Tone was decreased slightly in the left upper and lower extremities. He was unable to demonstrate upright head control and maintained his head in a position of left cervical spine lateral flexion and slight right cervical spine rotation. Hemodynamically, he displayed increases in his heart and respiratory rates when verbal and tactile input was provided, but his oxygen saturation remained stable throughout the examination. R.J. responded with a grimace to pain and was able to open his eyes upon verbal request in 3 of 5 attempts, but he was unable to make eye contact with the therapist. When his eyes were open, he maintained a strong left visual gaze.

Functional Limitations and Disability:

R.J. was examined with the Rancho Los Amigos Levels of Cognitive Functioning to determine his current level of coma recovery during the initial evaluation. He was found to be at a Rancho Level III, which is "Localized Response," indicating he turns away from/responds to sound, responds to physical discomfort, and exhibits inconsistent response to commands.

Diagnosis

Upon synthesis of the examination information, the following diagnoses were determined for R.J.: impaired arousal, attention, and cognition; impaired motor functioning; impaired sensory integration; and impaired functional mobility.

Prognosis

Because of the severity of R.J.'s initial Glasgow Coma Scale score of 5 (indicating a severe brain injury) and his extensive left femur fracture, his overall prognosis for recovery of function was guarded. As his injury occurred only 2½ weeks

Continued

CASE STUDY OF A CHILD WITH TRAUMATIC BRAIN INJURY—cont'd

prior to his transfer to an inpatient rehabilitation program, it was thought he would have the possibility of some motor recovery but likely have long-term cognitive impairments.

PLAN OF CARE

R.J.'s length of stay in the intensive rehabilitation program was estimated at the time of the examination to be approximately 8 to 12 weeks to best maximize his potential for motor and cognitive recovery. The following goals and outcomes for physical therapy were determined:

Goals:
1. R.J. will tolerate various types of stimulation without exhibiting signs of overstimulation or significant hemodynamic changes.
2. R.J. will maintain independent sitting at the edge of the bed or bench.
3. R.J. will maintain lower extremity weightbearing with assistance, once cleared by orthopedics to perform weightbearing as tolerated (WBAT).
4. R.J. will use all extremities in play.
5. R.J. will complete an activity following a two-step direction.

Outcomes:
1. R.J. will assist with his daily care with modifications and assistance.
2. R.J.'s mother and other family members will increase their understanding of traumatic brain injury and its effects, the anticipated goals, and the expected outcomes.
3. R.J. will participate in age-appropriate social interactions with modifications, as required.
4. R.J. will stand with assistance and ambulate short distances with or without an assistive device.

INTERVENTION

R.J. received extensive physical therapy services in an inpatient rehabilitation program for 12 weeks, with physical therapy services delivered twice daily Monday through Friday, daily on Saturdays, and no therapies on Sundays. Intervention included weekly staffing/care conferences and multidisciplinary rounds, reintegration of R.J. into child life activities 1 to 2 times daily, and extensive family training.

The focus of treatment was on increasing modulated arousal, attention and focus, trunk and extremity muscle strengthening, postural stability, improving motor control of his extremities with functional play activities, and reestablishing mobility options. Because of his weightbearing restrictions initially, no standing activities were done until the order was changed by the orthopedic surgeon to weightbearing as tolerated. Often, physical therapy sessions were in co-treatment with both occupational and speech therapy. R.J. responded well to the focus on increasing modulated arousal and attention and began to vocalize and communicate with single words, especially during movement activities. R.J. was evaluated for a customized pediatric manual wheelchair with tilt-in-space features and was also evaluated for specialized bath equipment, both of which were submitted to his insurance for approval. He also was evaluated for and received bilateral ankle-foot orthoses (AFO), which assisted in providing both knee and ankle/foot control during standing and ambulation activities and helped maintain his range of motion.

OUTCOMES

R.J. was discharged from the inpatient rehabilitation program after a 12-week stay. He was discharged home to his mother and then began attending a day rehabilitation program 5 days a week for 4 hours a day to continue his rehabilitation progress.

At the time of discharge, R.J. was able to independently roll from prone to supine, independently sit at the edge of a mat table or bench with upper extremity propping, transfer from sit to stand with moderate assistance, complete a stand-pivot transfer with minimal to moderate assistance, and ambulate 5 feet with moderate assistance and a posterior rolling walker. He exhibited anti-gravity movement of his right upper and lower extremity, although strength limitations persisted. He was able to tolerate increased environmental stimulation without exhibiting

CASE STUDY OF A CHILD WITH TRAUMATIC BRAIN INJURY—cont'd

signs of overstimulation, although with increased environmental stimulation, R.J.'s attention to task would decrease significantly. Verbal cuing and redirection were required in those situations to assist R.J. to stay on task. He continued to exhibit increased impulsivity and decreased safety awareness, requiring direct supervision at all times when in his wheelchair. He was able to self-propel his wheelchair 150 to 200 feet with use of bilateral upper extremities for propulsion and was able to communicate his basic wants and needs. His mother and other family members stated they were very pleased with the progress he made while in the intensive inpatient rehabilitation program and were looking forward to future progress with the continuation of therapy services in the day rehabilitation setting.

ANALYSIS OF CASE USING THE ICF MODEL (AT DISCHARGE):

Body functions: Recovering from traumatic brain injury, decreased strength in all extremities and trunk, decreased attention span, decreased cognitive processing.

Activity limitations: Requires constant supervision and monitoring, limited ambulation and wheeled mobility skills, limited endurance.

Participation restrictions: Decreased independence, limited ability to participate in age-appropriate community athletic activities, requires wheeled mobility to participate in community events and family outings.

Environmental factors: Required special-education learning environment, special recreation programming, calm and quiet environment for optimal interactions.

Chapter Discussion Questions

1. List three possible causes of traumatic brain injury.
2. How are traumatic brain injuries classified?
3. What are the possible effects on a child's long-term health and quality of life?
4. On the Glasgow Coma Scale, as the scores increase in the motor response category, what does this indicate about the child's level of function?
5. If a person is a 3 on the verbal skill portion of the Glasgow Coma Scale, what would you expect to see?
6. On your home health caseload, you receive a referral for a 12-year-old boy who has been at home for 3 days. He was an inpatient for 32 days, which included 15 days on the rehabilitation unit. He currently demonstrates the following abilities:
   - Propels a manual wheelchair with his feet
   - Responds inconsistently to yes and no questions
   - Cannot complete a two-step self-care–related task
   - Can walk 50 steps, but cannot climb stairs to access his bedroom
   a. What is the classification on the Rancho Los Amigos Levels of Cognitive Functioning?
   b. What might be four challenges associated with direct care delivery? Give one strategy to overcome each challenge.

REFERENCES

1. American Physical Therapy Association: *APTA guide to physical therapy practice*, Alexandria, Va, 2001, APTA.
2. Greenes DS, Madsen JR: Neurotrauma. In Fleisher GR, Ludwig S, editors: *Textbook of pediatric emergency medicine*, ed 4, Philadelphia, 2000, Lippincott Williams & Wilkins.
3. Zafonte RD, Hammond FM, Mann NR, and others: Relationship between Glasgow coma scale and functional outcome, *Am J Phys Med Rehabil* 75:364, 1996.
4. Wyszynski ME: Shaken baby syndrome: identification, intervention, and prevention, *Clin Excell Nurse Pract*, September 1999.

5. Kraus JF, Rock A, Hemyari P: Brain injuries among infants, children, adolescents, and young adults, *Am J Dis Child* 144(6):684, 1990.

6. McLean DE, Kaitz ES, Keenan CJ, and others: Medical and surgical complications of pediatric brain injury, *J Head Trauma Rehabil* 10:1, 1995.

7. Michaud LJ, Duhaime AC, Batshaw ML: Traumatic brain injury in children, *Pediatr Clin North Am* 40:553, 1993.

8. Pang D: Pathophysiologic correlates of neurobehavioral syndromes following closed head injury. In Ylviasaker M, editor: *Head injury rehabilitation*, Austin, Tex, 1985, Pro-Ed.

9. Bijur PE, Haslum M, Golding J: Cognitive and behavioral sequelae of mild head injury in children, *Pediatrics* 86(3):337, 1990.

10. Sohlberg MM, Mateer CA: Training use of compensatory memory books: a three stage behavioral approach, *J Clin Exp Neuropsychol* 11(6):871, 1989.

11. AAP Committee on Quality Improvement: The management of minor closed head injury in children, *Pediatrics* 104(6):1407, 1999.

12. Hurvitz EA, Mandac BR, Davidoff G, and others: Risk factors for heterotopic ossification in children and adolescents with severe traumatic brain injury, *Arch Phys Med Rehabil* 73:459, 1992.

13. Citta-Pietrolungo TJ, Alexander MA, Steg NL: Early detection of heterotopic ossification in young patients with traumatic brain injury, *Arch Phys Med Rehabil* 73:258, 1992.

14. Cusick BD, Stuberg WA: Assessment of lower extremity alignment in the transverse plane: implications for management of children with neuromotor dysfunction, *Phys Ther* 72:3, 1992.

15. Developed by the Mild Traumatic Brain Injury Committee of the Head Injury Interdisciplinary Special Interest Group of the American Congress of Rehabilitation Medicine: Definition of mild traumatic brain injury, *J Head Trauma Rehabil* 8(3):86, 1993.

16. Jackson PL, Vessey JA: *Primary care of the child with a chronic condition*, ed 2, St Louis, 1996, Mosby.

RESOURCES

Brain Injury Association of America (Support groups can be found on the BIA website)
www.biausa.org

Centre for Neuro Skills Website (Go to the "TBI Bookstore" on neuroskills.com for all the latest texts for professionals)
www.neuroskills.com

National Resource Center for Traumatic Brain Injury
www.neuro.pmv.vcu.edu

Traumatic Brain Injury National Data Center (TBINDC)
www.tbindc.org

Coping with Mild Traumatic Brain Injury, by Diane Stole

Brainlash, ed 2, by Gail Denton

Over My Head, by Claudia Osborn

I'll Carry the Fork!, by Kara Swanson

Where Is the Mango Princess?, by Cathy Crimmins

A Winner in Every Way, by Jewel Claude Allen

Neurological Rehabilitation, ed 5, by Darcy Umphred

Dizziness and Balance Disorders, edited by I. Kaufman Arenberg

Traumatic Brain Injury Rehabilitation, ed 2, edited by Mark J. Ashley and David K. Krych

Chapter 7

Ann W. Jackson, PT, DPT, MPH

Shaken Baby Syndrome

Guide Pattern 5A: Primary Prevention/Risk Reduction for Loss of Balance and Falling

key terms

Child abuse

Computerized tomography (CT)

Glasgow Coma Scale

Intracranial pressure

Magnetic resonance imaging (MRI)

Retinal hemorrhage

Shaken baby syndrome

outline

Definition
Pathology
Clinical Signs
Medical Treatment

Intervention
    Physical Therapy Assessment
    Physical Therapy Intervention

learning objectives

At the end of the chapter the reader will be able to do the following:

1. Identify five traits of classic shaken baby syndrome.

2. Identify five warning signs of possible shaken baby syndrome.

3. Discuss steps used to diagnose shaken baby syndrome.

4. Identify four potential health-related problems associated with diagnosis of shaken baby syndrome.

5. Identify parent education strategies that would help prevent shaken baby syndrome.

6. Describe the conditions under which the event is likely to occur and initial presentation of the victim.

7. Discuss a child's predisposition to injury in the shaken baby syndrome spectrum.

8. Describe hallmark signs of shaken baby syndrome and ways they are diagnosed.

9. Identify short- and long-term health-related issues associated with the diagnosis of shaken baby syndrome.

10. Describe three potential long-term problems that a physical therapist/physical therapist assistant may encounter.

DEFINITION

Injuries are the leading cause of death in children, and brain injury is the most common cause of death in this population.[1-3]

Often the scenarios are not linked by race, ethnicity, culture, or socioeconomic background, but rather by life stressors.[4-7] In this text, shaken baby syndrome, although a form of traumatic brain injury (TBI), is not included as part of the TBI chapter. This is because shaken baby syndrome is abusive and not accidental in nature.

Shaken baby syndrome is a highly preventable disorder (Box 7-1). Shaking occurs repeatedly and rapidly with the child being thrown into a surface, creating an increased impact. When the baby is shaken, the brain is jolted back and forth inside the skull, creating first acceleration then deceleration of movements inside the skull. The trauma may impact the development of the victims in many ways for many years into their future (Figure 7-1).

Infants, because of their disproportionate head-to-body ratio, weak neck muscles, and shallow, horizontally oriented cervical facet joints, are very susceptible to injury.[9] Circulatory structures in and around the brain are damaged, and bleed into structures inside and surrounding the brain. As previously stated,

in the most extreme cases, the shaking can result in death.[2,10] There is a great deal of variety in the clinical presentation of these children.

PATHOLOGY

In 1972 pediatric radiologist John Caffey first described a particular type of injury sustained in young children as "whiplash shaken baby syndrome."[2,11] These initial cases all had similar clinical profiles, including retinal, subdural, and/or subarachnoid hemorrhages with little to no signs of external head trauma.[2,6,11] Later work by other investigators examined the effects of the accompanying rapid deceleration of the infant brain inside a shaken head when it struck a surface such as a bed or pillow.[2,6]

Shaken baby syndrome is a form of **child abuse** and requires a multidisciplinary approach to its prevention.[6] First identifying the risk potential and possible triggers for abuse is an excellent start. Often as clinicians work with families with very sick, multiple-needs children under stressful situations, they may recognize the warning signs early. Typical stressors include anger, frustration, or sadness.

Other stressors can include the following[2]:
- An inadequately prepared parent
- A caregiver under stress
- Multiple births (e.g., twins)
- Having multiple children under 18 months of age
- A child with a disability
- Teenage parents
- A caregiver with poor coping skills
- Substance abuse in the home
- Economic strains and poverty
- Difficulty soothing or calming a crying infant

Children are especially susceptible to traumatic brain injury (TBI). Bike, skateboard, sports, and recreational injuries are common in the general pediatric population. Motor vehicle accidents account for the largest number of injuries to this group. A child's biologic response

---

Box **7-1**   Preventing Child Abuse

Child abuse, along with accidental injuries, can be found throughout the world. Prevent Child Abuse America cites this as a caregiver guide for behavior with small children and infants[8]:

"It is never OK to shake a baby or child. Shaking a baby or child can cause shaken baby syndrome. Children under age 2 are at greatest risk for shaken baby syndrome. Shaking a baby or child can cause lasting harm, even death.

"That's because they have weak neck muscles and heavy heads, and their brain and blood vessels are still growing. Shaken baby syndrome is the name for the health problems that shaking a baby can cause. It can result from any shaking of a child."

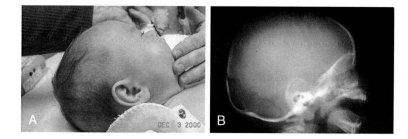

Fig. 7-1 Shaken baby syndrome. **A,** Subtle bruising is seen over the right frontotemporal area in this infant. **B,** Her skull radiograph shows a fracture and subdural hematoma. (From Zitolli BJ, Davis HW: *Atlas of pediatric physical diagnosis*, ed 5, Philadelphia, 2007, Mosby.)

to head trauma is somewhat different from an adult's. A higher resting cerebral blood flow is present, and this may lead to increased cerebral swelling after trauma. Issues such as small systematic blood volume, temperature instability, and difficulty with intubations of this population may also be contributing factors to outcome.[6] These variables make it imperative that **intracranial pressure** be monitored closely after suspected TBI. In some cases the intracranial pressure may rise as much as 60%. This is especially problematic for children under 1 year of age.[3,12]

Shaken baby syndrome has the potential to affect the development of all systems of the body. One third of infants with shaken baby syndrome will suffer some form of paralysis, retardation, or blindness. Another third will die from their injuries.[13] There are classical skeletal, neurologic, and ophthalmologic signs linked to repeated trauma.[6,10] These findings suggest that long-term ramifications exist for victims, their families, perpetrators, and the society at large. For the victim, it appears that even one incident of this whiplash-like movement can have long-term consequences, and there may be a very short time span between the incident and the onset of signs/symptoms.[14]

Through a study of long-term ramifications of shaken baby syndrome, Duhaime found that in a group of 14 children who were diagnosed at an approximate age of 6.6 months with shaken baby syndrome the following occurred: 6 children were lethargic or irritable, 3 children experienced seizures without being in a coma, 5 presented in a coma either with or without seizure activity, and 12 developed **retinal hemorrhage**. All infants' brain scans were abnormal and indicated the presence of blood in subarachnoid or subdural spaces of the brain. Seven were intubated in the acute phase for apnea, seizures, and/or unresponsiveness. All 14 infants were treated in the intensive care unit.[15] During a retrospective phase of the study 9 years later, the following had occurred:

- One child in a vegetative state had passed away from respiratory complications.
- Six children remained severely impaired and vegetative. Two were moderately impaired.
- Five were reported to have good outcomes.
- Three were legally blind, nonverbal, and wheelchair bound.
- One was legally blind and mentally impaired and had a seizure disorder. Two children had hemiparesis, severe learning impairments, and behavioral problems.
- Two were categorized as moderately impaired, experienced visual impairments, and had difficulties in cognition that required special education. One of the two also had mild hemiparesis.
- Five who were labeled as good outcomes were attending regular schools, but three out of the five repeated a grade or received tutoring to supplement their school day. Two of these children also had behavioral issues.

These data led the author to conclude that children diagnosed with shaken baby syndrome will have long-term functional impairments.[2]

The child's prognosis is also influenced by the details of the statistics that resulted in the diagnosis. These details are varied and can involve all members of the family. Was the child hurt by the parent? Caregiver? Friend of the family? Does the child return to the home setting? Are there other siblings at risk in this situation? Was the perpetrator found? Prosecuted? Was the parent not implicated in the actual incident prosecuted also? What are the long-term psychosocial ramifications for all of the individuals involved?[2,5]

CLINICAL SIGNS

The initial clinical presentation of a child with suspected shaken baby syndrome may be as described in the Clinical Signs box, with no external evidence of abuse. Signs of shaken baby syndrome can be hard to see and may also signal other health problems. However, an infant could still be suffering from internal injuries, such as to the brain and other organs.

Shaken baby syndrome is often diagnosed using **computerized tomography (CT)** and **magnetic resonance imaging (MRI)** scans.[8] Children who experience substantial repeat traumatic incidents may have cerebral damage, neurologic deficits, blindness, and cognitive impairments. These are often found without external evidence of head trauma. Hallmark signs of this condition are subdural and retinal hemorrhages accompanied by absence of external signs of abuse.[14,16]

Shaken Baby Syndrome Clinical Signs

- Trouble breathing
- Pale or bluish skin
- Convulsions or seizures
- Coma
- Irritability
- Sleepiness or lethargy
- Vomiting
- Poor feeding

MEDICAL TREATMENT

If a child with shaken baby syndrome is seen in the emergency room, the highest initial priorities are assessing airway, breathing, and circulation. It is also important to stop hemorrhaging, support the respiratory process, and stabilize blood pressure.[9] Once the patient is stabilized, the physician may perform an in-depth evaluation to determine whether fractures or internal damage are present. A neurologic examination and periodic assessments will be conducted to monitor level of consciousness and determine if brain swelling has occurred. Hemorrhages in the retina of the eye may be associated with subdural hematoma and are usually associated with child abuse.

In an acute setting the child can exhibit neurologic complications such as seizures, difficulty breathing, limp arms and legs, excessive drooling, and lethargy. Initially the need to medically stabilize the child is imperative. Establishing an open airway, stabilizing vital signs, and preserving the circulatory system are addressed in the first minutes of care. If the child is unconscious, the **Glasgow Coma Scale** (see Table 6-1 in the previous chapter) can be used to assess level of alertness and give some indication of long-term prognosis. The eye-opening, verbal response, and best motor response components of the scale are used to determine the severity of the diagnosis. When the scale is used in the first 6 hours after the injury, scores typically vary from 0-15, with 15 being highest achievable score and indicative of the best prognosis.

Shaken baby syndrome cannot be determined by examination only. Radiologic features on CT scans and MRIs are important in making a definitive diagnosis, and MRIs may help to establish incidence of repeated abuse, as well as extent of damage (Figure 7-1, *B*).[1,10] Once medical stability is established, the child should also be checked for signs of past abuse, especially bruising. Signs may or may not be present, which is why a radiologic workup is so important.

Ocular examination is also necessary in these situations. Retinal hemorrhage is a hallmark sign of shaken baby syndrome.[1] Hemorrhage inside the intraocular space is caused by a sudden increase in venous pressure in the head. This rise in pressure is communicated by the optic nerve sheaths. Ultimately blood leaks through damaged vessels, causing retinal edema. Severe damage to the eyes may cause permanent, partial, or total blindness. Wilkinson and colleagues observed that the severity of intraocular hemorrhage was found to have a direct and high correlation with the severity of intracranial hemorrhage in infants who have been shaken. Laboratory tests must be used to rule out the presence of other disorders that may also be present and cause retinal hemorrhaging. Menkes disease, a genetic disorder that regulates copper metabolism in the body, must also be ruled out, because both conditions present with similar hematomas.[17]

Neurosurgical consultation is recommended for all children who sustain more than mild head trauma.[12] Children with epidural and subdural hematoma may require surgery to prevent or treat increased intracranial pressure. Diagnosis of intracranial hemorrhage and swelling may also require surgical intervention. Seizures are also prevalent in this population, making CT scans and MRIs important tools for determining the type and extent of acute and residual brain damage.

Most children in TBI-induced comas regain consciousness. A small number do remain in a vegetative state. Regaining consciousness can occur slowly or quickly. Initially the child's responses may be limited to opening the eyes or responding to verbal commands.[10]

INTERVENTION

At this time an interdisciplinary approach to shaken baby syndrome is most often used. Issues dealing with medical, legal, and nursing/long-term care and preventive health perspectives must be addressed.[5,13]

PHYSICAL THERAPY ASSESSMENT

Physical therapists and physical therapist assistants may encounter these patients in the acute phase for posttraumatic intervention. Settings may include rehabilitation and long-term care facilities for progressive functional intervention or settings that offer a long-term maintenance program. They may also include community settings, such as an infant or early childhood program or school setting. Services exist across the life span to meet the challenges of daily living as children mature into adults. In each situation the approach must be the same: identify the immediate barriers to function based on pest practice and the *Guide to Physical Therapy Practice.*

The pediatric patient may have one or a combination of conditions. A clearer clinical profile can be created based on the findings of further diagnostic examinations or through tests and measures. Assessments in the following areas may be indicated:
- Aerobic capacity and endurance
- Arousal, attention, and cognition
- Assistive and adaptive devices
- Community reintegration
- Cranial nerve integrity
- Environmental, vocational, and avocational barriers
- Gait, locomotion, and balance
- Integumentary integrity (skin)
- Joint integrity and mobility
- Muscle performance
- Neuromotor development and sensory integrates
- Orthotic, protective, and supportive devices
- Pain
- Posture
- Range of motion
- Reflex integrity
- Self-care
- Sensory integrity
- Ventilation, respiration, and circulation

All of these systems have the potential to be altered by shaken baby syndrome.

PHYSICAL THERAPY INTERVENTION

Physical therapy is guided by the goal of achieving the highest functional level for all individuals. As an individual's needs change because of setting, community, and vocational needs, so might the intervention. Often with a diagnosis of shaken baby syndrome, many patients have an extensive team of medical specialists and an ancillary care team. If warranted, assistive technology and vision therapy may be provided as well. Most importantly, survivors must be empowered to focus on obtaining the greatest system functionality possible.[2,5,11,13]

Acute rehabilitation includes range-of-motion exercises, positioning, and splinting of limbs. This will help prevent deformities and development of contractures. Skin integrity and body positioning are also essential. Throughout the process, muscle tone, movement quality, spasticity, rigidity, and ataxia/tremors are the most common motor abnormalities. Medication and surgery may be needed to address these issues.[10] Children may have sensory, communication, cognitive, and psychologic or behavioral impairments. They may also have feeding issues or require modification in their academic environment.

It is important for healthcare providers to be aware of personal values and biases that may interfere with the ability to focus on the needs of children and family members dealing with the sequelae to shaken baby syndrome. Often professionals must handle conflicting personal feelings when a relationship with the perpetrator is part of providing care to the pediatric patient. The Interventions box lists physical therapy goals for the physical therapist assistant to focus on when caring for a child with a diagnoses of TBI secondary to shaken baby syndrome. One author describes the importance of support groups for the mother, and another suggests the parent's need to de-stress and build stronger support networks.[5,18]

Shaken Baby Syndrome Interventions

- Avert complications that arise from immobilization, disuse, and neurologic dysfunction.
- Augment the use of abilities regained as a result of recovery from coma.
- Teach adaptive compensation for impaired or lost function.
- Alleviate the effect of chronic disability on the process of growth and development.

CASE OF A CHILD WITH SHAKEN BABY SYNDROME: NINA

EXAMINATION

History

Nina was an eight-month-old Latino female accompanied to her initial physical therapy assessment by her foster mother. The infant had been recently released from a 3-month inpatient stay in the hospital secondary to shaken baby syndrome and was in need of community services for rehabilitative therapy.

General Demographics

Primary language: English is spoken in the foster home.

Race/ethnicity: Child is Hispanic, but is currently placed in African-American foster care situation.

Social History

Cultural impact: Prior to her injury, Nina lived at home with her mother, age 18, and her father, age 26. The couple had not married, but the father generated family income and set family rules.

Family support: Both parents were estranged from their families and alternately assumed responsibility for the infant's care.

CASE OF A CHILD WITH SHAKEN BABY SYNDROME: NINA—cont'd

Social interaction: Since the child was removed from the parents' home, no information was available regarding the birth family. The foster family has extended family activities and support.

Growth/development: Prior to the TBI incident, Nina was developing in a typical pattern. Right-handedness had been observed during feeding and activity initiation.

Living environment: At the time of the incident, Nina lived in a rental home with her parents and half-sister from her father's side.

Medical History

In September 2002, immediately prior to her hospitalization for TBI secondary to shaken baby syndrome, Nina's mother had taken Nina to the pediatrician because she had been exhibiting increased irritability and a decreased appetite. When the pediatrician examined Nina, her head size was an immediate concern. Nina and her mother were sent immediately to an area hospital for assessment. Neurologic findings were:

- Head circumference of 45 cm
- Bilateral subdural hematomas, s/p burr holes
- Macrocephaly
- Multiple rib fractures (healed)
- Ulnar fracture
- Failure to thrive (FTT)

A CT scan confirmed shaken baby syndrome, and Nina was hospitalized for acute rehab for approximately 3 months, until she was placed in foster care.

At the time of the physical therapy assessment, the foster mother was concerned about:

- Size of head and Nina's inability to control her head against gravity
- Poor sitting abilities
- No interest in standing
- Generalized muscle tightness in all extremities

Nina had received PT services during her extended inpatient and rehabilitation hospitalization, but she had been without any formal services for 3 weeks at time of the assessment. The foster mother had been educated on strategies to use with Nina by the physical therapy team in the rehabilitative setting. The physical therapist had taught her techniques to encourage rolling, supportive sitting, and prone position.

Medication: None.

Functional Status/Activity Level

General appearance: Well-developed female infant with disproportionate head-to-body size. (Foster mother reports no size increase in cranium since surgical evacuation.) Nina is tracking sounds and voices, especially the voice of the foster mother. She is freely using upper extremities when held in supportive sitting.

Balance/self-righting responses: Primitive reflexes integrated into system. Self-righting present in all directions, easiest to elicit to right and forward and to sides. Posterior righting is still emerging.

Muscle Tone/Range of Motion

Muscle tone: Nina presents with increased tone in all weightbearing joints proximally. Upper body tone is greater than lower body. She has forward-elevated shoulders. Left elevation greater than right and head slightly rotated to left approximately 10 to 15 degrees from midline.

Range of motion: All extremities have full passive mobility. The cervical region has increased difficulty rotating away from left side, but full range achieved. Movement pattern appears normal; no abnormal synergies present.

Strength

Nina spontaneously moves her upper body and extremities against gravity. She was unable to move her lower extremities against gravity, even with facilitation.

Posture/Mobility

Supported sitting: Nina sits with minimal posture support, head is found slightly rotated to left and fixed on body, spine is C-curved, and hands are positioned outside abducted legs. Reaching occurs 1% with right hand.

Unsupported: Self-stabilized extremities do not change, but Nina is not able to sustain herself longer than 15 seconds. Limiting factors are head righting and maintaining midline.

Side-lying: Infant reaches with bilateral upper extremities; minimal leg movement observed.

Rolling: Infant rolls independently supine to prone and returns.

CASE OF A CHILD WITH SHAKEN BABY SYNDROME: NINA—cont'd

Prone: Infant enjoys being prone and props spontaneously. She is able to hold for 45 to 60 seconds, but is not able to shift to reach for object of interest.

Quadruped: Nina will initiate weightbearing through arms but no weightbearing observed through lower extremities. When forced, she becomes fussy.

Standing: Initially collapsed; when guarded facilitation offered, she was able to stand with moderate assistance at lower trunk.

Stepping: When secured posteriorly, stepping responses were elicited.

Medical Diagnostic
- CT scan confirmed hemorrhage
- Vision specialist found no evidence of ocular hemorrhages
- No seizure activity

Family History

At this time Nina is separated from her parents and living in a different cultural environment. In order for the mother to regain care of Nina, she must separate from and never have contact with the father, who investigators believe is the perpetrator of the incident that caused TBI. Nina's mother must also begin counseling and secure a source of income to support herself and Nina.

PLAN OF CARE

- Nina will independently sit without need for support and reach for objects of interest.
- While prone, Nina will reach for objects of interest 2 to 4 inches away with right and left hands.

- Searching for objects to the right and left will occur with ease of neck rotation in horizontal and vertical positions.
- Nina will begin accepting weight through lower extremities in prone and standing positions for 45 to 90 seconds.

INTERVENTION

The foster mother demonstrates a vested interest in Nina's program. Nina's biological mother has communicated through the social worker that she wants to see her baby get better, but cannot help now because of legal issues.

Physical therapy is recommended weekly to focus on goal resolution for 6 months with emphasis on:
- Use of therapeutic handling to facilitate righting response challenges
- Positional play opportunities with sitting, prone, and standing, using varying levels of support
- Use of rolls, Swiss balls, and age-appropriate toys to encourage child and initiate movement.

ANALYSIS OF CASE USING THE ICF MODEL:

Body functions: Increased tone in all extremities, decreased cervical active movement, decreased head righting.

Activity limitations: Child cannot sit unsupported, child will not take weight through her lower extremities.

Participation restrictions: Nina has decreased ability to interact with her environment and peers.

Environmental limitations: Nina currently resides with a foster family and has no contact with her biological parents at this time.

CASE OF A CHILD WITH SHAKEN BABY SYNDROME: ROGER

EXAMINATION

History

Roger is a 3½-year-old boy recovering from TBI secondary to shaken baby syndrome. His injury was reportedly sustained at the age of 4 months while in the care of a paid home caregiver. According to the record, Roger was in a deep sleep

when his father picked him up from daycare and did not arouse on the ride home. The parents contacted the pediatrician, who instructed them to take Roger immediately to the hospital emergency room. Extensive medical evaluation determined that Roger had sustained a subdural hematoma, with active bleeding still evident. Roger was

CASE OF A CHILD WITH SHAKEN BABY SYNDROME: ROGER—cont'd

rushed to surgery for intervention and later required a shunt placement. He received speech, physical, and occupational therapies in an early intervention (0 to 3 years) program and is presently eligible for admission to the early childhood program at a neighborhood school.

General Demographics
Age: 3½ years
Primary language: English
Race/ethnicity: Caucasian
Sex: Male

Social History
Cultural impact: Roger lived at home with his mother and extended maternal family prior to injury. After inpatient stay and criminal investigation, Roger was allowed to return home.

Family support: Roger is the first child of college-aged parents, and from all investigative reports has apparently been well cared for his entire life.

Caregiver support: Due to his parents' need to work and continue their educations, the toddler had been placed in a home caregiver situation for 3 to 4 hours daily on average, but up to 8 hours daily, depending on parents' school and work schedules. Whenever possible, the grandparents also provided caregiver support.

Growth/development: At his initial physical therapy assessment, Roger exhibited atypical growth and development because of the TBI secondary to shaken baby syndrome that occurred when he was approximately 4 months old.

Medical History
Anti-seizure medications are given on a daily basis. Anti-spasticity medications were tried, but the family did not like the impact on Roger's level of alertness.

Range of motion: Left upper extremity is activated in small gross patterns with inclusions of trunk in many movements. At the elbow, full passive range is achieved only after extended stretching. Active movements at the elbow are achieved in side-lying position, working primarily in 30% of available range. At wrist and hand, there is no active movement. Passively, joints are influenced by hypertonicity and cannot be positioned passively for weightbearing.

Right upper and right lower extremities: Without range limitations, but weakness is noted at right ankle during gait cycle. Left lower extremity hypertonicity present in foot; ankle weakness and hypertension at base.

Equipment
Roger has a manual wheelchair, adaptive bath chair system, and Rifton chair at home. At school Roger will bring Rifton gait trainer and manual wheelchair. He wears a supramalleolar orthotic (SMO) on his right side and an articulating ankle-foot orthosis (AFO) on his left side.

Postures/Mobility
Sitting: Roger is able to "W" sit independently and long-sit with minimal posterior support. If in ring, sitting pattern is with arms outside of legs and back flexed (curved spine).

Dynamic sitting: Roger can reach for objects in all postures, but is most secure in W-sitting. Long sitting is the most difficult.

Quadruped: Roger rolls and crawls independently. Crawl pattern does not consistently exhibit reciprocal patterning of all extremities. Lower extremities are often carried in a hop-like mode. When cued, Roger can use reciprocal pattern.

Standing: In orthotics, Roger can stand with minimal assistance from wheelchair or other seated surface. In free standing, Roger is not confident and will maintain self for less than 15 seconds.

Ambulate/stepping: From free space, Roger has attempted independent steps, but has difficulty maintaining trunk fully erect. Arms are kept at high guard. When hand-held assistance or the use of walls is given, Roger is able to go 30 to 75 feet on occasion. Ambulation in gait trainer is slow but functional. Using the gait trainer, Roger is able to move independently in all directions for 30 to 50 feet within 15- to 20-minute time span.

Medical Diagnostics
School-based team does not have any formal medical reports. The mother has provided the PT team with the names of the medical specialists Roger sees. They include:
• Neurologist
• Orthopedic specialist
• Gastrointestinal consult as needed

CASE OF A CHILD WITH SHAKEN BABY SYNDROME: ROGER—cont'd

The mother provided medical history and diagnosis at time of intake into early childhood program. The team was also given copies of evaluations done by the 0-3 program and the team therapists.

Family Risk

At the time of intake, Roger's parents, who are both nearing the end of their college careers, verbalized a desire for Roger to be "all better" now. They also shared that after a long investigation, the perpetrator in Roger's case happened to be the caregiver's assistant at the in-home daycare. Roger's mother went on to say that Roger was a "colicky" baby and could be difficult to comfort.

The parents also discussed their concern about Roger's long-term prognosis in all developmental areas. The family in general is stable, with plans for a future caregiver system for Roger distributed among family members.

PLAN OF CARE

In the school setting, goal emphasis is on improved functionality and eliminating barriers to inclusion in school-based activities.

The team will work toward eliminating wheelchair use at school and possibly eliminating the need for a wheelchair-lift bus. Increasing ambulation distance and quality and reducing Roger's level of support are other goals. Improved righting responses and inhibition of tonal hand fluctuations in Roger's left hand will be encouraged through exercise and positioning.

INTERVENTION

The team goals for physical therapy for a 6- to 9-month time period (1 school year) include the following:

- Roger will increase distance that he ambulates about the school building to 150 to 300 feet with hand-held assistance or with use of walls.
- Roger will discontinue use of wheelchair at school and ambulate about building with hand-held assistance or using gait trainer 100% of the time.
- Roger will independently use environmental assistance to transition self from sit to stand at table in classroom with distant supervision only.
- Roger will sit on floor in long sit or circle sit without instability and be able to self-right when challenged for 15 minutes.

ANALYSIS OF CASE USING THE ICF MODEL:

Body functions: Decreased upper extremity passive and active range of motion, increased tone in left lower extremity, right ankle weakness.

Activity limitations: Roger tends to W-sit for stability, does not have any other independent stable sitting postures, bunny hops for mobility, but can use reciprocal pattern when cued. He has decreased independent standing skills.

Participation restrictions: Roger requires a wheelchair for long-distance mobility and has decreased interactions with peers and limited opportunities to join community-based programs.

Environmental limitations: Relatively young parents, special-education school placement, requires wheelchair accessibility.

Chapter Discussion Questions

1. What factors distinguish the diagnosis of shaken baby syndrome from other classified traumatic brain injuries?
2. Babies and children who are victims of shaken baby syndrome often go untreated for what reason? How is the condition ultimately diagnosed?
3. What specific medical and/or social consideration must be taken into account when treating a classic case of shaken baby syndrome?
4. List four possible areas of a child's development that may be altered after an injury caused by shaken baby syndrome.

5. How does shaken baby syndrome differ from other head traumas?
6. What comorbidities may result from shaken baby syndrome?
7. What are the PT foci of the acute rehabilitation phase for a child with shaken baby syndrome?
8. What is the percentage of recovery for children with shaken baby syndrome?
9. Who is the most common perpetrator of shaken baby syndrome?
10. What type of team is recommended to intervene with a child diagnosed with shaken baby syndrome?

REFERENCES

1. Committee on Child Abuse and Neglect: Shaken baby syndrome: inflicted cerebral trauma 1993-1994, *Del Med J* 69(7):365, 1997.
2. Helfrich CA: *Domestic abuse across the lifespan: the role of occupational therapy*, Binghamton, NY, 2001, Haworth.
3. Ward JD: Pediatric issues in head trauma, *New Horiz* 3(3):539, 1995.
4. Conway MD, Peyman GA, Recasens M: Intravitreal tPA and SF6 promote clearing of premacular subhyaloid hemorrhages in shaken and battered baby syndrome, *Ophthalmic Surg Lasers* 30(6):435, 1999.
5. D'Lugoff MI, Baker DJ: Case study: shaken baby syndrome–one disorder with two victims, *Public Health Nurs* 15(4):243, 1998.
6. Lancon J, Haines DE, Parent AD: Anatomy of the shaken baby syndrome, *Anat Rec* 253(1):13, 1998.
7. Sinal SH, Petree AR, Herman-Giddens M, and others: Is race or ethnicity a predictive factor in shaken baby syndrome? *Child Abuse Negl* 24(9):1241, 2000.
8. Prevent Child Abuse America: *Preventing shaken baby syndrome*, South Deerfield, Mass, 2003, Prevent Child Abuse America Publications.
9. Lavelle JM, Shaw KN: Evaluation of head injury in a pediatric emergency department, *Arch Pediatr Adolesc Med* 152(12):1220, 1998.
10. Batshaw ML: *Children with disabilities*, Philadelphia, 2002, Brookes.
11. Goldberg KB, Goldberg RE: Review of shaken baby syndrome, *J Psychosoc Nurs Ment Health Serv* 40(4):38, 2002.
12. Loh JK, Lin CL, Kwan AL, and others: Acute subdural hematoma in infancy, *Surg Neurol* 58 (3-4):218, 2002.
13. Cox LA: The shaken baby syndrome: diagnosis using CT and MRI, *Radiol Technol* 67(6):513, 1996.
14. Chiocca EM: Shaken baby syndrome: a nursing perspective, *Pediatr Nurs* 21(1):33, 1995.
15. Duhaime A, Christian C, Moss E, and others: Long-term outcomes in infants with shaking-impact syndrome, *Pediatr Neurosurg* 24:292, 1996.
16. Levine LM: Pediatric ocular trauma and shaken infant syndrome, *Pediatr Clin North Am* 50(1):137, 2003.
17. Nassogne MC, Sharrard M, Hertz-Pannier L, and others: Massive subdural hematomas in Menkes disease mimicking shaken baby syndrome, *Childs Nerv Syst* 18(12):729, 2002.
18. Duhaime A, Christian C, Rorke L, and others: Nonaccidental head injury in infants—"The shaken baby syndrome," *New Engl J Med* 338(25):1822, 1998.

RESOURCES

Child Help USA National Child Abuse Hotline
1-800-4-A-CHILD
(1-800-422-4453)

Parents Anonymous
www.parentsanonymous.org
1-909-621-6184

Prevent Child Abuse America
www.preventchildabuse.org
1-312-663-3520

Support and Referral Service on Shaken Baby Syndrome
2955 Harrison Blvd #102
Ogden, UT 84403
Telephone: 801-393-3366
Fax: 801-393-7019

Chapter 8

Roberta Kuchler O'Shea, PT, PhD
Colleen Sullivan, PT, MS

Rheumatic Disorders

Guide Pattern 4H: Impaired Joint Mobility, Motor Function, Muscle Performance, and Range of Motion Associated With Joint Arthroplasty

key terms

Autoimmune disease
Iridocyclitis
Joint inflammation

Micrognathia
Pauciarticular JRA
Polyarticular JRA

Scleroderma
Systemic JRA

outline

Definition
Pathology
Clinical Signs
   Pauciarticular JRA
   Polyarticular JRA
   Systemic JRA

Secondary Factors
   Skeletal Abnormalities
   Ophthalmic Considerations
Intervention
Other Rheumatic Diseases

learning objectives

At the end of the chapter the reader will be able to do the following:

1. Identify the different types of juvenile arthritis.

2. Identify intervention techniques for juvenile arthritis.

3. Identify appropriate long- and short-term treatment objectives.

DEFINITION

Juvenile rheumatoid arthritis (JRA) is a disorder causing **joint inflammation** and stiffness for more than six weeks in children less than 16 years of age (Figure 8-1). It is estimated that between 30,000 and 50,000 children in the United States have JRA, making it the most common rheumatic disorder among this age group.[1]

PATHOLOGY

Like adult rheumatoid arthritis, JRA is an **autoimmune disease,** in that the body mistakenly identifies some of its own cells and tissues as foreign.[2] The immune system, which normally helps to fight off harmful invaders such as bacteria or viruses, begins to attack healthy tissues. The result is inflammation marked by redness, heat, pain, and swelling.[2] The cause of JRA may vary in different children. Doctors do not yet understand what causes the immune system to malfunction, but genetic factors and viruses have been suggested as playing a role.

CLINICAL SIGNS

There are three types of JRA: pauciarticular, polyarticular, and systemic. The determination of diagnoses between types is made within the first 6 months of onset.

Rheumatic Disorders Clinical Signs
Pauciarticular JRA
• Affects 4 or fewer joints
• Affects large joints, most commonly the knees
• Risk for iridocyclitis in subtype 1
• Affects 5 times as many girls as boys
Polyarticular JRA
• Affects 5 or more joints
• Affects both large joints and smaller joints
• Often affects the same joint on both sides of the body
• RF antibodies in subtype 1
• Affects 3 times as many girls as boys
Systemic JRA
• High-spiking fevers
• Rash on chest and thighs
• Joint involvement
• Internal organs can be affected
• Affects girls and boys in equal numbers

PAUCIARTICULAR JRA

Pauciarticular JRA affects four or fewer joints in a child. Pauciarticular JRA is also known as *oligoarthritis.* This type of JRA is five times more prevalent among girls than boys and is the most common JRA form, seen in about half

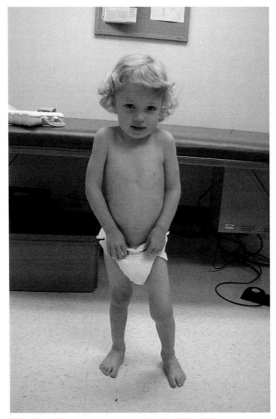

Fig. 8-1 A 2-year-old girl with arthritis of the left knee. (From Zitelli BJ, Davis HW: *Atlas of pediatric physical diagnosis,* ed 5, Philadelphia, 2007, Mosby.)

of all children diagnosed with JRA. There are three subtypes of pauciarticular JRA:

- First subtype: children test positive for antinuclear antibodies and have a high risk for **iridocyclitis** (inflammation of the eye)
- Second subtype: affects the spine, although possibly not until late teens, and the children

may test positive for the gene identified with adult ankylosing spondylitis (rheumatoid arthritis of the adult spine)

- Third subtype: joint involvement is the extent of the disease

Pauciarticular disease usually affects large joints, most commonly the knees (Figure 8-2).

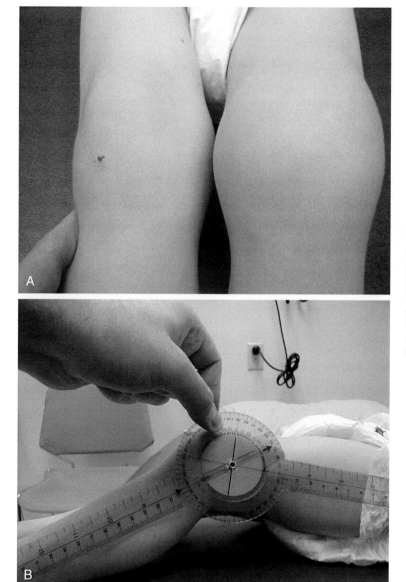

Fig. 8-2 Pauciarticular juvenile rheumatoid arthritis. **A,** A close look at this child's knees reveals left knee swelling. **B,** The left knee can only be extended to 35 degrees (secondary to a flexion contracture). (From Zitelli BJ, Davis HW: *Atlas of pediatric physical diagnosis*, ed 5, Philadelphia, 2007, Mosby.)

Involvement of other parts of the body is unusual, with the exception of the eyes. About 20% of children affected with pauciarticular JRA also develop eye disease. While many of the children with pauciarticular disease outgrow arthritis by adulthood, eye problems can continue, and joint symptoms may recur in some people.

Certain children with pauciarticular JRA have special proteins in the blood called *antinuclear antibodies* (ANAs). Up to 80% of those with eye disease also test positive for ANA, and the disease tends to develop at an earlier age in these children. To prevent serious vision and eye problems, regular eye examinations are imperative.

POLYARTICULAR JRA

Polyarticular JRA affects about one third of all children with JRA, with three times more girls than boys affected. In this type of JRA, five or more joints are involved. The arthritis typically involves large joints, such as knees, wrists, elbows, and ankles, but can also affect the smaller joints of the hands and feet (Figure 8-3). Polyarticular JRA often affects the same joint on both sides of the body. There are two subtypes of polyarticular JRA. In the first subtype, children possess a special kind of serum antibody known as *rheumatoid factor* (RF) and often suffer a more severe form of JRA. In the second subtype, children only experience joint involvement, which is potentially less severe than the first subtype.

SYSTEMIC JRA

The third type of JRA is known as **systemic JRA**. This type of JRA is characterized by high-spiking fevers off and on for weeks and a distinctive rash on the chest and thighs. Systemic JRA is also known as *Still's disease* and accounts for about 20% of cases of JRA. It is seen equally in boys and girls. In addition to joint involvement, internal organs such as the heart, liver, spleen, and lymph nodes can be affected.

SECONDARY FACTORS

Regardless of the type, there are several secondary factors associated with juvenile rheumatoid arthritis.

SKELETAL ABNORMALITIES

Skeletal abnormalities may be seen in the extremity joints, spine, or jaw. Chronic hyperemia (excess blood flow) in an inflamed joint can

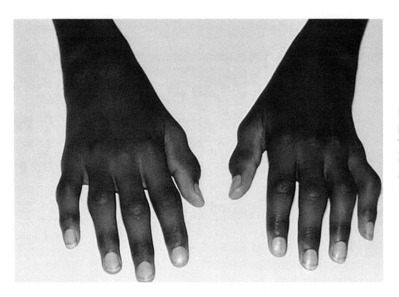

Fig. 8-3 The hands of a patient with polyarticular JRA. Note the inability to fully extend the fingers. (From Zitelli BJ, Davis HW: *Atlas of pediatric physical diagnosis*, ed 5, Philadelphia, 2007, Mosby.)

stimulate accelerated maturation of the epiphyseal plates, which leads to skeletal overgrowth in the affected extremity. This overgrowth can result in a leg-length deformity. Associated lower-extremity involvement includes limitations in hip flexion, hip abduction, and hip rotation as a result of iliopsoas and adductor spasms. Additionally, a valgus deformity in the knee may lead to resultant valgus of the hindfoot and varus of the forefoot.

In the jaw, **micrognathia** (abnormally small jaw), mandibular underdevelopment, and malocclusion are often related to JRA. These conditions may lead to issues in oral care and oral motor function.

In the spine, apophyseal joint disease is associated with poor development of the vertebrae and eventual fusing of the involved vertebrae. Early signs of polyarticular JRA are pain and stiffness in the cervical spines with a rapid loss of extension and rotational movements. Scoliosis is also a related pathology in children with JRA.

OPHTHALMIC CONSIDERATIONS

Regardless of the type of JRA, all children with JRA need to be followed by an ophthalmologist for eye involvement and uveitis, also known as *iridocyclitis*, which is an inflammation of the iris and ciliary body. Children must also be followed closely for proper nutrition to ensure that they are receiving appropriate caloric intake. Children with JRA also may experience anemia. Either poor nutrition or anemia may cause increased fatigue, so children with JRA should be closely monitored for both.

INTERVENTION

Therapeutic interventions for children with JRA include a multidisciplinary team approach.[2,3] The team should include the family and the pediatric rheumatologist, pediatrician, physical therapist, occupational therapist, speech therapist, nutritionist, ophthalmologist, social worker, recreational therapist, nurses, pharmacist, and educators. All team members may not be involved in every case, however. The primary goals of treatment for JRA include relieving pain, reducing swelling, maintaining movement and joint mobility, and slowing the progression of the disease.

Some of the medications used to treat adult rheumatoid arthritis are used to treat JRA as well. Children may respond differently to drugs than their adult counterparts, and dosage adjustments are necessary, based on the age and weight of the child. Medications used in treating JRA can be broken into four categories (Table 8-1). Nonsteroidal antiinflammatory drugs (NSAIDs) are the drugs of choice for treating children with JRA. Disease-modifying antirheumatic drugs (DMARDs) may be prescribed if NSAIDs fail to adequately relieve symptoms. DMARDs can slow the progression of JRA, but because they may take weeks or months to alleviate symptoms, often they are used in conjunction with an NSAID. Methotrexate is a DMARD prescribed for some children with JRA whose symptoms are not relieved by other medications. Small doses of this medication are used to relieve the arthritis symptoms. Etanercept (Enbrel) is a biologic response modifier that works by blocking the action of tumor necrosis factor, an inflammation-promoting substance produced by the body. Enbrel is used to treat children with polyarticular JRA who have not responded sufficiently to other

TABLE **8-1** Medications Used to Treat JRA

DRUG CATEGORY	EXAMPLES
Nonsteroidal antiinflammatory drugs	Ibuprofen
	Naproxen
Disease-modifying antirheumatic drugs	Gold
	Hydroxychloroquine
	Sulfasalazine
	D-penicillamine
	Methotrexate
Biologic response modifier	Etanercept (Enbrel)
Corticosteroids	Prednisone

drug therapies. In children with very severe JRA, corticosteroids such as prednisone may be added to the treatment plan to control the child's symptoms. However, corticosteroids can interfere with a child's normal growth and cause weakened bones. Once the medication successfully controls the more severe symptoms, the physician may reduce the dose gradually and eventually stop administering it completely.

Physical therapy interventions are important to the overall care and well-being of the child with juvenile rheumatoid arthritis.[3] Typically PT interventions focus on pain relief, maintaining and regaining passive and active range of motion, maintaining and increasing strength and endurance, improving the child's mobility and independent functioning, educating the child and family about the musculoskeletal effects of the pathology processes and secondary damage from the medications, and increasing community awareness about JRA. This may include a visit to the child's daycare center or school to provide information about the disease and any assists or precautions that may be needed for the child.

Rheumatic Disorders Interventions

- Relieve pain
- Reduce swelling
- Maintain movement and mobility
- Slow disease progression

OTHER RHEUMATIC DISEASES

In addition to JRA, there are several other rheumatic diseases that affect children. **Scleroderma** is a connective tissue disease involving the skin, blood vessels, and the immune system. Scleroderma is also known as *systemic sclerosis*. In its systemic form internal organ involvement can occur. Scleroderma translates as "hard skin." The disorder is thought to be driven by a local inflammatory/immune response. Thickening and tightening of the skin occurs from a buildup of collagen and other natural skin proteins. Collagen, a fibrous protein made by cells, provides firmness in the skin, forms the lining of organs, and is the basic structural protein in bones, tendons, ligaments, and joints.

It is believed there are thousands of cases of juvenile scleroderma worldwide. Since it is likely that juvenile scleroderma commonly goes undiagnosed or misdiagnosed, the number of children affected may be greater than suspected. There are two types of scleroderma: localized and systemic.

Localized scleroderma does not normally involve internal body systems, but may affect joints, the nervous system, and the eyes. The localized type is much more common in children than adults. Children with localized scleroderma may display different types of skin involvement known as *linear morphea* or *general morphea*. Morphea are patches of thickened, waxy, ivory or yellow-white shiny skin. Linear morphea describes markings in which the affected skin forms a line pattern down an arm or a leg. In this case the morphea changes the skin and can interfere with the growth of a limb. Generalized morphea occurs when the lesions of morphea and linear morphea involve almost the entire skin. A distinct type of localized scleroderma is called *en coup de sabre*. In this condition there is an indentation on the forehead or at the frontal hairline. The area of thickened skin can spread to the entire face. Atrophy of the lower part of the face is known as *Parry-Romberg syndrome*. There is no known cure to stop the atrophy progression. The prognosis varies; in some cases it is limited to only a cosmetic issue, whereas in other cases the atrophy may stop before involving the entire face.[4]

Systemic juvenile scleroderma involves the internal organs and occurs less often in children than the localized version. There are two types of systemic juvenile scleroderma:

limited and diffuse. The limited type is characterized by later involvement of the internal organs. It is also known as "CREST," denoting areas of involvement (Box 8-1).

Diffuse juvenile scleroderma is characterized by general skin involvement and early internal organ involvement, especially of the lungs and gastrointestinal system. This results in potential esophageal dysmotility, poor food absorption, and constipation. Additionally, Raynaud phenomenon (localized ischemia) is very common. Involvement of the heart, kidneys, muscles, and joints also occurs. In any case, it is important to remember that localized juvenile scleroderma does not overlap with systemic scleroderma.

There is no known cause or cure for juvenile scleroderma. Few patients are treated at individual centers, which limits well-controlled studies. Treatment of the disease remains a dilemma, especially when determining which children should receive treatment and how the treatment should be monitored. The impact of a chronic illness on a growing child is very different from the impact of a similar disease in the adult population. Children affected by scleroderma require the care of experienced pediatricians who are willing to use a skilled and coordinated approach.

Box **8-1**   CREST
Calcinosis (calcium deposits in the skin) **R**aynaud phenomenon (fingers and toes turn white, blue, red in response to cold temperatures or stress) **E**sophageal dysmotility (frequent heartburn and difficulty swallowing) **S**clerodactyly (thickening of the skin of the fingers, causing contractures into flexion) **T**elangiectasias (areas of red, prominent blood vessels in the skin)

CASE STUDY OF A CHILD WITH A RHEUMATIC DISORDER

EXAMINATION

History
General demographics: Christopher is an 11-year-old Hispanic boy who is bilingual. He attends fifth grade at his neighborhood parochial school.

Social: Chris lives with his mother, father, and two younger siblings. He enjoys swimming, diving, and building things. His large extended family lives nearby and helps with childcare. Chris's family travels extensively during the summer.

Growth and development: Chris is right-hand dominant. Although shorter than average in stature, he was healthy until recently. He achieved all developmental milestones at the appropriate time.

General health: Chris has been generally healthy. He succumbed to a virus 3 to 4 months ago, which may be related to current complaints.

Family history: There is no family history of JRA.

Medical history: Chris has not had any previous hospitalizations or surgeries.

History of current condition: Chris's mother reports he had a virus 3 to 4 months ago. Upon recovery, Chris complained of pain and stiffness in his joints. His physician ordered blood work and subsequently diagnosed Chris with polyarticular JRA.

Functional status and activity level: Chris had difficulty ambulating during the recent exacerbation. He also had difficulty performing ADL activities. (See Tests and Measures for more detailed information.)

Medications: Nonsteroidal antiinflammatory drugs (NSAIDs).

Lab and diagnostic tests: Blood test positive for Rh factor.

Systems Review
Cardiovascular/pulmonary: Normal

Integumentary: See Tests and Measures

Musculoskeletal: See Tests and Measures

Neuromuscular: See Tests and Measures

Communication and cognition: Chris speaks fluent English and Spanish. He is studying Japanese at school. His cognition appears to be typical of a fifth grader. He does well in school and does not require additional assistance.

Continued

CASE STUDY OF A CHILD WITH A RHEUMATIC DISORDER—cont'd

Tests and Measures

Endurance: Chris's endurance is within normal limits. He doesn't complain of fatigue at this point.

Anthropometric characteristics: Chris has relatively short stature for a boy his age. He has moderate bilateral swelling in his knees, wrists, and fingers 2, 3, and 4.

Assistive/adaptive devices: Chris uses a button holer and shoehorn as necessary.

Nerve integrity: All nerves are intact.

Environmental barriers: If in pain, Chris has difficulty climbing steps. In his house there is a staircase leading to the basement.

Gait, locomotion, and balance: Chris's gait is affected by his decreased range of motion. He demonstrated decreased knee extension bilaterally and diminished lateral weight shift as well. He prefers a slower cadence. His dynamic balance reactions of the lower extremities are diminished.

Integumentary: There is increased warmth and redness bilaterally in Chris's knees, wrists, and fingers 2, 3, 4.

Muscle performance:
Strength: All ranges within functional limits (WFL) except:
Bilateral knee extension: 3/5
Bilateral knee flexion: 3/5
Bilateral wrist flexion: 3/5
Bilateral wrist extension: 3/5
Bilateral radial deviation: 3/5
Bilateral ulnar deviation: 3/5
Grip strength bilateral: 3/5

Activities of daily living: Prior to the current episode, Chris was independent in all IADLs and ADLs. At this time he requires assistance for buttons and donning and doffing his shoes and socks.

Pain: Chris reports moderate to severe pain and stiffness in bilateral knees, wrists, and fingers. This may be a limiting factor in his strength testing.

Posture: Chris's postural alignment is good, and no asymmetries are noted at this time. He has slightly winging scapulas bilaterally.

Range of motion: All ranges within normal limits except:
Knee extension: Right −15 degrees; left −10 degrees
Knee flexion: Right −120 degrees; left −130 degrees

Wrist flexion: Right 75 degrees; left 60 degrees
Wrist extension: 0 degrees bilaterally
Wrist radial deviation: 5 degrees
Wrist ulnar deviation: 5 degrees
Finger #2: Flexion: MCP 15
Extension: MCP −5 right −10 left
Finger #3: Flexion: MCP 15
Extension MCP −5 right −10 left
Finger #4: Flexion MCP 15
Extension MCP −5 right −10 left

EVALUATION

Christopher is an 11-year-old boy with a new onset of polyarticular JRA. Joint involvement includes bilateral knees, wrists, and fingers. He is reporting pain and stiffness in these joints. There is noticeable swelling and tenderness in these joints as well. At this time, Chris is having difficulty with his ADLs and ambulation.

Diagnosis

Guide to Physical Therapy Practice Pattern 4H.

Prognosis

Chris should demonstrate optimal joint mobility, ROM, and independence in ADLs.[2] He and his family will also learn how to manage his care, to include pain management, joint protection, and energy conservation techniques. Expected number of visits: 18 over a 6-week period.

INTERVENTIONS

Coordination, Communication, Documentation

Coordination will need to occur between Chris's teachers, pediatrician, rheumatology team, and family. At this time he does not require any academic modifications. Communication between service providers will need to be consistent. Additionally, Chris's teachers will need to be aware of joint protection strategies and exercise/activity precautions. Chris and his family will need to be in communication with the rheumatology team regarding changes in pain, swelling, and activity level.

Patient Instruction

Chris and his family received a written home exercise program (HEP) and also a recorded video of his HEP. The HEP included directions on how to gently and safely complete ROM and strength activities, energy conservation activities (don't let Chris become fatigued, frequent rest periods, use

CASE STUDY OF A CHILD WITH A RHEUMATIC DISORDER—cont'd

backpack or cart with wheels to carry heavy objects), joint protection strategies (no hyperextension, proper body mechanics for bending and lifting), and pain management strategies (self-calming and visualization, medication if needed, heat at home as needed).

Direct Intervention

Therapeutic exercise: Chris's PT program consisted of PROM initially. As his pain symptoms subsided, ROM was advanced to include active assisted ROM and active ROM. Chris was also given a low-impact exercise program. Chris enrolled in a weekly aquatics program at the local hospital's therapeutic pool. At the pool group, he also met other children with arthritis.

Functional training: Chris learned about joint protection strategies and energy conservation techniques. He received a video of himself performing his exercise and stretching program, as well as performing activities using joint protection strategies.

Physical agents: To decrease stiffness, Chris's program included hot packs for his knees and Fluidotherapy for his upper extremities. The family purchased a paraffin unit for home use.

GOALS

1. Chris's ROM will return to the normal range so that he can dress himself.
2. Chris's pain will decrease so that he can play with his friends.
3. Chris and his family will learn his HEP so that he can stay healthy.
4. Chris's strength will return to normal so that he can participate in age-appropriate activities.
5. Chris will have an optometry evaluation.
6. Chris will be independent in performing his home program so that he can maintain his ROM and strength.

REEXAMINATION

Chris will return to rheumatology clinic in 6 weeks for a follow-up examination.

ANALYSIS OF CASE USING THE ICF MODEL:

Body functions: Polyarticular JRA affecting bilateral knees, wrists, and fingers. Pain and swelling in these joints. Loss of ROM bilaterally in knees, wrists, and fingers.

Activity limitations: Decreased ambulation, decreased independence in ADLs and IADLs, decreased fine motor skills and gross motor skills.

Participation restrictions: Cannot ride on skateboard, cannot participate in age-appropriate sports as desired, difficulty changing into gym clothes at school, difficulty carrying books and supplies at school.

Environmental factors: Use backpack with wheels to manage books and schoolwork, wear gym clothes under school uniform/clothes to ease donning/doffing gym uniform at school, add modalities into home environment.

Chapter Discussion Questions

1. What is the disease process that causes juvenile rheumatoid arthritis?
2. Compare and contrast pauciarticular JRA, polyarticular JRA, and systemic JRA.

	Pauciarticular	Polyarticular	Systemic
Subtypes			
Joints involved			
Gender prevalence			

3. Why is it important for a child with JRA to be followed by an ophthalmologist?
4. What are the four medication categories for children with JRA?
5. What are the general PT intervention goals for children with JRA?
6. What is "CREST," and what pathology is associated with it?
7. Compare and contrast localized and systemic scleroderma.
8. What is the translation for *scleroderma*?

REFERENCES

1. Arthritis Foundation: *Raising a child with arthritis: a parent's guide*, Atlanta, 1998, Arthritis Foundation.
2. Tucker LB, DeNardo BA, Stebulis JA, and others: *Your child with arthritis: a family guide for caregiving*, Baltimore, 2000, Johns Hopkins University.
3. Hafner R, Truckenbrodt H, Spamer M: Rehabilitation in children with juvenile chronic arthritis, *Baillieres Clin Rheumatol* 12(2):329, 1998.
4. National Institute of Neurological Disorders and Stroke: *NINDS Parry-Romberg information page* (website): www.ninds.nih.gov/disorders/parry_romberg/parry_romber.htm. Accessed August 1, 2005.

RESOURCES

The Arthritis Foundation
www.arthritis.org
RheumMates
www.RheumMates.com
BrainPOP
www.BrainPOP.com
Healthtalk Interactive
www.healthtalk.com
Mayo Clinic
www.mayoclinic.com
National Institutes of Health
www.nih.gov/naims/healthinfo/rahandout
University of Washington Orthopaedics & Sports Medicine
www.orthop.washington.edu/arthritis.
Enbrel/etanercept
www.enbrel.com/conditions

Part THREE

Congenital Disorders

9

Roberta Kuchler O'Shea, PT, PhD

Arthrogryposis Multiplex Congenita (AMC)

Guide Pattern 4I: Impaired Joint Mobility, Motor Function, Muscle Performance, and Range of Motion Associated with Bony or Soft Tissue Surgery

key terms

Club foot deformity
Joint contractures

outline

Definition
Pathology
Clinical Signs

Intervention
    Physical Therapy Assessment
    Physical Therapy Intervention

learning objectives

At the end of the chapter the reader will be able to do the following:

1. Describe the underlying pathology associated with AMC.

2. Understand the two common forms of AMC.

3. Recognize and describe associated comorbidities.

4. Formulate a treatment plan based on clinical signs and functional impairments.

DEFINITION

Arthrogryposis multiplex congenita (AMC) describes a nonprogressive syndrome of multiple congenital **joint contractures** involving a symmetric pattern in all four extremities. It is also known as *multiple congenital contractures (MCC)*.[1]

PATHOLOGY

This pathology of unknown origin occurring in approximately 1 in 3000 live births,[1] AMC is purely a motor syndrome.[2] It seems to occur within the first trimester of fetal development. Several factors are thought to contribute to the atypical fetal development, including environmental, genetic, and other unknown factors. Maternal fevers, infection, vascular compromise, and limited room in the uterus or low amounts of amniotic fluid may compromise fetal development.[3] The basic pathophysiologic trigger for AMC seems to be lack of fetal movement.[4] Four causes for limited joint movement before birth have been identified[5]:

1. Muscle atrophy
2. Insufficient room within the uterus for normal fetal movement
3. Central nervous system and spinal cord deformities
4. Atypical development of tendons, bones, joints, or joint linings

CLINICAL SIGNS

The deformities of AMC are apparent at birth and include multiple severe joint contractures, dislocations, decreased muscle strength (secondary to atrophy and sometimes absence of muscle groups), lack of normal skin creases, and diminished reflexes (although sensation may be intact).[1,6] Classically there is much variation between children; however, extremity joints typically affected are the hands, wrists, elbows, ankles, knees, and hips

(Figure 9-1). Occasionally a child only has a few affected joints and nearly full range of motion.[5]

There are two commonly seen variations of AMC. In one type the child exhibits abducted and laterally rotated hips, flexed knees, clubfeet (also known as *talipes equinovarus*), medially rotated shoulders, extended elbows, and wrists in flexion with ulnar deviation. The other type of AMC manifests as flexed and dislocated hips, extended knees, clubfeet, medially rotated shoulders, flexed elbows, and flexed and ulnarly deviated wrists.

AMC Clinical Signs

- Multiple involvement of joints with severe contractures
- Dislocations
- Decreased muscle strength secondary to atrophy
- Possible absences of muscle groups
- Lack of normal skin creases
- Diminished reflexes, although sensation may be intact
- Extremity joints typically affected are hands, wrists, elbows, ankles, knees, and hips

---

INTERVENTION

A transdisciplinary team consisting of the child, family, orthopedic surgeon, physical therapist, and occupational therapist should create functional goals for the child. Surgeries should be timed to be developmentally appropriate.

There is discussion about how and when to surgically correct the skeletal deformities and malalignments. Hence foot alignment surgery must occur prior to the age when the child will begin to assume or maintain standing and begin ambulating.

Children with AMC frequently have club feet. Typically the **club foot deformity,** a condition in which the heel of the affected foot points downward and the forefoot turns markedly inward, is surgically corrected between

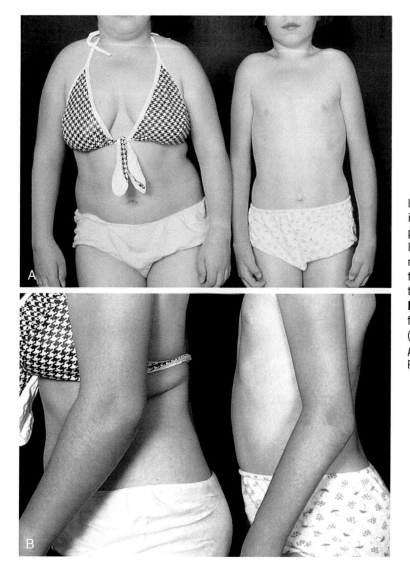

Fig. 9-1 Two sisters with the generalized form of AMC. **A,** Note the stiff posture and tubular appearance of the limbs. Motion of all joints is limited as a result of failure in the development of or the degeneration of muscular structures. Their stature is short.
B, The lateral view highlights the flexion contractures of the elbows. (From Zitelli BJ, Davis HW: *Atlas of pediatric physical diagnosis*, ed 5, Philadelphia, 2007, Mosby.)

6 and 12 months of age.[1] Oleksak, Fernandes, and Saleh found that surgical correction of the knee and foot using circular fixators (external adjustable hardware to correct bony deformities) had longer-lasting correction effects than solely using soft tissue surgical correction.[7] Children with AMC also have an increased incidence of dislocated hips. If both hips are dislocated, surgical reduction is usually not considered, because the pelvis will be relatively level, but if only one hip is dislocated,

surgery may be considered to balance out the pelvis and prevent scoliosis.[4]

PHYSICAL THERAPY ASSESSMENT

Physical therapy assessment should include:
- Measurement of passive and active range of motion of all extremities and neck and trunk
- Strength assessment of all extremities, neck, and trunk
- Evaluation of protective and equilibrium reactions forward, laterally, and backwards

- Evaluation of age-appropriate gross motor skills, including transitional movements and mobility
- Evaluation of age-appropriate activities of daily living skills.

PHYSICAL THERAPY INTERVENTION

The primary motor impairments for the child with AMC are limitations in joint movement and decreased strength and muscle bulk. Intensive stretching and strengthening interventions that assist in gaining and sustaining range and strength are vital. Interventions should be age-appropriate and family-centered.

In the upper extremities, functional independence must be at the forefront of desired treatment outcomes. Elbow flexion and extension are paramount for independence in activities of daily living skills. If bilateral extremities cannot gain motion in both flexion and extension, Tecklin recommends that one arm gain in elbow flexion and the other arm gain in elbow extension, thus allowing functional tasks to be mastered unilaterally.[1]

AMC Interventions

- Strengthening
- Stretching
- Motor control

Infant

Infant intervention will incorporate techniques for the caregiver to use when holding the child and positioning the child for sleep and feeding. Effective interventions will assist the child in gaining range, but also can occur as part of the family's daily routine and interactions with the child. Additionally, serial casting for deformities of the foot, knee flexion contractures, and wrist contractures may be implemented. Extreme care must be taken not to stretch the child's joints past end range and then maintain the stretch using splints or serial casting. Long-term splinting and orthotic use will assist in maintaining joint range of motion and appropriate position. Early mobility is important and sometimes difficult. Rolling may not be optimal when lower-extremity dislocations and contractures are present. Children may learn to sit well but have difficulty transitioning into and out of this position. Many learn to scoot while sitting because quadruped mobility may be complicated by joint contractures and decreased muscle strength.

Toddler

Strengthening and stretching during the toddler years should be incorporated into play schemes. Similarly, functional tasks such as self-feeding, beginning dressing, and ambulation/mobility should be embedded into the routines of the family and not set aside as separate therapeutic activities done in isolation. For example, the child should work on object manipulation and pincer grasp to secure food while eating with the family. Range of motion exercise and dressing can be combined when the child is completing donning and doffing tasks throughout the day. Mobility practice can be built into the task of moving about the environment (instead of being carried). Transition from the floor to standing and standing activities can occur during playtime and dressing time.

An important point to remember is that the physical therapy provider can help the child's caregivers figure out when a child would most likely be doing stretching or strengthening activities during the day and then embed the PT intervention into the family's routines. A home exercise program is far more likely to be carried over if it harmonizes with something the family and child are already doing. To ask a family to add an isolated routine of stretching and strengthening activities onto the beginning or end of their day may result in noncompliance and added family stress.

Preschool and School-Age

As the child develops, intervention activities and goals should reflect age-appropriate skills. These children are typically fully included in the regular education system, with adaptive physical education and therapies outlined on the individualized educational plan (IEP). Preschoolers and school-age children need to strive to be independent in toileting, mobility, and self-care tasks.

The child should become independent in orthotic care and using adaptive equipment during this time as well. Orthotic intervention helps to maintain the joints in optimum alignment, and while orthotics may allow the child to be more functional, they also may contribute to a lack of strength development. The team must be careful to balance the two interventions so that the child can develop optimal strength and motor control but also maintain as much independence as possible.

Strengthening should be system-wide but focused on increasing and maintaining abdominal, hip, and knee strength. Hip and quadriceps strength will be vital for ambulation, ascending and descending steps, and moving through transitional positions. Abdominal strength is also crucial for maintaining upright positions, transitional movements, and ambulation. The therapist may consider offering an intensive strengthening program to the school-aged child with AMC, meaning the child would attend therapy 3 to 5 times during the week for several hours to work intensively on stretching and strengthening activities. Research studying intensive resistance training in children with neuromuscular involvement suggests that a 4-hour session 3 times a week will build strength and endurance without damaging the motor units. Children with AMC need to learn to strengthen and use their muscles. Often, due to weakness and lack of experience, a child will initially require motor planning and sequencing intervention to learn motor skills. After becoming familiar with the movement pattern and learning when to recruit muscle fibers and muscle groups, the child can build on this knowledge to increase strength and endurance.

Children with AMC should be able to gain ambulation skills, perhaps using orthotics and walkers or crutches. As the child ages, decisions concerning ambulation and mobility should take into account the distance needed to be traveled, the speed necessary to be functionally mobile, and the child's energy expenditure. Often older children and young adults will use ambulation within the home or school environment, but opt for wheeled mobility for longer community distances. The goal for all therapeutic and mobility decisions should focus on continued independence and maintaining social and work interaction with peers.

CASE STUDY OF A CHILD WITH ARTHROGRYPOSIS MULTIPLEX CONGENITA

EXAMINATION

History

Sam, the youngest of seven children, was born via cesarean section. His mother, Lynn, reports that at birth, his legs were "folded up and crumpled." A sonogram showed that the fetus's skeletal system had deformities. At birth, Sam was diagnosed with AMC. Sam is now 3 years, 9 months old. He lives at home with his parents, 5 siblings, and a dog. One sibling lives out of the home. Lynn reports that Sam is loved and well cared for by all the family and he adores his older siblings, who love to do activities with him.

Current Condition

Sam has participated in several sessions of pool therapy and therapeutic horseback riding and currently receives weekly PT and OT services through his early childhood program. Sam attended a 3-week intensive transdisciplinary therapy program that included 4 hours a day, 5 days a week, of stretching, strengthening, fine and gross motor skills training, and mobility skills. The protocols also included massage and Suit Therapy program to augment the aforementioned program.

Continued

CASE STUDY OF A CHILD WITH ARTHROGRYPOSIS MULTIPLEX CONGENITA—cont'd

Systems Review

Cardiovascular/Pulmonary: Sam does not have any pathology in his cardiac or pulmonary systems.

> Integumentary: See Tests and Measures
> Musculoskeletal: See Tests and Measures
> Neuromuscular: See Tests and Measures

Functional Status

At his initial evaluation, Sam was an engaging youngster who appeared to be able to charm his way into or out of any situation. He had normal hearing and vision capabilities. He did not exhibit any sensory integration issues. His primary language is English.

Tests and Measures

Sam's skeletal build was typical of a child with arthrogryposis multiplex congenita (AMC). He had undergone bilateral clubfoot correction in the past; the skin was well healed and intact. He had no muscle activation in his lower extremities bilaterally, and muscle atrophy was apparent in both legs. He had normal strength in his proximal upper extremities and trunk; his wrists and hands were weaker. He had intact balance reactions and protective extension of his trunk and upper extremities. His range of motion was within normal limits in his trunk, neck, and upper extremities. He tended to hold his hands in an ulnar drift pattern (hand positioned medially toward the ulna), primarily due to distal weakness. His left hip was limited in extension −15 degrees), but he had full flexion. He had full external rotation, abduction, and adduction of the hip. He could not get to neutral internal rotation. His right hip had full range of motion. Hip radiographs revealed well-seated hips without subluxation or dislocation. Bilaterally his knees lacked passive range. On the left he lacked 35 degrees of full extension, on the right he had movement between −15 degrees and 100 degrees of flexion. He could achieve 5 degrees of passive plantar flexion on the left; all other foot and ankle movement was stuck at neutral.

In order to ambulate Sam wore bilateral KAFOs (knee, ankle, foot orthotics) with drop lock knees and bilateral anterior knee pads. He ambulated using a swing-through gait and a reverse walker at very fast speeds. He had minimal overall poor gait pattern. With his braces on, Sam could transition from the floor to standing with minimal assistance and back again, primarily using his walker and upper extremities. Without orthotics he was unable to maintain weightbearing through his lower extremities. Holding onto the walker he could maintain standing balance for 5 to 8 seconds maximum. If displaced even slightly, he would exhibit overresponsive balance reactions to maintain an upright position. He was unable to manage small perturbations quietly.

Sam could roll independently, he assumed prone position on hands masterfully, but he could not flex his lower extremities under him to assume 4-point position. For floor mobility, he chose to pull himself along using his upper extremities, with the lower extremities dragging behind. He could not attain or maintain 4-point position without assistance. He could floor-sit independently, tending to sacral-sit and use his upper extremities to change his position. He had difficulty maintaining a neutral pelvis in sitting without upper extremity support. He required maximum assistance to transition and maintain tall kneeling and to shift his weight when in tall kneeling. He complained of knee pain when in tall kneel. He could not attain a half-kneel position.

EVALUATION

Sam is a 3¾-year-old male with AMC. He has significant muscle atrophy and muscle weakness in his bilateral lower extremities. He currently ambulates with bilateral long-leg braces (KAFOs bilaterally) and a reverse walker. He can move quickly using a swing-through gait. He demonstrates good balance. Sam should gain strength and more efficient mobility in an intensive therapeutic exercise program.

Diagnosis

4A Prevention/Risk Reduction–Skeletal Demineralization & 4C Impaired Muscle Performance

Prognosis

The prognosis for improving Sam's ambulatory functioning and increasing his strength is good.

INTERVENTION

Coordination, Communication, Documentation

During his intensive PT training, it was important to maintain communication with Sam's physician and community- and school-based therapists.

CASE STUDY OF A CHILD WITH ARTHROGRYPOSIS MULTIPLEX CONGENITA—cont'd

Patient Instruction

Sam and his family received a written home exercise program (HEP) with pictures of Sam completing his exercise routine. The PTs also made a DVD of Sam completing all the exercise routines. Sam can use this at home while exercising.

Direct Intervention

During his 3 weeks of intensive therapy, Sam underwent daily massage and hot packs and gentle passive stretching. These warm-up activities were followed by donning the suit therapy garment. (See Chapter 3 for details on the TheraSuit. The child receives facilitation of weak movement patterns and resistance of dominant movements when in the suit.) While in the suit, Sam completed a series of isometric exercises, including hip extension exercise when prone and dangling his legs off the end of a plinth. Sam also completed trunk extension exercise by hanging his trunk and head over the end of the plinth and attempting to complete repetitions of trunk extension. Sam required maximum stabilization to achieve 1 to 2 repetitions of these exercises. Sam practiced transitioning using typical movement patterns through the developmental sequence: sit to tall kneel, half-kneel to standing, and the reverse. He worked on isolating lower extremity muscles so they would activate when appropriate and not randomly. He practiced improving his standing balance outside of the reverse walker and ambulating with bilateral Lofstrand crutches or hands held.

GOALS

Sam's therapy goals for the 3-week intensive session were: achieve independent ambulation 750 to 1000 feet with the least restrictive device; recruit and activate appropriate muscles in lower extremities to accomplish age-appropriate tasks; decrease the number of verbal cues needed to remind Sam to maintain good and safe hand position.

TERMINATION

Sam made significant gains during his 3-week intensive session. Sam can exhibit spontaneous muscle activity in his lower extremities. He is able to transition from sit to stand using half-kneeling when verbally cued. He ambulates independently and safely with bilateral loft stand crutches using a reciprocal 4-point gait pattern and full weight-bearing through both extremities. This case demonstrates that intensive strengthening and motor therapy can positively impact a child's life.

ANALYSIS OF CASE USING THE ICF MODEL:

Body functions: Muscle atrophy and severe weakness of bilateral lower extremities; significant decreased range of motion in bilateral lower extremities.

Activity limitations: Ambulates with KAFOs and walker; cannot stand or ambulate with assistive technology.

Participation restrictions: Cannot participate in age-appropriate community-based activities.

Environmental limitations: Requires modified access to steps at home and in the community.

Chapter Discussion Questions

1. What are the four potential causes of AMC?
2. Describe the two types of AMC.
3. Typically, who are the members of the transdisciplinary team for a child with AMC?
4. Why would intensive therapy be recommended for a child with AMC?
5. Tecklin recommends what strategy to achieve independence if bilateral upper extremities cannot achieve full range of motion?
6. What are two areas to work on with parents of infants with AMC?
7. What three areas should be the focus of consistent strength training?
8. When is it recommended to perform hip surgery on a child with AMC?
9. Identify three play-based activities that could be used to increase strength.
10. Identify two potential community-based activities appropriate for a child with AMC.

REFERENCES

1. Tecklin JS: *Pediatric Physical Therapy*, ed 3, Philadelphia, 1999, Lippincott Williams & Wilkins.
2. Accardo PJ, Whitman BY: *Dictionary of developmental disabilities terminology*, ed 2, Baltimore, 2002, Paul H. Brookes.
3. Ratliffe KT: *Clinical pediatric physical therapy: a guide for the therapy team*, St Louis, 1998, Mosby.
4. Campbell S, Vander Linden DW, Palisano RJ: *Physical therapy for children*, ed 3, Philadelphia, 2006, Saunders.
5. Avenues, 2004. *What is arthrogryposis?* (online): www.sonnet.com/avenues/pamphlet.html. Accessed May 19, 2004.
6. Akazawa H, Oda K, Mitani S, and others: Surgical management of hip dislocation in children with arthrogryposis multiplex congenita, *J Bone Joint Surg* 80(4):436, 1998.
7. Oleksak M, Fernandes JA, Saleh M: The use of circular fixators for the treatment of joint deformities in arthrogryposis in children, *J Bone Joint Surg* 85:269, 2003.

RESOURCES

Avenues: National Support Group for Arthrogryposis Multiplex Congenita
www.sonnet1.sonnet.com/avenues

National Organization for Rare Diseases
55 Kenosia Ave.
PO Box 1968
Danbury, CT 06813-1968
800-999-6673
203-744-0100

Roberta Kuchler O'Shea, PT, PhD

Down Syndrome

Guide Pattern 4C: Impaired Muscle Performance

learning objectives

At the end of the chapter the reader will be able to do the following:

1. Understand the causes and developmental effects of Down syndrome.

2. Formulate an appropriate treatment plan for a child with Down syndrome.

3. Advocate services for a child with Down syndrome and the child's family.

DEFINITION

Down syndrome (Figure 10-1) was named for and originally described by John Langson Down in 1866. The genetic error responsible for the syndrome was isolated in 1959 when Jerome Lejeune demonstrated the atypical chromosome count.[1,2]

PATHOLOGY

Three types of chromosomal abnormalities can lead to Down syndrome: (1) trisomy 21, occurring in 95% of cases; (2) translocation, making up 4% of cases; and (3) **mosaicism** (some of the body's cells have trisomy 21 and some do not), causing 1% of cases. **Trisomy 21**

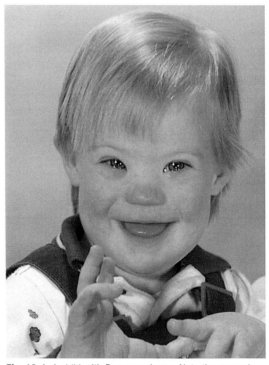

Fig. 10-1 A child with Down syndrome. Note the upward slanting palpebral fissures and epicanthal folds, flat nasal bridge, small ears, and small hands. (From Zitelli BJ, Davis HW: *Atlas of pediatric physical diagnosis*, ed 5, Philadelphia, 2007, Mosby.)

results in an extra chromosome 21. Individuals with trisomy 21 have 47 chromosomes instead of the typical 46. Translocation occurs when the long arm of the extra chromosome 21 attaches to chromosome 14, 21, or 22. Individuals with mosaic trisomy display some of the characteristics of the syndrome, but not all of the characteristics. They tend not to have as significant cognitive delays as individuals with trisomy 21.[2]

Incidence of Down syndrome is approximately 1 in 660 live births—1 in 1500 to 2000 for mothers younger than 30 years, and 1 in 20 to 25 for mothers over age 45.[1,2] Interestingly, trisomy 21 Down syndrome occurs more frequently in males, and translocation Down syndrome occurs more frequently in females.[2]

CLINICAL SIGNS

Some of the most common physical features of Down syndrome are **hypotonia** (low muscle tone), short stature (including short digits), flat facial profile, epicanthal folds and an upward slant to the eyes unusual in the child's ethnic group, small ears, a single transverse palmar crease, and some degree of cognitive limitation. Other abnormalities may include cardiac defects, duodenal atresia, **atlantoaxial instability** (excessive movement in the joint between the atlas [C1] and the axis [C2]), thyroid disorders, conductive hearing loss, Brushfield spots (speckling of the iris), and nutritional concerns.

Down Syndrome Clinical Signs
• Hypotonia
• Short stature
• Flat facial profile
• Epicanthal folds
• Upward slanting palpebral fissures
• Small ears
• A single transverse palmar crease
• Cognitive limitations
• Additional related medical conditions

INTERVENTION

As mentioned previously, there are several related medical conditions associated with Down syndrome. Congenital heart defects occur in 66% of individuals. The most common defect is an endocardial cushion defect. During normal fetal heart development, the inner cardiac tissues (collectively known as *endocardial cushions*) separate into chambers. If this process fails, holes may remain and allow mixing of oxygenated blood with deoxygenated blood. This problem is often compounded by defects in the heart valves regulating blood flow volume to the lungs. As a result, many individuals with Down syndrome experience a rapid decline with congestive heart failure.[2]

Individuals with Down syndrome have specific nutritional issues. Research has demonstrated that children with Down syndrome burn 15% fewer calories per day than their typically developing peers.[3,4] Rather than limit their caloric intake, it is recommended that these children be encouraged to exercise more each day. Exercise opportunities must be built into daily routines (e.g., take the stairs instead of the elevator, walk to a destination instead of driving, or get involved in a physical activity instead of watching TV).

Children with Down syndrome are at risk for many orthopedic comorbidities. This may be in large part from central hypotonia (floppiness without weakness) and ligament laxity. Atlantoaxial instability must be carefully screened for and monitored. This upper spinal segment may dislocate in approximately 15% of individuals with Down syndrome; however, only 1% becomes symptomatic. Symptoms of subluxation include becoming easily fatigued, abnormal gait and/or difficulty ambulating, neck pain, decreased neck mobility (including torticollis), decreased hand function, sensory changes, new onset of incontinence, or clumsiness.[2] Because of their greater likelihood of sustaining orthopedic injuries, children with Down syndrome should be cautious when thinking about playing sports that involve heavy physical contact.

Cognitive limitations are also a concern for individuals with Down syndrome. Early in life, children with Down syndrome tend to be significantly delayed in gross and fine motor skills. As they age and gain skills and experience, motor delays may become less significant. The cognitive delays may be more persistent and influential across the child's life span. Early intervention for motor, cognitive, and social skills can assist the child in learning new tasks and aptitudes. It is imperative that a child with Down syndrome learn the correct way to accomplish a task, be it motor or cognitive. Once the child has mastered a strategy to overcome an obstacle, strong dependence on that strategy is maintained. Children with Down syndrome have difficulty unlearning and relearning a skill or transitioning through the developmental sequence. For example, children with Down syndrome may roll as a primary means of mobility for significantly longer than their typically developing peers. Rolling is fast, energy efficient, and easily mastered. Mastery of four-point crawling is often perceived as a nuisance, because it initially consumes more energy and effort than rolling. Thus the child is less likely to transition from rolling to four-point crawling for mobility when rolling is working well. Eventually, however, the child with Down syndrome walks, runs, and masters higher-level balance activities.

Research shows that 85% of children with Down syndrome have mild to moderate cognitive delays.[2,5] Newer research demonstrates that 100% of adults with Down syndrome who are over the age of 50 exhibit deteriorating brain changes, including the markers for Alzheimer's disease.[2] The educational program for a child with Down syndrome should provide optimal learning and stimulation for the child to grow and develop. A hybrid mix of special education and regular education classes and activities might be most appropriate. Recently several Illinois students with Down syndrome completed high school without enrolling in any special education curricula.[6] This demonstrates a great cooperative effort among the educational district, the family, and the child.

PHYSICAL THERAPY INTERVENTION

Physical therapy interventions should focus on assisting the child to become as independent and functional as possible. Early intervention should focus on improving the child's developmental and coordination skills. Hence activities should promote stability at proximal joints and co-contraction of the joint. Also, activities that promote early development of motor skills and perambulation following the developmental sequence are important.

To improve lower extremity alignment and stability, orthotics may be considered. The rule of thumb is to provide as minimal orthotic intervention as possible to attain the goals. The SureStep flexible supramalleolar orthotic (SMO) usually works very well with children with low tone. This SMO design uses a flexible plastic that provides stability by compressing the tissues of the foot. Thus the foot's intrinsic muscles continue to be recruited and develop. The child is helped to develop typical balance and equilibrium reactions, which are often not fully developed when the child wears traditional orthotics.

SureStep also fabricates a small knee cage to prevent hyperextension. It is based on the manufacturing process of the SureStep SMO, so it is flexible and comfortable. The children who use it gain significant knee stability, because the orthotic prevents hyperextension of the knee joints. Often a soft dynamic orthosis such as TheraTogs can be used to help maintain good skeletal alignment and promote improved function and participation.

Early therapy should focus also on engaging and supporting the family as they adjust to their child with a disability. This may involve locating resources for the family and giving them printed information about Down syndrome, as well as support group information. These families, like other families of children with disabilities, will need to adjust their dynamics to incorporate handling, positioning, and developmental strategies into their everyday routines. The family may potentially need assistance with managing several coexisting medical and social service programs that often come with having a child with a disability.

Down Syndrome Interventions
• Focus on function and independence
• Promote early development of motor skills
• Engage and support family

CASE STUDY OF A TEEN WITH DOWN SYNDROME

EXAMINATION

History

Julian is a 15-year-old boy born with Down syndrome diagnosed at birth. He did not have cardiac involvement and was a healthy newborn. Julian was immediately enrolled in an early intervention program for children. Three years ago, Julian was in a serious motor vehicle accident (MVA) that resulted in a perforated spleen and internal bleeding. Julian underwent emergency surgery. After a hospital stay, Julian was discharged to recover fully at home. He has no remaining issues from the MVA.

Current Condition

Julian is currently referred to PT for conditioning and wellness. He is interested in competing on the high school basketball team. Julian has stable cervical spine, based on current x-ray results.

Systems Review

Cardiovascular/pulmonary: No atypical findings
  Integumentary: No atypical findings
  Musculoskeletal: See Tests and Measures
  Neuromuscular: See Tests and Measures

CASE STUDY OF A TEEN WITH DOWN SYNDROME—cont'd

FUNCTIONAL STATUS

Tests and Measures

Tone: Julian has moderate hypotonia in his trunk and all extremities. He can independently rise from the floor.

Range of Motion: Julian has excessive range of motion in bilateral knees and elbows.

Strength: Julian has 4/5 strength in his distal extremity musculature (wrists, ankles, knees, and elbows) and 5/5 strength in his proximal joints (hips and shoulders)

Sensation: Julian has intact sensation to sharp/dull and light touch.

Balance: Julian has good balance. He can maintain sitting with eyes open and closed with large perturbations. In standing, Julian can maintain static standing with eyes open and large perturbations. He is a bit more unstable in standing with eyes closed, swaying but not losing his balance with moderate perturbations. While balancing on one foot, Julian must keep his eyes open to maintain his balance. He was unable to maintain single leg stance with eyes closed for more than 5 seconds.

Posture: Julian has erect standing and sitting posture. He can easily maintain upright against gravity.

Gait: Julian demonstrates pronated feet bilaterally and knee valgus bilaterally when ambulating. He has a wider than normal base of support but can ambulate forward well. He has difficulty with side to side lateral gait. He can ambulate backwards. When running, Julian has minor difficulties with tripping over his feet.

Endurance: Julian has good endurance for day-to-day activities. He has difficulty completing 20 minutes of aerobic exercise.

EVALUATION

Julian is a 15-year-old boy with Down syndrome. He currently wants to play basketball for his high school team. At this time he demonstrates decreased strength in distal muscles, decreased exercise endurance, and decreased high-level coordination skills.

Diagnosis

4C Impaired Muscle Performance

Prognosis

The prognosis for improving Julian's functioning and increasing his strength, coordination, and endurance is good.

INTERVENTION

Coordination, Communication, Documentation

Julian was given an extensive training and conditioning program. The PT staff communicated with the high school training staff prior to discharging Julian. The athletic trainer employed by the school district would monitor Julian's conditioning program.

Patient Instruction

Julian was taught to monitor his heart rate by taking a pulse count. He was taught to monitor his exertion using the perceived rate of exertion (PRE). He was to work at a PRE of 8-9 when exercising.

Direct Intervention

Julian participated in an outpatient exercise program with peers from school. He had a circuit training program on the weight machines that he completed 2-3 times per week. On alternate days he rode the exercise bike or ran on the treadmill.

GOALS

LTG: Julian wants to be a member of his high school basketball team.

STG: Julian will be able to safely use the weight machines for 20 minutes.

STG: Julian will be able to complete aerobic activity for 20 minutes at a PRE of 9.

STG: Julian will be able to run 4 laps on a basketball court and dribble the ball with less than 2 turnovers.

STG: Julian will be able to shoot the basketball from the free throw line with 70 percent accuracy.

TERMINATION

Julian will be re-examined in 6 weeks. At that time his need for ongoing monitoring will be determined.

ANALYSIS OF CASE USING THE ICF MODEL:

Health condition: Down syndrome

Body functions: Low tone, excessive joint play, decreased strength, overweight.

Activity limitations: Decreased motor skills, limited peer interactions, decreased endurance

Participation restrictions: Cannot be successful in high school sports program, limited opportunities to be friends with peers

Chapter Discussion Questions

1. What are some of the related medical conditions associated with Down syndrome that might interfere with exercise?

2. Because of central hypotonia associated with this syndrome, what types of positioning might be used to assist a parent with the development of head control for improved feeding?

3. Children with Down syndrome frequently have hearing impairments that interfere with learning. What types of activities might be included in an early intervention situation as you work to improve motor skills?

4. You are working in a developmental kindergarten program. A child with Down syndrome is having difficulty with activities that require one-foot standing balance, because his forefoot rolls medially. What therapeutic activities might be helpful for this child?

5. As children with Down syndrome age through early childhood, what types of physical activity would you recommend to parents to improve general strength, coordination, and flexibility?

6. Families with children who have Down syndrome often seek support and information through different stages of development. What are some resources to assist families?

7. Before referring a child with Down syndrome to the local park district tumbling/gymnastics program, which musculoskeletal comorbidity should be screened for?

8. Long-term and positive participation in physical activity is the aim for all children. It is critical for this population that movement experiences be enjoyable, as well as enhance balance and motor skills. How can PTAs assist with programming so the child with Down syndrome will choose to be physically active?

9. Describe the physical characteristics of Down syndrome that may restrict participation in playground activities.

10. Susie is a 9-year-old in second grade. She has mosaic Down syndrome. One-foot standing balance is difficult for Susie, and yet the class is playing kickball during physical education/gym. What adaptations can be made so that Susie can participate in the activity?

REFERENCES

1. Accardo PJ, Whitman BY: *Dictionary of developmental disabilities terminology*, ed 2, Baltimore, 2002, Paul H. Brookes.
2. Roizen N: Down Syndrome. In Batshaw M, editor: *Children with disabilities*, ed 5, Baltimore, 2002, Paul H. Brookes.
3. Luke A, Roizen NJ, Sutton M, and others: Energy expenditure in children with Down syndrome: correcting metabolic rate for movement, *J Pediatr* 125:829, 1994.
4. National Center on Physical Activity and Disability (website): www.ncpad.org. Accessed August 1, 2005.
5. Wisniewski KE: Down syndrome children often have brain with maturation delay, retardation of growth, and cortical dysgenesis, *Am J Med Genetics* 37(S2):274, 2005.
6. Shannon, Anne: Personal communication from director of Aspire, Westchester, Ill, March, 2007.

RESOURCES

National Down Syndrome Society
800-221-4602
www.ndss.org

National Association for Down Syndrome
PO Box 4542
Oak Brook, IL 60522
630-325-9112
www.nads.org

National Down Syndrome Congress
800-232-6372
www.ndscenter.org

March of Dimes
1275 Mamaroneck Ave
White Plains, NY 10605
www.marchofdimes.com

**Health Care Guidelines for Individuals
with Down Syndrome**
   www.denison.edu/collaborations/dsq/
   health96.html
My gift: The Magic of a Special Child, by
   Daniela Geracitano Vance
*My Word Book: Words and Tools for Writing and
   Spelling*, by Dale Marilyn
*The Down Syndrome Nutrition Handbook:
   A Guide to Promoting Healthy Lifestyles*,
   by JE Guthrie Medlen

*Understanding Down Syndrome: An
   Introduction for Parents*, by C. Cunningham
*A Parent's Guide to Down Syndrome:
   Towards a Brighter Future*, by S. Peuschel
*Down Syndrome: Birth to Adulthood: Giving
   Families an Edge*, by JE Reynolds &
   JM Horrebin

Chapter 11

Roberta Kuchler O'Shea, PT, PhD

Spina Bifida

Guide Pattern 5B: Impaired Neuromotor Development
Guide Pattern 5C: Impaired Motor Function and Sensory Integrity Associated with Nonprogressive Disorders of the Central Nervous System—Congenital Origin or Acquired in Infancy or Childhood

key terms

Hydrocephalus	Myelomeningocele	Spina bifida occulta
Meningocele	Neural tube defect	Tethered cord syndrome

outline

Definition	Clinical Signs
Pathology	Intervention

learning objectives

At the end of the chapter the reader will be able to do the following:

1. Describe the different types of spina bifida.

2. Formulate an appropriate treatment plan for a child with spina bifida.

3. Advocate for assistive technology for a child with spina bifida.

DEFINITION

Spina bifida, literally meaning cleft spine or incomplete closure of the spinal column,[1] is a congenital condition caused by the neural tube not fully closing and forming at about 4 gestational weeks in utero (Figure 11-1). It is the most common **neural tube defect**.[1,2]

PATHOLOGY

Spina bifida can be detected prenatally using imaging diagnostic tools or laboratory tests. At about 4 months gestation, a maternal blood test can check for the presence of *alpha-fetoprotein (AFP)*. Elevated maternal serum AFP levels indicate potential presence of spina bifida in the fetus. Additionally, an amniocentesis may be used to detect elevated AFP levels in the amniotic fluid.[3] Immediate aggressive medical and surgical intervention is the current best practice philosophy. Surgical closure of the lesion will help to prevent infection and further trauma to the spinal cord and surrounding neural tissues. Surgery will not, however, repair any damage to the spinal cord or prevent paralysis.[4] Currently surgery is being performed in utero; however, this is still experimental.[3]

There are several levels of spina bifida (occulta, meningocele, and myelomeningocele), each with its own implications and deficits. Generally the systems affected are the neuromuscular and genitourinary systems.[1] The incidence of spina bifida is 1 in 1000 newborns in the United States.[3]

CLINICAL SIGNS

Spina bifida occulta describes the condition where the neural arches do not connect, but there is no neural material located outside of the spinal canal. This is the most common form of spina bifida, characteristically involving the lower lumbar spine. It is also the most benign, with typically no resultant neurologic effects or abnormalities.[1,2] Approximately 40% of the population may have a spina bifida occulta malformation but be asymptomatic.[5]

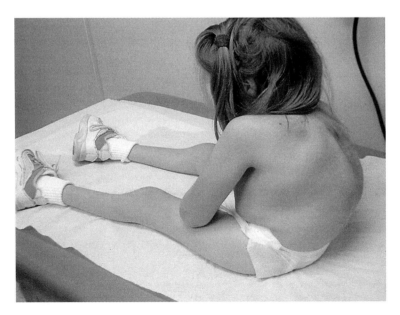

Fig. 11-1 This girl with spina bifida has an obvious kyphotic deformity. The scars on her back are from surgical closure of her myelomeningocele. (From Zitelli BJ, Davis HW: *Atlas of pediatric physical diagnosis*, ed 5, Philadelphia, 2007, Mosby.)

In a **meningocele**, the neural arches do not connect, and the meninges (the three protective membranes covering the brain and spinal cord) protrude through the opening in the child's spinal column. The spinal cord is not trapped, and these children often do not exhibit any neurologic symptoms.[1,2]

In a **myelomeningocele**, both the spinal cord and meninges protrude through the vertebral defect into a sac or open area in the back. The spinal cord and surrounding tissues may be visible and exposed to the environment, which places the child at high risk for infection. The spinal cord is malformed, and defects may extend below the level of the primary herniation. The skin at the lesion is rarely intact, and there may be dura mater fused to the edges of the skin defect, with the sac being covered exclusively by arachnoid membrane. The child exhibits atypical development, including flaccid lower extremities and loss of sensation below the level of the meningomyelocele. The defect can occur at any spinal level, but is often seen in the lumbosacral area. There are several other neurologic sequelae that may accompany myelomeningocele, including abnormalities of the brain, abnormal migration of neurons, and Arnold-Chiari malformation.

Hydrocephalus is found in more than 80% of children with myelomeningocele. **Hydrocephalus** is the enlargement of the ventricular system in the brain due to an increase in cerebrospinal fluid.[3] Interestingly there is little correlation between the degree of hydrocephalus and intellectual functioning.[3] Children with extensive hydrocephalus have demonstrated typical intelligence. Hydrocephalus may be a result of the Arnold-Chiari malformation.[1,3] Type 2 Arnold-Chiari defect associated with myelomeningocele is a malformation in which the base of the brain (cerebellum, pons, medulla) is elongated and protrudes into the foramen magnum.[3] The child's hydrocephalus requires immediate treatment and correction by the medical team. This correction usually is in the form of a ventriculoperitoneal (VP) shunt,[4] a narrow tube that is surgically inserted into the ventricle, threaded under the skin, behind the ear, under the clavicle, and into the peritoneal area. The shunt drains cerebrospinal fluid out of the brain and into the gut. An extra length of tubing is typically placed into the gut to allow for growth of the child without needing to replace the shunt. Caregivers should be taught the warning signs of shunt malfunction in the child, which include irritability, personality changes, increased sleepiness, "sunset eyes" (the child's eyes assume a downward gaze, mimicking a sunset), or headaches. The child should return to the physician if a shunt malfunction is suspected.

Bowel and bladder dysfunction also become significant issues in individuals with meningocele and myelomeningocele spina bifida. Incontinence can usually be managed with clean catheterization. Children should be taught to independently and safely catheterize themselves as soon as developmentally possible.

Latex allergies are present in up to 73% of children with spina bifida. This may be attributable to the early and constant exposure to rubber/latex products (therapy equipment, catheterization equipment) that children with spina bifida experience as infants and young children.[6]

Due to the nature of the resultant disabilities, children with spina bifida often have difficulties in social and emotional development. Purposeful thought must be given to this aspect of client management. All therapists and team members should be highly alert to the quality of the child's social and emotional growth and adjustments. Children need to be given opportunities to interact with other children in age-appropriate social settings, be it at home, at school, or within the community.

An associated impairment of spina bifida is **tethered cord syndrome**. This occurs when the spinal cord is fixed caudally because of pathology. The tethered spinal cord becomes stretched, distorted, and ischemic. The child with tethered cord may show atypical neurologic signs that include decreased strength, increased spasticity in the lower extremities, changing urologic patterns, back pain, or scoliosis. Surgery to free the cord is usually performed, and success of the surgery is measured by a return of neurologic function.

The clinician should be aware of a related form of spina bifida, occult spinal dysraphism (OSD). OSD is a condition in which there is a noticeable abnormality of the child's lower back. This abnormality may be a birthmark (perhaps red in color), tufts of hair, a small opening in the skin, a small lump, or a sacral dimple. This sacral dimple is suspicious if it is not in the midline, is above the sacral region, is large, or does not have a visible bottom. In OSD, the spinal cord may be directly exposed to infection and bacteria via a slit in the skin. The spinal cord may also be tightened down in certain areas. Babies with a sacral dimple should be further evaluated using imaging techniques to determine if pathology is present.[1,2]

Spina Bifida Clinical Signs

Spina Bifida Occulta
- Skin depression or dimple
- Dark tufts of hair
- Telangiectasis
- Soft subcutaneous lipomas at the site
- Asymptomatic in 40% of cases

Meningocele
- Neural arches unconnected
- Herniation of meninges through spinal opening
- Asymptomatic
- Possible bowel and bladder dysfunction

Myelomeningocele
- Herniated sac containing spinal cord, meninges, and tissues protrudes through a congenital cleft in vertebral column
- Flaccid lower extremity
- Loss of sensation below myelomeningocele
- Other abnormalities possible
- Hydrocephalus in 80% of cases
- Possible bowel and bladder dysfunction

INTERVENTION

Physical therapy should focus on assisting the child to become independent in functional skills—including mobility, transfers, and recreational activities—to enhance the child's ability to participate with all peers. Therapy programs may include active stretching and strengthening of musculoskeletal tissues, increasing endurance for mobility, developing independent transfer skills, and teaching motor activities that improve the child's performance in everyday life routines.

A child with a lumbosacral myelomeningocele may exhibit any or all of the following: flaccid paralysis, muscle weakness, muscle wasting, atypical tendon reflexes, atypical sensation, incontinence, and hydrocephalus. Comorbidities for the individual with myelomeningocele would include skin breakdown in weightbearing areas, severe vasomotor changes, osteoporosis, soft tissue contractures, cognitive delays, and social delays. Additionally, there may be other congenital abnormalities related to the abnormalities of the spinal vertebrae, such as cleft palate or skeletal malformations.[1] Interventions should address the child's functional deficits and capitalize on the child's strengths.

The family must be educated in the proper care and nutrition of the infant/child with spina bifida. This will include teaching optimal positioning for the child, reminding about the importance of weightbearing and upright positioning, reiterating shunt care and signs and symptoms of shunt malfunction, and providing information on how to safely construct the child's environment to compensate for decreased sensation. The family should be allied with a medical and therapeutic team familiar with children with spina bifida. The family should also be referred to a relevant support group.

Intervention will always depend on the child's lesion level, functional abilities, and age. Children with myelomeningocele will develop gross motor skills more slowly than their peers. Strengthening and range of motion of all extremities and the trunk is an integral portion of the child's rehabilitation program. It is easier to prevent contractures than reverse them. Strengthening and range of motion exercises should be embedded into the family's ordinary daily routines as much as possible.

The child with spina bifida should be positioned in the upright posture as soon as feasibly possible. This will assist in developing strong abdominal muscles and good trunk alignment. Supported standing will also promote bone density development and good structural alignment. Practice will be needed to develop strong balance and equilibrium reactions in sitting and standing to be able to play and become independently mobile. The child with spina bifida and motor impairments often uses orthotics and will need good balance reactions to be mobile while using the orthotics so as not to fall over when ambulating or participating in age-appropriate activities. For example, the young child with independent sitting balance is free to play on the floor with friends or sit in a chair and interact with classmates and peers. Good standing balance can enable the child to participate in more activities independently. If a child can maintain standing, then the child can participate in board activities in the classroom or sports activities at some level. The child with good static and dynamic balance will also be able to be more mobile within his or her environment.

Orthotics will play an important role in the medical management of the child with spina bifida. Ankle-foot orthoses may be needed to maintain proper foot, ankle, and knee position during standing and ambulation. The child might also benefit from a reciprocal gait orthosis (RGO). The RGO, designed to assist in ambulation, is essentially a dynamic HKAFO (hip, knee, ankle, foot orthosis) with a trunk component incorporated into its design. When the user leans backward leading with one shoulder, the contralateral hip flexes, and that

lower extremity is advanced. This pattern of movement—lean back, advance leg, lean back on other side, advance other leg—allows the user to gain forward upright mobility. Typically the child uses the RGO in conjunction with a walker or crutches to maintain balance. An orthosis to support the trunk may also be worn independently of lower extremity orthotics. This orthosis will be named for the body area it covers. If the orthosis encompasses the entire trunk from the inferior spine of the scapula to the pelvis, it is called a *thoracic-lumbar-sacral orthosis (TLSO)*. If it only encompasses the lower back, it is referred to as a *lumbar-sacral orthosis (LSO)*.

Prior to recommending wheeled mobility, the team should evaluate the child for orthotics, ambulation potential, and energy expenditure with self-propelled mobility. If it is determined that the child would benefit from wheeled mobility, a referral to an assistive technology team is worthwhile. Most children with spina bifida can propel a manual wheelchair without difficulty. Depending on the child's trunk and lower extremity strength, the child may need a contoured seating system. The child may also require a pressure-relief cushion to maintain skin integrity. There is a complete discussion of seating and mobility equipment in Chapter 17.

The prognosis for individuals with spina bifida is improving with advances in medical technology. Ninety percent of babies born with spina bifida survive into adulthood, 80% have normal intelligence as measured by IQ testing, and 75% participate in sporting activities.[3]

Spina Bifida Interventions

- Focus on independence in functional skills
- Stretching and musculoskeletal tissue strengthening activities
- Address functional deficits
- Care and nutrition education
- Range of motion exercises
- Promote good static and dynamic balance
- Address mobility

CASE STUDY OF A CHILD WITH SPINA BIFIDA

EXAMINATION

History

General demographics: Angelica (Annie) is a 3-year-old child with spina bifida. She was diagnosed with spina bifida 1 week prior to birth. She lives at home with her mother, father, paternal grandparents, and three older siblings.

Growth and development: Annie has not determined hand dominance yet. She had delays with mastery of developmental milestones, but can independently roll, sit, and transition to standing now.

General health: Annie underwent surgical closure of the spina bifida lesion (at level L3) when she was 2 days old. No shunt placement was necessary. Her overall health has been excellent. She has never had a bladder infection.

Family history: There is no family history of spina bifida.

Medical history: With the exception of the postnatal surgery, all other medical history is unremarkable. Annie has received therapy services (PT, OT, and developmental therapy) through the early intervention program.

History of current condition: Annie's condition was diagnosed via ultrasound 1 week prior to birth. She was delivered at full term by cesarean section and immediately transferred to the neonatal intensive care unit (NICU). Following surgery she was monitored in the NICU for several days before being discharged home.

Functional status and activity level: Annie is a very happy and active child who moves around her home independently without assistive devices. She will use assistive devices when out in the community. See Tests and Measures for more detailed information.

Medications: Annie does not take any medications. She does take nonprescription vitamins daily.

Systems Review

Cardiovascular/pulmonary: No abnormalities reported.

Integumentary: See Tests and Measures

Musculoskeletal: See Test and Measures

Neuromuscular: See Tests and Measures

Communication and cognition: Annie speaks fluent English, her primary language. She does not have any cognitive limitations at this time, although occasionally she has difficulty solving novel complex-task problems.

Tests and Measures

Endurance: Annie fatigues more quickly than her peers if walking long distances. She prefers to be carried or ride in a stroller or wagon for walks around her neighborhood.

Pain: No evidence of pain or discomfort.

Integumentary: Well-healed scar on posterior lower trunk at the level of L3-4. Callusing noted on bilateral medial and lateral foot borders. Mild redness noted at left lateral malleoli; however, this dissipated after 6 minutes.

Range of motion: Passive range of motion in all extremities and trunk. Head is held in midline, and there are no spinal asymmetries noted.

Strength: Trunk and bilateral upper extremities 4+/5; bilateral hips all planes 3+/5; bilateral knee flexion and extension 3/5; bilateral ankle strength, all planes, 3−/5, 1/5 in bilateral feet, all planes.

Sensation: Decreased sensation in distal lower extremities and feet.

Environmental barriers: Annie lives in a single story ranch house. There are no stairs inside the home. There is a small step at both the front entranceway and back door, which Annie can maneuver over if she concentrates.

Balance: Annie demonstrates initial self-righting responses when sitting. When standing she uses a hip strategy, but does not demonstrate an ankle strategy. When standing, Annie uses her upper extremities for support and stability.

Transitional skills: Annie independently transitions from supine to standing by progressing through half-kneeling without assistance.

Gait/locomotion: Annie ambulates with a wide stance and significant lateral sway. She maintains her upper extremities in the low guard position.

Assistive/adaptive devices: Annie does not use any assistive devices at home. If ambulating outdoors, she may choose to use Lofstrand crutches. If she is feeling particularly tired, she may ask to use her walker, but that is not a typical request.

Activities of daily living: Annie can assist with donning and doffing her AFOs. She assists with her

CASE STUDY OF A CHILD WITH SPINA BIFIDA—cont'd

dressing of the lower extremities; however, she has some difficulty donning and doffing shoes and socks. Her siblings work with her to improve her skills and speed. Annie can feed herself, comb her hair, and brush her teeth. She drinks from a cup, typically without a lid, and uses a spoon or fork to eat.

Posture: Annie sits erectly and stands with a slight lordosis.

Gross Motor Function Measure summary:
- Lying and rolling—mastered all 17 items, 100%.
- Sitting—mastered all 19 items, 100%
- Crawling and kneeling—completed 12/13 tasks, 92%. Annie had minimal difficulty with walking and tall kneeling.
- Standing—completed 10/12 tasks, 83%. Annie had minimal difficulty when attempting to stand on one foot for up to 10 seconds. She was able to maintain unilateral stance for 3 to 6 seconds.
- Walking, running, jumping—completed 20/23 tasks, 87%. Annie had difficulty stepping over a bar raised 6 to 8 inches off the floor and jumping horizontally or vertically. Annie also had minimal difficulty walking backwards. She can run and ride a tricycle short distances.

EVALUATION

Annie is a happy, mobile, 3-year-old preschooler. She wears bilateral hinged AFOs and typically only ambulates with Lofstrand crutches for long distances outdoors. She has significant weakness in her lower extremities and difficulty performing some high-level gross motor skills. Her skin is intact, and there are no integumentary concerns at this time.

Diagnosis
PT Guide Practice Pattern: 5B, 5C

Prognosis
Annie's strength and endurance should continue to improve. She is at risk for comorbidities of spina bifida as she ages, and these should be monitored. She should be able to learn and master bowel and bladder routines in the future. Expected number of visits: 24 over the next 6 months.

INTERVENTION

Coordination, Communication, Documentation
Coordination will need to occur between Annie's family, school therapists and teachers, clinic therapists, and physicians.

Patient Instruction
Annie and her family received a written home program for working on endurance and community ambulation skills. Activities included Annie keeping a journal of how far/number of steps she walked while at home and changing Annie's chores to include retrieving the mail, helping to walk the family dog, or any activity that involved walking medium to long distances. Annie was shown how to check her skin after taking off the orthotics. Annie's family was encouraged to stay connected with the local support groups for spina bifida.

Direct Intervention
Therapeutic exercise: Strengthening exercises for the lower extremities using latex-free Thera-Band. Aerobic exercise, including walking on the treadmill in the clinic.

Functional training: Annie was also enrolled in a local age-appropriate swimming program to help increase her overall strength and endurance. Dynamic balance and climbing activities were offered in PT to focus on higher-level gross motor skills. These included standing on a balance board and varying the balance point, walking on unstable surfaces (soft foam cushions covering the floor), jumping on a mini-trampoline with a rail support, and climbing playground equipment.

GOALS

1. Annie will improve lower-extremity strength one grade so she can safely ascend and descend the school bus steps.
2. Annie will increase her endurance so she can walk two blocks to the park to play with her friends.
3. Annie will maintain good skin conditions and be reevaluated for new AFOs as she grows.
4. Annie will be able to dress herself with occasional assistance so she can be more independent.

Continued

CASE STUDY OF A CHILD WITH SPINA BIFIDA—cont'd

REEXAMINATION

Annie will be reassessed in 6 months by her hospital-based clinic team.

ANALYSIS OF CASE USING THE ICF MODEL:

Body functions: Spina bifida L3 level, no shunt. Significantly decreased strength in bilateral lower extremities. Decreased endurance. Decreased high-level gross motor skills. Ambulates with bilateral AFOs, uses crutches when ambulating outdoors.

Activity limitations: Difficulty playing with peers outdoors, not independent in dressing, difficulty ascending and descending steps, fatigues easily.

Participation restrictions: Requires assistance for activities of daily living, requires assistance on and off the school bus, has difficulty playing at the park with peers and walking around her neighborhood.

Environmental limitations: Requires single-story home and ramps to access buildings and park equipment.

Chapter Discussion Questions

1. Describe the warning signs of VP shunt malfunction in a toddler with spina bifida and hydrocephalus.
2. What types of assistive walking devices when playing at the park might be used for an 18-month-old toddler with spina bifida, functioning at the L4 level?
3. Juan is a 4-year-old boy with spina bifida. He uses bilateral AFOs and crutches to ambulate. His early childhood classroom is going on a field trip to the local firehouse. What other types of mobility might be used to increase his efficiency and reduce fatigue?
4. Fran is a 15-month-old girl with spina bifida, functioning at the T12 level. She was fitted for a vertical stander to support her in standing. Plan a program incorporating the stander into her daily routines. What types of therapeutic exercise could be encouraged with this piece of equipment?
5. Jackson attends first grade at the local public school. He is receiving PT per his IEP. He uses AFOs and crutches for mobility. You notice a change in his gait pattern. You remove the right orthotic and note a very reddened area at the lateral calcaneus. What is your plan of action?

6. Children with spina bifida are at higher risk for latex sensitivities. What type of exercise equipment might need to be modified/adapted so these children are not excluded from participating in physical education or conditioning programs?
7. Joe had surgery to lengthen soft tissue restrictions and returned to school using bilateral KAFOs and a walker. Prepare a program for Joe that includes standing transfers to/from wheelchair to walker. What problems might he encounter using a walker in a school environment?
8. Tess is a sophomore in high school. She was born with spina bifida and wears a TLSO to assist alignment for a structural scoliosis. She functions at the L5 motor level. Tess uses a manual wheelchair for school, but will walk with bilateral AFOs and forearm crutches in the community setting. Tess is a straight-A student, president of the debate club, and class secretary. She recently fell and fractured her arm. Surgical intervention resulted in 10 weeks in an above-elbow cast with strict restrictions on weightbearing through the fractured extremity. How can Tess achieve independent mobility at school?

REFERENCES

1. Shepard RB: *Physiotherapy in pediatrics*, ed 3, Oxford, 1999, Butterworth-Heinemann.
2. Liptak GS: Neural tube defects. In Batshaw M, editor: *Children with disabilities*, ed 5, Baltimore, 2002, Paul H Brookes.
3. Columbia University Medical Center: Department of Neurological Surgery: *Spina bifida* (website): http://columbianeurosurgery.org/ct/spina_bifida.html. Accessed September 18, 2004.
4. Umphred D: *Neurological rehabilitation*, ed 5, St Louis, 2007, Mosby.
6. Spina Bifida Association of America (website): www.sbaa.org. Accessed June 1, 2004.
5. Accardo PJ, Whitman BY: *Dictionary of developmental disabilities terminology*, ed 2, Baltimore, 2002, Paul H Brookes.

RESOURCES

Easter Seals
230 W. Monroe Street #1800
Chicago, IL 60606-4802
800-221-6827
www.easter-seals.org

March of Dimes Birth Defects Foundation
1275 Mamaroneck Avenue
White Plains, NY 10605
888-663-4637
www.marchofdimes.com

Spina Bifida Association of America
www.sbaa.org

National Rehabilitation Information Center (NARIC)
4200 Forbes Boulevard, #202
Lanham, MD 20706
800-346-2742
www.naric.com

National Resource Center on Spina Bifida
4590 MacArthur Boulevard NW, Suite 250
Washington, DC 20007
800-621-3141/ 202-944-3285

Spina Bifida Association of Canada
220-388 Donald Street
Winnipeg MB CAN R3B 2J4
1-800-565-9488
www.sbhac.ca
French: www.sbhac.ca/sbhfrbo.html

International Federation for Hydrocephalus and Spina Bifida
www.ifglobal.org

Children with Spina Bifida
www.waisman.wisc.edu/~rowley/sb-kids/

Chapter 12

Margaret O'Shea, OTR/L

Autism and Autism Spectrum Disorders

Guide Pattern 5B: Impaired Neuromotor Development

key terms

Asperger syndrome
Autism
Autism spectrum disorders

Childhood disintegrative disorder

Rett syndrome

outline

Definition
Pathology
Clinical Signs
    Other Autism Spectrum Disorders

Intervention
    Physical Therapy Assessment
    Physical Therapy Intervention

learning objectives

At the end of the chapter the reader will be able to do the following:

1. Identify autism and the various autism spectrum disorders.

2. Understand the social, communication, cognitive, and other issues associated with autism and autism spectrum disorders.

3. Identify intervention techniques for children with autism and autism spectrum disorders.

4. Identify appropriate long- and short-term treatment objectives for children with autism and autism spectrum disorders.

DEFINITION

Autism is the most common of a series of related neurobiological disorders known collectively as **autism spectrum disorders** or *pervasive developmental disorders*. Other autism spectrum disorders include Rett syndrome, Asperger syndrome, childhood disintegrative disorder, and pervasive developmental disorder not otherwise specified (PDD/NOS).

PATHOLOGY

Autism was first identified in 1943 and until the 1970s was generally treated as a psychologic disorder caused by poor parenting. Now autism is recognized as a neurobiological disorder. Researchers have yet to identify a clear, single cause of autism, although most researchers now believe that genetics play a leading role. Some research indicates that autism may have environmental, viral, or metabolic causes, while other research supports the theory that autism may stem from a genetic predisposition meeting certain environmental or other triggers. Whatever the cause, the number of diagnosed cases of autism has risen sharply in recent years.

According to the Autism Society of America, diagnoses of autism have risen from 1 in 10,000 births in 1943 to 4 in 10,000 births in 1990 to 1 to 2 in 1000 births in 2007.[1] The Centers for Disease Control estimates that 1.77 million Americans suffer from an autism spectrum disorder.[2] It is unclear whether there is an actual increase in the incidence of autism or whether increased attention to and improved diagnosis of the disorder accounts for the rise in number of cases reported.[3] The prevalence of autism is four times higher in boys than it is in girls; however, girls with autism often have more severe impairments than boys.[2]

Children with autism often may have one or more other disorders, including ADD or ADHD, anxiety disorder, deafness, depression, obsessive compulsive disorder, and Tourette syndrome.[4] Between 26% and 68% of children with autism have mental retardation,[4] although accurate IQ testing on children with autism can be difficult. Many autistic children do have highly developed "splinter skills," but generally not to the savant level portrayed in movies like *Rain Main* and *Mercury Rising*. Approximately 35% of individuals with autism will develop seizures, often around the onset of puberty.[5]

New legislation has been enacted that mandates autism-specific activities. The Children's Health Act of 2000, the New Freedom Initiative of 2001, and the Combating Autism Act of 2006 all promote awareness and increase the availability of services to children with disabilities, including autism. The Combating Autism Act of 2006 enhances research, surveillance, and education for autism spectrum disorders (Box 12-1).

Box 12-1 Combating Autism Act of 2006

The Act authorizes the Secretary of Health and Human Services to:
- Provide information and education on ASD and other developmental disabilities to increase public awareness of developmental milestones
- Promote research into the development and validation of reliable screening tools for ASD and other developmental disabilities and disseminate information regarding those screening tools
- Promote early screening of individuals at higher risk for ASD and other developmental disabilities as early as practicable
- Increase the number of individuals who are able to confirm or rule out a diagnosis of ASD and other developmental disabilities
- Increase the number of individuals able to provide evidence-based interventions for individuals diagnosed with ASD or other developmental disabilities
- Promote the use of evidence-based interventions for individuals at higher risk for ASD and other developmental disabilities as early as practicable

From Office of the Press Secretary: Fact Sheet: Combating Autism Act of 2006, December 19, 2006 (online): http://www.whitehouse.gov/news/releases/2006/12/20061219-3.html. Accessed October 17, 2007.

CLINICAL SIGNS

A variety of impairments in social interaction can be indicative of autism. Individuals with autism often demonstrate poor eye contact when interacting with others. They may make no or only cursory eye contact, may make eye contact in an unorthodox manner (such as turning their head to the side and looking obliquely at the individual with whom they are interacting), or in a group may look at someone who is not speaking.

Individuals with autism may also demonstrate marked impairment in facial expressions, body postures, and gestures. Whereas children without autism learn intuitively to understand and then use appropriate facial expressions and other physical cues to reflect their own feelings and needs and understand nonverbal cues from others, children with autism generally demonstrate flat affect and show marked impairment in their ability to interpret facial or gestural cues from others.

Children with autism also typically fail to form successful peer relationships. They often prefer to be alone and will choose activities that have no social component, such as watching videos. They often will ignore others in the area or even may react negatively to attempts to "intrude" upon their isolating activities. They generally do not share their interests or accomplishments. Whereas a child without autism often wants to share an accomplishment with parents or peers ("Mommy, look at the picture I drew!"), a child with autism typically shows little or no interest in such interactions.

Individuals with autism exhibit limited or no joint attention (engaging another to interact) and frequently have difficulty shifting attention from one item or task to another. Whereas children without autism readily learn to share attention (i.e., respond to a request or directions from a parent or peer to look at something else) or devote the communal attention necessary to complete a social task, children with autism will often resist or not even understand such requests. Children with autism also will frequently devote an inappropriate amount of attention to a particular object or activity (Figure 12-1).

Social reciprocity is another area where children with autism generally show deficits. All children must learn basic reciprocal behaviors that make social congress possible (e.g., waiting in line, taking turns, and sharing). And while such behaviors are often somewhat

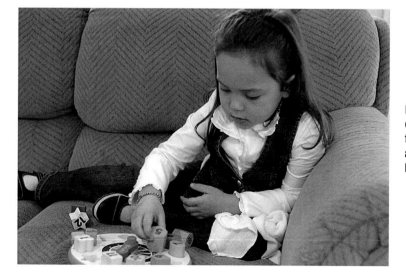

Fig. 12-1 Children with autism often demonstrate a preference and skill for relating objects in construction activities and puzzles. (Courtesy Shay McAtee.)

problematic for all young children, they are especially difficult for those with autism. The less concrete the rules for behavior are, the more problematic they are likely to be for someone with autism. For example, a child with autism might be able to learn to wait in a formal line, but likely would have more difficulty dealing with the informal queuing up involved in, say, boarding a train.

Delay in or lack of language skills development is a key diagnostic indicator for autism. Not only is language often delayed or diminished, but children with autism generally do not substitute mime, gesture, or other alternative communication strategies to compensate, as would a child with a limitation like deafness.

Even in cases where a child has developed language skills, there is often a marked deficit in the ability to initiate or maintain a conversation. Because of the autistic individual's social impairments and the attendant lack of motivation to engage in normal social exchange, language for the autistic child is often limited to meeting concrete wants and needs, even in cases where the child has fluent language skills. He or she might ask for something to eat, but is unlikely to tell you about his or her day. Children with autism also frequently use stereotyped or repetitive language. They often may have standard rote responses to certain questions or situations, or may perseverate (uncontrollably repeat) a word or phrase.

Autistic children generally do not engage in spontaneous or imitative play. Whereas children without autism are able to generalize and abstract information, children with autism have limited abilities in these areas. Thus they are unlikely to transfer the experience of watching an activity into imitative or spontaneous play.

A child with autism often will demonstrate abnormally intense interest in unusually narrow areas of interest. For example, one might encounter a child with autism who has memorized the entire cable television schedule and could readily tell you the date and time for any program, even those of no particular interest. Another child with autism might go to a mall and want to do nothing but ride in all the elevators. This intense interest in a narrow area can manifest as an abnormal fear (e.g., a fear of elevators instead of a desire to ride them).

Autistic children often rigidly adhere to routines or rituals with no apparent functional purpose. For example, a child with autism might insist on always sitting in the same seat or always opening and closing the door to the room twice when entering. Although the purpose of the rituals is not apparent, a child with autism is likely to become upset if these routines are interrupted or interfered with.

Stereotyped motor behaviors also are common among children with autism. Examples of such behaviors could include constant rocking and flapping of the hands or fingers. Such behaviors often are self-stimulatory in nature.

Finally, children with autism may be abnormally preoccupied with certain objects—anything from pencils to paper clips to pot lids. If they encounter such an object, they may remain focused on it for hours.

Odd or exaggerated responses to sensory stimuli are common in autistic children. They often are very sensitive to sound, sometimes even seeming to find normal levels of sound painful or intrusive. They may overreact to being touched or have difficulty with tags in their clothing or certain textures of cloth. Many dislike bright lights and often will choose dark, enclosed spaces. They also may have exaggerated reactions to odors or other stimuli, but sometimes demonstrate an unusually high tolerance for pain.

For the diagnosis of autism, onset of symptoms must have occurred prior to age three. In addition, Rett syndrome and childhood disintegrative disorder should be ruled out as more likely causes of developmental problems before arriving at a diagnosis of autism.

Autism and ASD Clinical Signs

- Does not babble or coo by 12 months
- Does not gesture (point, wave, grasp) by 12 months
- Does not say single words by 16 months
- Does not say two-word phrases on his or her own by 24 months
- Has any loss of any language or social skill at any age
- Does not respond to his or her name
- Cannot say what he or she wants
- Language is delayed
- Doesn't follow directions
- Appears deaf at times
- Seems to hear sometimes but not at others
- Doesn't point or wave goodbye
- Used to say a few words, but now doesn't
- Doesn't smile socially
- Seems to prefer to play alone
- Gets things for himself or herself
- Is very independent
- Does things "early"
- Has poor eye contact
- Is in his or her own world
- Tunes other people out
- Is not interested in other children
- Has tantrums
- Is hyperactive, uncooperative, or oppositional
- Doesn't know how to play with toys
- Gets stuck on things regularly
- Toe walks
- Has an unusual attachment to toys
- Lines things up
- Is oversensitive to certain textures or sounds
- Has odd movement patterns

OTHER AUTISM SPECTRUM DISORDERS

Rett Syndrome

Like autism, **Rett syndrome** has an early onset (prior to age 4) and features impairments in communication and socialization. Unlike autism, which affects males four times more frequently than females, Rett syndrome has only been diagnosed in girls. It is a genetic condition associated with an abnormality on the X chromosome.[6] Children with Rett syndrome develop normally through the first few months of life, and then around 5 months of age lose hand function and develop stereotyped hand movements that resemble hand wringing or hand washing. Head growth slows, and social impairments similar to those in autism emerge. Children with Rett have difficulty—often severe difficulty—with walking and trunk movements. There is severe learning disability, little or no language development, and no pretend play. Unlike autism, the social impairments associated with Rett syndrome often ease in late childhood or adolescence.

Childhood Disintegrative Disorder

Childhood disintegrative disorder is a condition occurring in 3- and 4-year-olds who have developed normally to age 2. Over several months a child with this disorder will deteriorate in intellectual, social, and language functioning from previously normal behavior. The cause of childhood disintegrative disorder is unknown, but it has been linked to neurologic problems. An affected child shows a loss of communication skills, has regression in nonverbal behaviors, and demonstrates significant loss of previously acquired skills. The condition is very similar to autism.

Asperger Syndrome

Asperger syndrome is a neurobiological disorder. Children with this disorder have average or above-average IQs, whereas children with autism usually have below-average IQs. Asperger syndrome can be evidenced by marked deficiencies in social skills, difficulties with transitions or changes, obsessive routines, and preoccupation with a particular subject of interest. Affected children often demonstrate many autistic symptoms, including elevated sensitivities to certain sounds, tastes, textures, or light. Whereas individuals with autism generally have significant delays and deficits in speech, language development in individuals with Asperger syndrome generally seems normal, although they may have difficulties with pragmatic language and can be overly literal or have problems with idiom and using language in a social context.

Pervasive Developmental Disorder—Not Otherwise Specified

Pervasive developmental disorder—not otherwise specified (PDD-NOS) is a subthreshold condition in which the individual meets some, but not all, the diagnostic criteria necessary for a diagnosis of autism. Generally children diagnosed with PDD-NOS demonstrate issues with socialization and behavior similar to but less severe than those behaviors evidenced by persons with autism. They have fewer if any language issues.

INTERVENTION

Symptoms of autism can begin to emerge as early as 12 to 18 months and are almost always evident between 24 months and 6 years of age. Numerous studies have demonstrated that early diagnosis and treatment of autism results in substantially improved outcomes. Although differences in methods and interventions exist, there is a growing consensus about the elements that are most important and effective in early childhood intervention (Box 12-2).

PHYSICAL THERAPY ASSESSMENT

Autism is a developmental disability that by its nature emerges gradually. In many cases parents, through their intense daily experience with their child, will have noticed important but subtle issues and raise those issues with the child's healthcare provider. Pediatricians or other clinicians may dismiss parents' concerns, because the signs are not readily evident during a brief visit within a clinical setting. By the time the developmental issues in question become obvious, important time has been lost, so it becomes vital that clinicians not dismiss a parent's express concerns out of hand.

Once diagnostic issues have been raised, the preferred option for pursuing an appropriate diagnosis is through a multidisciplinary team composed of some or all of the following disciplines: development pediatrician, psychiatrist,

---

| Box **12-2** | Effective Early Childhood Intervention for Children with ASD |

1. Entry into intervention as soon as an autism diagnosis is seriously considered, rather than delaying until a definitive diagnosis is made.
2. Provision of intensive intervention, with active engagement of the child at least 25 hours per week, 12 months per year, in systematically planned, developmentally appropriate educational activities designed to address identified objectives.
3. Low student-to-teacher ratio to allow sufficient amounts of 1:1 and very small group instruction to meet specific individualized goals.
4. Inclusion of a family component, including parent training when appropriate.
5. Promotion of opportunities for interaction with typically developing peers to the extent that these opportunities are helpful in addressing specified educational goals.
6. Ongoing measurement and documentation of the individual child's progress toward educational objectives, resulting in adjustments in programming when indicated.

7. Incorporation of a high degree of structure through elements such as predictable routine, visual activity schedules, and clear physical boundaries to minimize distractions.
8. Implementation of strategies to generalize learned skills to new environments and situations.
9. Use of assessment-based curricula addressing the following:
   a. Functional, spontaneous communication.
   b. Social skills, including joint attention, imitation, reciprocal interaction, initiation, and self-management.
   c. Functional adaptive skills that prepare the child for increased responsibility and independence.
   d. Reduction of disruptive or maladaptive behavior through empirically supported strategies, including functional assessment.
   e. Cognitive skills, such as symbolic play and perspective-taking.
   f. Traditional readiness skills and academic skills.

From Johnson CP, Myers SM: Autism spectrum disorders. In Wolraich ML, Drotar DD, Dworkin PH, and others: *Developmental-behavioral pediatrics: evidence and practice,* pp. 519-577, Philadelphia, 2008, Mosby.

psychologist, occupational therapist, speech therapist, and physical therapist. This team can draw on a number of diagnostic instruments presently available to assist in screening and evaluating a child for autism. They include the following:

- The Ages and Stages Questionnaire, Second Edition (ASQ)
- The Autism Screening Questionnaire
- Bayley Scales II
- BRIGANCE Screen II
- Childhood Autism Rating Scale (CARS)
- The Checklist for Autism in Toddlers (CHAT)
- The Child Development Inventories
- The Parents' Evaluation of Developmental Status
- The Wechsler Preschool and Primary Scale of Intelligence, Revised Edition (WPPSI-R)

This is a representative list of some of the more commonly used instruments, but there are a variety of other instruments available. Different professionals often have different preferences.

PHYSICAL THERAPY INTERVENTION

If a diagnosis of autism is appropriate, the next step is developing a comprehensive treatment plan. There is no cure for autism, nor is there any universally adopted approach to its treatment. The treatment plan should be based on the needs of each individual child and must continually be reevaluated and adjusted based on results and emerging needs. Consider too that the level of functioning varies widely among individuals with autism, and therefore the level and direction of the treatment plan must be tailored.

An ideal treatment plan will address a wide range of issues, including communication, behavior, social skills, sensory integration, fine and gross motor skills, and activities of daily living.

An initial focus should be the development of both receptive and expressive language. Children with autism who develop verbal language skills have a significantly better prognosis than those who do not. However, many autistic children develop no or limited verbal language, and even those who do frequently also rely on various augmentative communications tools and programs. A good treatment plan will identify each individual's strengths and utilize those tools that best exploit them.

A variety of behavioral issues, including tantrums, aggression, and personal boundaries, are common to autistic children. Because most of these individuals depend on strict routine to understand and work within their environment, carefully designed and consistently followed behavior programs are an essential element of any treatment plan. Medications also can play a key role in behavior management.

Difficulties understanding and acting within appropriate social roles are a root issue. Lack of attention to or understanding of the environment also raises key personal and community safety concerns, so particular attention must be paid to helping children understand critical concepts. Role-playing exercises, guided community activities, symbol or picture scripts, and a variety of other tools and techniques can be helpful in this area.

Children with autism frequently have exaggerated or otherwise atypical reactions to vestibular, proprioceptive, auditory, visual, tactile, olfactory, or other sensory input. Those reactions can exacerbate behavioral issues, interfere with appropriate attention to the environment, and leave the child in a state of under- or over-arousal or otherwise interfere with the ability to organize sensation for use. A variety of techniques have proven helpful in assisting autistic children to more appropriately process and integrate sensory input and better understand and react to their environments.

Motor skill impairments often go hand in hand with autism, so a specific evaluation of the individual's motor capabilities and a treatment plan to address impairments is vital. Interventions can include both specific stretching exercises and general exercise activity, such as horseback riding or swimming.

Helping each individual develop the highest possible level of competency with daily activities such as personal hygiene, eating, and dressing should be a key focus of any treatment plan. Special care should be taken to make the child more receptive to hygiene activities; a long-handled, soft bath brush or a mechanical toothbrush may help the child become more independent.

Autism and ASD Interventions

- Develop language skills
- Create a consistent behavior program
- Develop social skills
- Use techniques for processing and integrating sensory input
- Address motor impairments
- Develop competence in daily activities

CASE STUDY OF A CHILD WITH AUTISM SPECTRUM DISORDER

EXAMINATION

History: Nicholas is a 12-year-old boy with a history of autism, ADHD, and controlled seizures. His birth history is complicated with a wrapped umbilical cord causing respiratory problems and a mother with infections in the lungs during pregnancy. He received OT, PT, and ST services through the early intervention program as a baby and continued to receive these services through the school system. He attends the local public elementary school. He has a history of generalized weakness, toe walking, and oral and tactile sensitivity. His caregivers began noticing turning in of both feet 3 months ago, and his teachers at school voiced concern about decreased function and complaints of pain in the left foot. He showed decreased ability for running and bike riding at that time. His mother reported trying an arch support insert that didn't help foot position or pain, but high-top shoes showed some improvement.

Nicholas is a very mild-mannered boy who showed some difficulty following directions, requiring 1 to 2 requests, demonstration, and physical prompting. He communicated and interacted with this therapist, but with noticeable decreased attention and eye contact. He showed decreased attention to tasks and toys as well.

Nicholas's mother verbalized concern with the position of his feet and would like for him to return to a more normal walking pattern and have no complaints of pain in his foot. She would also like him to be able to return to running and bike riding so that he can keep up at school.

Systems Review

Cardiopulmonary: No concerns at this time

    Musculoskeletal: Concerns

Neuromuscular: Concerns

Integumentary: No concerns at this time

Test and Measures

Range of motion: Nicholas presented with normal PROM in all joints except bilateral dorsiflexion was limited to 0°. He also showed some limited AROM due to weakness and soft tissue approximation due to obesity.

Strength (manual muscle testing): These measurements may not represent Nicholas's true muscle strength as he had difficulty following MMT directions and isolating joint motions.

	RIGHT LOWER EXTREMITY	LEFT LOWER EXTREMITY
Ankle dorsiflexion	3/5	2/5
Plantar flexion	2+/5	2+/5
Hip flexion	2/5	2/5
Hip abduction	2/5	2/5
Knee flexion	3/5	3/5
Knee extension	3/5	3/5
Straight leg raise	+ x1	-

Tone: Nicholas showed no increased in muscle tone with quick stretches, but suspect decreased muscle tone throughout as evidenced by sitting and standing posture being slouched with genu valgum and bilateral foot pronation.

Pain: Nicholas had no complaints of pain during the evaluation session, but his mother reported complaints of pain in the left foot or ankle at school and at home in the evenings. She stated that Nicholas is unable to pinpoint exact area of pain.

Endurance: Nicholas showed decreased muscle endurance with fatigue during active range of motion and manual muscle testing. Cardiovascular

CASE STUDY OF A CHILD WITH AUTISM SPECTRUM DISORDER—cont'd

endurance was not tested, but suspected to be low based on his mother's report of decreased ability to walk long distances.

GROSS MOTOR SKILLS/FUNCTIONAL MOBILITY

Sitting: Nicholas sat independently at the edge of a mat table with kyphotic posture and frequent use of arms to support. With reaching greater than 90° he showed decreased equilibrium reactions in the trunk as evidenced by increased trunk lean and use of opposite arm to support. He also sat independently in long sitting, but showed increased kyphosis and posterior pelvic tilt.

Standing: Nicholas stood independently with kyphotic posture, genu valgum, and bilateral foot pronation with forefoot abduction causing out-toeing. He performed single leg stance (SLS) on each foot for 1-2 seconds for multiple trials. He required increased prompting and demonstration to complete SLS on the left foot.

Ambulation: Nicholas ambulated independently with multiple gait deviations. He showed decreased arm swing, a wide base of support, excessive lateral hip rotation, genu valgum, heel strike, and rocker motion over the lateral edge of the foot and toe off with forefoot adduction. These deviations were noted to be greater in the left foot when compared to the right. He ran 25 feet with decreased speed, decreased arm swing with elbows fixed into extension, minimal to no knee flexion, decreased stride length/LE dissociation, and minimal to no flight phase. His mother reported his running to be decreased in coordination since foot pain and deviation began.

Stairs: Nicholas went up and down 4 steps independently with alternating pattern and no assist of rails.

EVALUATION

Diagnosis
PT Guide Practice Pattern: 5B

Prognosis
Nicholas should show improvement in functional skills with direct PT to address balance and gait training, core strengthening, and a stretching program.

Intervention
Please note: This PT intervention took into account Nicholas's behavioral needs secondary to his ASD. However, Nicholas also had musculo-skeletal and neuromuscular impairments that required direct PT services. Nicholas did not tolerate orthotics well due to his sensory issues. Nicholas required discussions and explanation of the interventions planned prior to beginning each session. He tended to have a consistent schedule of appointments and therapy routine. He did not tolerate changes in schedules or changes in routine well.

Coordination, Communication, Documentation
Coordination occurred between Nicholas's family, school therapists and teachers, clinic therapists, and physicians. Nicholas's family received education in how to increase his exercise program by incorporating more walking activities into the family routine, including daily walks after school.

Patient Instruction
Nicholas and his caregivers would benefit from a home program focusing on plantar flexor stretching and desensitization of both feet. It is also recommended that they be educated in the incorporation of physical exercise into their daily routine such as increased walking distances, using stairs instead of elevator, etc. His mother was educated today in the use of a mesh sponge over the medial plantar surface of the foot for desensitization.

Direct Intervention
Nicholas's program should include:
- High-level balance activities such as activities on a balance beam, balancing on one foot alternating with eyes open and closed, standing on a mini-trampoline while catching and throwing balls
- Jumping and hopping activities
- Core strengthening exercises including resistance training using TheraBand, Swiss ball activities
- Swimming to help increase proprioception and improve overall strength
- Lower-extremity stretching program

Continued

CASE STUDY OF A CHILD WITH AUTISM SPECTRUM DISORDER—cont'd

- Taping of soft tissues followed by shoe orthotics to help align Nicholas's foot position and decrease foot pain

GOALS

Nicholas will ambulate without foot pain for the entire school day.

Nicholas will increase his bilateral hip muscle strength 1 muscle grade to decrease wide base of support and waddling gait deviation.

Nicholas will improve ankle strength 1 grade to improve push off during gait.

Nicholas's overall strength and endurance will improve so that Nicholas can climb 3 flights of stairs and arrive to class without being late.

Nicholas will be able to ride his bike 12 miles to participate in family bike rides.

REEXAMINATION

Nicholas received 8 weeks of direct PT services 2 times per week. He has begun a weekly swimming program that seems to have positively impacted his endurance and overall strength. At the end of the 8-week session, Nicholas was able to ambulate at school without complaints of pain. He can ascend 3 flights of stairs at a faster pace, but is occasionally late for class, especially at the end of the day. On observation, Nicholas achieved consistent pushoff, but his mother reports that he requires verbal cueing on occasion to correct gait deviations.

ANALYSIS OF CASE USING THE ICF MODEL

Body functions: Significantly decreased strength in bilateral lower extremities, decreased endurance, decreased high-level gross motor skills, foot pain.

Activity limitations: Difficulty playing with peers outdoors, difficulty ascending and descending steps, fatigues easily.

Participation restrictions: Some of Nicholas's restrictions are secondary to his autism behaviors. However, Nicholas is also limited in participating in age-appropriate sporting activities and bike riding activities with family members.

Environmental limitations: None. Nicholas's family was encouraged to have Nicholas walk more and take the elevator at school and in the community less. They were encouraged to walk short distances within the neighborhood instead of driving.

Chapter Discussion Questions

1. Identify 2 characteristics of children with autism.
2. What legislation improved services for children with autism spectrum disorder?
3. What communication techniques might a child with autism use?
4. Identify varying social patterns used by children with autism.

REFERENCES

1. Autism Society of America: *Facts and statistics* (website): http://www.autism-society.org/site/PageServer?pagename=FactsStats. Accessed October 8, 2007.
2. Centers for Disease Control and Prevention, Autism Information Center (website): http://www.cdc.gov/ncbddd/autism/index.htm. Accessed October 8, 2007.
3. Williams JG, Higgins JP, Brayne CE: Systematic review of prevalence studies of autism spectrum disorders, *Arch Dis Child* 91:8, 2006.
4. Johnson CP, Myers SM: Autism spectrum disorders. In Wolraich ML, Drotar DD, Dworkin PH, and others: *Developmental-behavioral pediatrics: evidence and practice*, Philadelphia, 2008, Mosby.
5. Deykin EY, MacMahon B: The incidence of seizures among children with autistic symptoms, *Am J Psychiatry* 136(10):1310, 1979.
6. Wing L: *The autistic spectrum: A guide for parents and professionals*, London, 1996, Trans-Atlantic.

SUGGESTED READINGS

1. American Psychiatric Association: *Diagnostic and statistical manual of mental disorders*, ed 4, text revision (DSM-IV-TR), Washington DC, 2000, American Psychiatric Association.

2. Boheme P: *Characteristics of autism spectrum disorders*, Naperville, Ill, 2003, Krejci Academy, Little Friends Inc.
3. Cowley G: Boys, girls and autism, *Newsweek*, September 8, 2003.
4. Zager D, editor: *Autism: Identification, education and treatment*, Mahwah, NJ, 1999, Lawrence Erlbaum.

RESOURCES

Autism Society of America
http://www.autism-society.org/site/PageServer
Autism Speaks Inc.
http://www.autismspeaks.org/

MAPP Services for Autism and Asperger Syndrome
http://www.asperger.org/index.html
National Autism Association
http://www.nationalautismassociation.org/
Reaching the Child With Autism Through Art: Practical, "Fun" Activities to Enhance Motor Skills and Improve Tactile and Concept Awareness, by Toni Flowers

Part FOUR

Other Pediatric Conditions

13

Stacy L. Bauer, PT, PCS

Pediatric Burns

Guide Pattern 7B: Impaired Integumentary Integrity Associated with Superficial Skin Involvement
Guide Pattern 7C: Impaired Integumentary Integrity Associated with Partial-Thickness Skin Involvement and Scar Formation
Guide Pattern 7D: Impaired Integumentary Integrity Associated with Full-Thickness Skin Involvement and Scar Formation

key terms

Chemical burn

Electrical burn

Escharotomy

Full-thickness burns

Hypertrophic scar

Partial-thickness burns

Rule of nines

Superficial burns

Thermal burn

Total body surface area (TBSA)

outline

Definition
Pathology
Clinical Signs
    Thermal Burns
    Chemical Burns
    Electrical Burns

Medical Treatment
Intervention
    Physical Therapy Assessment
    Physical Therapy Intervention

learning objectives

After reading this chapter, the reader will be able to do the following:

1. Differentiate between the different thicknesses of burns.

2. Identify medical complications that occur after a burn injury.

3. Formulate treatment activities appropriate for the patient's degree of burn and stage of recovery.

4. Differentiate acid burns from alkali burns.

5. Discuss what burns are most common in given pediatric age groups.

6. Describe how to measure total surface burn area in children and adults.

Burn injuries in infants and children can be quite devastating and are caused by a myriad of mechanisms and methods (Figure 13-1). In this chapter, mechanisms of injury, demographics, and the management and treatment of burn injuries in children will be the focus. Because of the often disfiguring effects of burns and the future growth many of these children will still undergo, burn, skin, and scar management is a lifelong process fraught with very difficult and sometimes painful procedures. Burns, especially those visible to others, can be extremely distressing to not only the child but also the family, including siblings, parents, and caregivers. Depending on the severity of the burns, the social and physical implications for a particular child can be quite dramatic. Understanding all the potential mechanisms and outcomes of burns is vital to the successful rehabilitation of these children and education of their families.

DEFINITION

Statistics show that burn-related injuries are the leading cause of accidental death in children under the age of 2 and the second leading cause of death in children under the age of 14.[1] According to the American Burn Association, approximately 1.2 million people seek treatment for burns each year in the United States. Of those, 30% to 40% are children.[2] Over the past 20 years, the incidence of burns in children has decreased, but still is an overly prevalent occurrence. Nearly 24,000 children are treated in hospital emergency departments each year for scald burn injuries,[3] and approximately 4000 children experience electrical injuries.[4] Between 25,000 and 100,000 chemical burns are reported each year, but the specific statistics on children in this group are lacking.[5]

The majority of burn accidents occur during the first 4 years of life.[6] In this time period the mechanism of injury is most often related to abuse and neglect.[7] The prevalence of scald burn injuries from hot liquids is extremely high in the first 2 years of life (nearly 95%[6]). As children get older the incidence of indoor-occurring burns decreases, and the type of burns they sustain are less likely to be due to a scald and more likely to be due to flame.[6]

Survival prognosis following burns in children is directly related to the percentage of

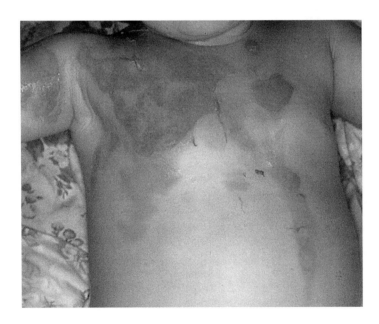

Fig. 13-1 This toddler grabbed a pot handle projecting out over the edge of a stove, spilling hot soup over her chest and shoulder. (From Zitelli BJ, Davis HW: *Atlas of pediatric physical diagnosis*, ed 5, Philadelphia, 2007, Mosby.)

skin affected by the burn, the skin thickness affected by the burn, the prevalence of infection, and the ability of medical personnel to provide adequate fluid replacement. According to Herndone and Rutan,[8] today there is only a 50% mortality rate in children younger than 15 with burns greater than 95% of total body surface area. Compare this to a 50% mortality rate in 1949 for children under the age of 14 with burns over 51% of the body (reported by Bull and Squire[9]).

PATHOLOGY

Burn injuries occur when energy is shifted from a heat source to the body. If the heat is not dissipated at a rate greater than it is absorbed, then the cellular temperature increases beyond the point at which cells can survive. This causes cell death and a myriad of other cellular-level destructions. The temperature to which the skin is exposed and the length of time the skin is exposed to the heat source determines the depth of the injury.[10] Burns are classically divided into four types: *thermal, chemical, electrical,* and *radiation* burns. For purposes of this chapter, radiation burns will not be discussed; they are extremely rare, especially in children.

Burn injuries are further classified as *superficial, partial-thickness,* or *full-thickness,* with full-thickness burns extending into the deeper tissues (Figure 13-2). Because the surface area of a 6-month-old infant differs considerably from that of an 8-year-old child, the infant will suffer deeper burns from heat of the same intensity that may cause only partial-thickness injuries in the older child.

CLINICAL SIGNS

Superficial burns, or *first-degree burns,* are limited to the epidermis. The most common type of superficial burn is sunburn; it is painful but self-limiting. Superficial burns tend not to lead to scarring. **Partial-thickness burns,** otherwise known as *second-degree burns,* are typically divided into superficial and deep partial-thickness burns. Superficial partial-thickness burns entail damage to the epidermis and a small part of the dermal layer of the skin. These burns exhibit increased sensitivity to pain and temperature, with a noted red coloration and large, thick-walled blisters. Involvement of the epidermis and a deeper portion of the dermal layer of the skin characterize deep partial-thickness burns. Increased sensitivity to pain and temperature, a marbled-white edematous appearance, and large, thick-walled blisters that typically will increase in size are also features of deep partial-thickness burns. **Full-thickness burns,** or *third-degree burns,* entail a total destruction of the epidermis and dermis, which may include deeper tissues, such as fascia, muscle, or subcutaneous fat. Temperature or pain sensation is not intact because of the destruction of the epidermal and dermal layers, which contain sensory nerve endings. The skin will have a white, brown-black, charred appearance and will feel leathery in texture. Blistering does not typically occur.[4,5]

The measurement of the extent of a burn injury can be estimated by using the "**rule of nines,**" although this is highly unreliable in children less than 15 years of age, because it overestimates the extent of burns to the legs and underestimates the extent of burns to the head and face.[11] This method divides the body surface into areas, each of which is considered to be 9% or a multiple of 9% of the total body surface area. Another method of burn surface area estimation, although less accurate, is to use the palm of the child's hand, which is roughly equivalent to 1% of the child's **total body surface area (TBSA).**[3] This is not recommended for use on large burns because of its limited accuracy. The most accurate and time-consuming method of burn surface area estimation is the Lund-Browder chart (Figure 13-3). The healthcare provider has an anterior and posterior diagram of the child

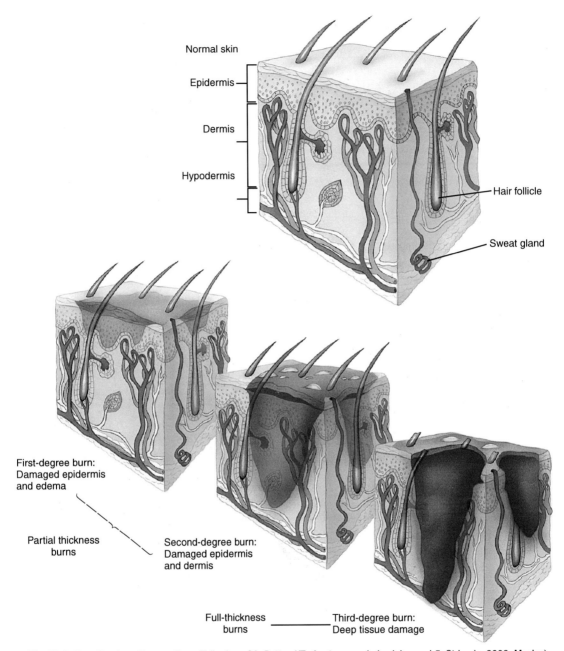

Normal skin

Epidermis

Dermis

Hypodermis

Hair follicle

Sweat gland

First-degree burn:
Damaged epidermis
and edema

Partial thickness
burns

Second-degree burn:
Damaged epidermis
and dermis

Full-thickness
burns

Third-degree burn:
Deep tissue damage

Fig. 13-2 Classification of burns. (From Thibodeau GA, Patton KT: *Anatomy and physiology*, ed 5, St Louis, 2003, Mosby.)

(available for different age groups) on which the clinician colors in both the anterior and posterior burned regions of the child's body. The sum of the colored area is the TBSA involved.[3] Most burn units follow the American Burn Association guidelines for assessment and treatment of burns. The burn unit is primarily involved in the care of moderate to severe burns that involve greater than 20% of a child's TBSA.

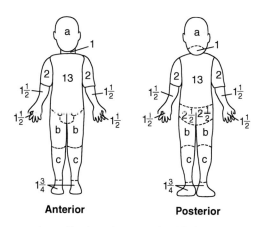

Relative percentage of body surface area (% BSA) affected by growth

Body Part	Age				
	0 yr	1 yr	5 yr	10 yr	15 yr
a = ½ of head	9 ½	8 ½	6 ½	5 ½	4 ½
b = ½ of 1 thigh	2 ¾	3 ¼	4	4 ¼	4 ½
c = ½ of 1 lower leg	2 ½	2 ½	2 ¾	3	3 ¼

Fig. 13-3 Lund-Browder chart for children for estimating the extent of burns. (Redrawn from Artz CP, Moncrief JA: *The treatment of burns*, ed 2, Philadelphia, 1969, Saunders.)

Burns Clinical Signs

Superficial Burns
Damage to epidermis

Superficial Partial-Thickness Burns
Damage to epidermis and small part of dermal layer
Increased sensitivity to pain and temperature
Red skin and large, thick-walled blisters

Deep Partial-Thickness Burns
Damage to epidermis and deeper portion of dermal layer
Increased sensitivity to pain and temperature
Marbled-white edematous appearance and large, thick-walled blisters that will increase in size

Full-Thickness Burns
Total destruction of epidermis and dermis
No temperature or pain sensation because of damaged sensory nerve endings
Leathery skin with a white, brown-black, or charred appearance

THERMAL BURNS

Thermal burn injuries are the most likely category to affect infants and children. The most common types of thermal injuries are scald- and flame burn injuries.

Scald burn injuries are extremely common in young children and can occur from spilled food and beverages (including grease), hot tap water, clothes irons, hair curling irons, space heaters, and ovens/ranges.[2] When assessing burns, especially in a child under the age of 4, there are prototypical locations for abuse-related burns. Burns on the feet, perineum, and back of the buttocks, but not on the posterior knees or anterior hip regions, are often indicators of a child dipped into a tub of scalding water.[12] Approximately 100,000 scald burn injuries result from spilled food or beverages, quite commonly a child pulling on a hanging cord or tablecloth while walking or using a baby walker. The incidence of burn injuries to children using baby walkers is quite high, despite safety warnings placed on the walkers.[13] Five thousand children are scalded from hot water every year, commonly occurring when an unattended child in the bathroom either turns on the hot tap or falls into a full tub of hot water. Often apartment building water heaters are set at higher temperatures to accommodate the increased volume of usage, and this can lead to accidental scald burns. Contact thermal burns result from contact with hot objects such as clothes irons and curling irons, which often cause hand burns, and ranges or ovens. Space heaters are a common cause of house fires, especially in the winter months in cold climates. Each year approximately 60,000 children are burned by contact with a hot surface.[2] At 52°C (126° F), it takes 2 minutes to cause full-thickness burns, compared to only 5 seconds of immersion at 60° C (140° F).[3]

Flame burns are a common cause of burn-related injuries to older children. These commonly occur in house fires, which often start at night and escape early detection because no one in the home is awake. During the winter months, space heaters, electrical failures, and oven heating are often to blame. A secondary injury that can occur with flame burns, especially during a house fire, is smoke inhalation injury. These, if severe enough, can cause brain damage as a result of the increase in carbon dioxide and decrease of oxygen in the blood.

CHEMICAL BURNS

Chemical burn injuries are divided primarily into two groups: acid and alkali. Several industrial-strength products are available to the general public, and these are often culprits in the occurrence of chemical burn injuries in children. To successfully assess and treat the presenting chemical burn injury, the physician requires a complete assessment of the "offending agent." This includes its composition and concentration, whether it is acid or alkali, the type of exposure (e.g., inhalation, cutaneous, ocular, or gastrointestinal), duration of exposure, and other events or injuries associated with the burn, such as an explosion, fall, or trauma.[4,5]

Acids produce coagulation necrosis by denaturing proteins upon tissue contact, and the development of this area of coagulation limits any extension of the injury. Common types of acids are toilet bowl or drain cleaners, tile cleaners, battery fluid, or engraving solution.

Alkalis cause a liquefaction necrosis, meaning the tissue is liquefied by the presentation of the alkali and then necroses as a result. These burns are potentially more dangerous than acid burns. In contrast with acid burns, alkali burns continue to penetrate to much deeper tissue levels.[4,5] Typically, younger children are exposed to these types of injuries accidentally because of inadequate childproofing.[5] Older children and young adults may experience exposure because of impetuous behaviors or experimentation. Often these are ingestion burns.[4,5] Common types of alkalis are drain or oven cleaners, ammonia-based cleaners and detergents, household bleach, and dishwashing and clothing detergents.

ELECTRICAL BURNS

Electrical burn injuries comprise a variety of mechanisms. Injuries range from the very mild, as seen with low-voltage household current, to the truly devastating, as seen with high-tension electrical injuries. No reliable statistics are available on the prevalence of lightning-strike injury to children. Electrical burn injuries affect approximately 4000 children every year, and the most common mechanism is low-voltage contact. Electricity involves the flow of energy along the path of least resistance toward a natural ground. All objects are either resistors or conductors. The skin acts as a natural resistor to flow. Standard household current in the United States and Canada is 110 V AC with a frequency of 60 Hz.[4,5] Skeletal muscle is stimulated into tetany by currents with frequencies of 40 to 110 Hz. Because most low- and high-tension electric currents are AC, AC produces tetany and the "locked-on" phenomenon.[4,5] As a result, an individual's grasp is uncontrollably locked onto the object, which can increase the length of time the current passes through the body and may result in greater injury.[1,5] Low-voltage injuries have very low morbidity and mortality. Both morbidity and mortality increase proportionally as voltage increases. Low-voltage injuries in toddlers often result from chewing on electrical cords or sticking objects into outlets; these injuries are most common in males.[4,5] Overall, prognosis with low-voltage electrical burn injuries is quite good.

MEDICAL TREATMENT

The burn unit functions as a very different sort of trauma unit compared to that of other acute care units. Typically a strong multidisciplinary approach is taken in most pediatric burn units, because the child's needs require that all aspects of care, development, and well-being be addressed. The pediatric burn team in the intensive care burn unit and many rehabilitation hospitals commonly includes burn-specialized surgeons/physicians, nurses, physical and occupational therapists, speech/language pathologists, infant development specialists (for children under the age of 3), clinical dieticians/nutritionists, social workers, psychologists or psychiatrists, child life specialists, and school teachers. Other personnel are consulted as needed. They may be orthotists, prosthetists, or medical sculptors. When assessing and treating infants and children with burns, the team approach and minimizing any further trauma to the infant or child are vital considerations.

Medical treatment of burns, albeit slightly different depending upon the mechanism, follows a standardized method of assessment. The initial assessment of the burn is focused on determining the extent of the burn injury, including an estimate of the TBSA involved,

and the child's overall condition. Immediate decisions are made about whether or not intubation, mechanical ventilation, and intravenous fluid therapy are required. Shock is a common aftereffect of burns and can even occur with very small burns when they are full-thickness in nature, as well as with increased TBSA burns.

Fluid replacement requirement is typically greater in children, because they experience more evaporative water loss compared with adults.[14] As a result, children have greater fluid requirements during resuscitation. As more water is lost, heat loss increases, and the ability to avoid hypothermia becomes more difficult. Fluid replacement becomes even harder to manage in infants younger than 6 months; these infants exhibit renal immaturity, which leads to increased difficulties with handling fluid overload.[4,5]

Once the pediatric burn victim is stabilized, a nasogastric tube is usually placed, because the child's caloric needs for wound healing will be far greater than the child can ingest orally. Following burn injury, there is a dramatic increase in the basal metabolic rate, which may increase to twice the baseline. As a rule, metabolic expenditures increase in proportion to the burn injury. Therefore a child with a 60% TBSA burn will require a 60% increase in the basal level of energy ingestion.[4,5]

Escharotomy, incisions through the burns, may be necessary to reduce the pressures within the burns caused by the ever-increasing edema during the initial stages of the burn progression. This is done to restore circulation when the tissue pressures increase beyond 40 mmHg.[12]

Thorough and aggressive wound care is necessary to promote the development of well-granulated tissue, which then promotes healing and closure. Often, skin grafting is required with full- and partial-thickness burns and promotes wound closure and healing. Various types of grafting procedures are available, but often with children, split-thickness skin grafts taken from the child are utilized as donor sites. Typically donor sites never extend across joints and therefore should not cause significant range of motion limitations. All areas of the body are possible donor sites, except for the face and the hands. Dressing changes are normally done daily, but following skin grafting, a period of 5 to 7 days lapses prior to the initial dressing change to allow the graft to grow into the wound bed.

Potential complications of burn injuries include heterotopic ossification, amputation, and peripheral nerve involvement. Heterotopic bone ossification is not common in smaller children, but can occur in adolescents, typically at the elbow joint. This complication occurs in 2% to 3% of the burned population. Aggressive range of motion is the treatment of choice. Amputations present a myriad of challenges in the child with a burn injury. Toleration of stump compression and weightbearing can be quite poor because of fragility of the newly grafted or healing skin, open wounds, and sensory impairments. Other amputations, such as of the fingers, also impact the child quite dramatically and create the need to relearn activities of daily living and play skills with the remaining digits. Peripheral nerve involvements occur as a result of compression of the nerve tissue or compartment, edema with elevated tissue pressures, and/or nutritional deficiencies.

Scarring and musculoskeletal deformities are the two greatest limitations to successful outcomes with children who have sustained burn injuries. The body's recuperative abilities after either a minor or significant burn injury are both amazing and problematic. As the body repairs its skin, especially deep dermal injuries, it produces massive amounts of fused, highly disorganized collagen that replaces the normal dermal elastic ground with a more inelastic substance. The microblasts begin to contract, and an inflammatory response causes increased vascularity and localized edema.[14]

The bonding of the twisted collagen and the inelastic substance, together with the contraction of the microblasts, contributes to the "thickness" of a **hypertrophic scar**. A child with darker skin exhibits a greater propensity for hypertrophic scarring.[15] The active inflammatory process of scarring typically lasts for 1½ to 2 years following burn injury. Redness, itching, irritation, and thickness are all indicators that the inflammatory process is still occurring and requires medical and pharmacologic management.

Pharmacologic management is highly varied and very physician-dependent. New research is examining the effects of using topical lotions with salicylic acid (aspirin) on scars to minimize inflammation, redness, itching, and further development of scarring.

Once an infant or child is medically stable in the burn unit, determining the most appropriate next step for that child's recovery and rehabilitation will be paramount. For children with larger partial- and full-thickness burn injuries or open areas that require closure, one option for furthering recovery is transitioning the child to an inpatient rehabilitation program specializing in burn care and rehabilitation. This option offers the child the benefits of intensive, comprehensive therapies that are highly important to the success of recovery. Depending upon the nature and extent of the child's injuries, the length of stay for this course of treatment is quite variable. Burn rehabilitation stays can range from 3 to 16 weeks and possibly longer if a child is on a pharmacologic regimen requiring weaning from a narcotic or if the skin is not adequately closing.

For children who experience less severe burns and do not require the intensive therapy of an inpatient rehabilitation program, other options include day rehab programs and outpatient therapies. Day rehab programs offer intensive, daily therapies in a clinic environment, but allow the child to be at home at night with caregivers and family. Day rehab programs are often a natural progression from inpatient rehabilitation for many children—less often for infants with burns, more often for children who require ongoing outpatient therapies. They are often appropriate for an infant or child with ongoing range of motion and/or functional limitations. Early intervention programs do not ordinarily involve themselves with burn rehabilitation; they are more developmentally focused.

INTERVENTION

PHYSICAL THERAPY ASSESSMENT

The physical therapy examination will typically begin immediately within the acute burn unit and again in an intensive inpatient rehabilitation program, usually in conjunction with occupational therapy. Early initiation of treatment ensures range of motion, flexibility, and muscle length are maintained. The physical therapy examination should include assessment of integumentary integrity, in particular, the burn, donor, and graft sites; joint integrity and mobility; muscle performance, including strength, power, and endurance; assessment of the need for any orthotic, protective, or splinting devices; pain levels; posture in all appropriate developmental positions; sensory integrity; functional mobility; and home and environmental requirements. For young children and infants, a thorough developmental assessment should be completed and compared to their pre–burn-injury status. A variety of standardized gross motor tests are available to the physical therapist for completion of this assessment.

As soon as all examinations are completed, the expected length of stay in the rehabilitation program, day rehabilitation program, or outpatient therapy program should be determined and discussed with the child and the family to anticipate the child's emotional, physical, and physiologic needs and ensure they will be met. Communication between the therapy staff and family is essential to the success of the rehabilitation program and can make certain the family is an active member of the rehabilitation team.

Based upon this thorough examination, the physical therapist completes the evaluation, synthesizes the data, makes clinical judgments, and determines a diagnosis. The primary dysfunctions are identified and become the focus of the direct interventions. Lastly, the plan of care is created, and through this the functional and measurable goals and expected outcomes are determined. It is of great importance to include the goals of the family/caregivers in this process, and even the child if appropriate, to ensure their participation in the child's recovery. The family and caregivers are vital to successful rehabilitation, especially with children and infants who have sustained burn injuries.

PHYSICAL THERAPY INTERVENTION

Physical therapy interventions will begin immediately within the acute burn unit to ensure range of motion, flexibility, and muscle length are maintained. As the skin heals, the loss of elasticity causes it to become tight and resistive to stretch, and this can produce contractures at joints across which the burns are located. The maintenance of range of motion of all joints affected by the burns, donor sites, and positional deformities, if present, is the main goal of burn rehabilitation. Restoration of function will return the child to baseline functional levels.

Several treatment interventions to address range of motion limitations are active, passive, and active assistive range of motion and splinting, including thermoplastic splinting and use of dynamic splinting systems such as Dynasplint Systems, knee immobilizers, or custommade orthotics and/or prosthetics, if required. Serial casting or splinting to increase range of motion can be quite effective and can be used for both upper and lower extremity contractures. The goal of serial casting or splinting is to provide gradual realignment of the collagen in a parallel and lengthened state.[15] This is accomplished by positioning the limb near the end range of movement and casting the limb to provide a slow, constant stretch. The cast is changed frequently (every 2 to 4 days) and a new cast applied until the desired range of motion has returned. In the case of serial splinting, the splint is adjusted to increase the stretch until the desired range of motion is achieved. Positional programs also are effective methods of improving and maintaining range of motion throughout the body. An advantage to creating a positioning program early in the rehabilitation process is that it helps to manage edema and inflammation, especially with the use of elevation.

Compliance with positioning and splinting programs is often a contentious experience with children because of their difficulty with seeing the long-term implications of joint contractures and scarring. Reward programs, such as sticker charts, sticker games, and point charts, are often effective methods of motivation for children. These programs should be based upon the child's chronological and cognitive age levels so they provide salient motivation for the child to perform and comply with splint-wearing programs.

As children with burn injuries begin to heal, they appear very "stiff-looking." This may be a result of the child's desire to not move their joints through any range of motion in an attempt to prevent pain and stretch of the burned tissue. It is the role of the physical therapist and physical therapist assistant to engage the child in appropriate therapeutic exercises to maintain range of motion, muscle strength, and functional abilities. Therapeutic exercises must have an element of relevant "fun" for the child, and this will vary depending on the child's age and cognitive level. Allowing the child to select an activity, then using that activity to promote therapeutic goals, gives the child an increased level of control in the rehabilitation process. The advancement of the therapy interventions must be made on a daily basis to continue the progression of regaining functional skills, range of motion, and overall recovery.

Pressure garments are commonly used to minimize scarring following burn injury. A variety of manufacturers create custom-made garments from highly detailed measurements taken of the child's affected areas. Staley and Richard[16] studied why the pressure garments are beneficial during the healing process and concluded that the pressure created by the garments enhances the skin maturation process. Because these garments are not only tight but create heat at the skin surface, initial research is exploring the role of the heat in minimizing scarring in those who have sustained burn injuries. Custom-made burn pressure garments are worn approximately 23 hours a day for up to 2 years following burn injury.

Fabrication of a custom-made, clear facemask can provide full contact to the child with extensive facial burns. Children and their parents are typically more compliant with use of the clear facemasks than they are with cloth facemasks.

As stated earlier, children who sustain burns are in need of both immediate and long-term therapy interventions to prevent the development of excessive scarring and the loss of range of motion and function. Family involvement and support of the therapy program is critical to the outcome of burn rehabilitation.

Burns Interventions
• Address range of motion limitations with splinting or positioning programs • Maintain range of motion, muscle strength, and functional abilities through therapeutic exercises • Minimize scarring with pressure garments

CASE STUDY OF A CHILD WITH BURNS

EXAMINATION

History

T.W. is a 9-month-old boy who was brought to a community hospital with significant burns over his entire body. His mother reports he was in the care of her boyfriend when she went to the store. When she returned to the hotel room in which they were living, T.W. was unresponsive and blistered over his entire body. Approximately 24 hours after the burn incident, T.W.'s mother took him to the community hospital. Upon initial examination in the emergency room, T.W.'s burns were estimated to involve over 76% of his body. His face was the only area not burned, according to the initial assessment. Due to the severity of his burn injuries, he was immediately intubated and placed on mechanical ventilation, given a nasogastric tube for nutrition, and started on intravenous fluid replacement. He was transferred by helicopter to a pediatric trauma center specializing in severe burn injuries.

At the trauma center, T.W. was mechanically ventilated for 4 weeks. The severity of his injuries and risk of infection led several times to the expectation that he would not survive. He underwent several surgeries for wound debridement, skin grafting, and compartment syndrome release of his left anterior-lateral compartment. After 4 weeks of intubation and mechanical ventilation, T.W. was removed from the ventilator and extubated. He remained in a medically induced coma for pain management, and plans for his rehabilitation phase of care began. It was determined he would be transferred to an intensive inpatient rehabilitation program for further therapies and wound care. Prior to his transfer, the court granted Child Protective Services custody of T.W. after it was established that the infant had been dunked in a bathtub full of scalding water by his mother's boyfriend as a punishment for wetting his diaper. The mother's delay in seeking medical treatment for T.W. made her culpable as well. Specialized foster placement will be required for T.W. when he is ready for discharge.

Upon arrival at the inpatient rehabilitation program, T.W. continued to be highly sedated and was seldom awake; this was required because of the extent of his injuries. Initial physical, occupational, and developmental therapy examinations were done, and a plan of care was determined.

No family was present at the time of the initial examination because of the removal of custody from T.W.'s mother.

Review of Systems

Upon initial examination of T.W., the following items were noted:

1. T.W. exhibited severely impaired skin integrity throughout his body, except for his face.
2. T.W. exhibited severely impaired range of motion throughout his trunk, neck, and extremities.
3. Due to the medically induced coma, T.W. was unresponsive to stimulation.
4. T.W. was unable to move his extremities actively.
5. T.W. was unable to communicate verbally.

Physical, occupational, and developmental therapies were involved in T.W.'s care from the onset of the admission. Once his sedative medications were decreased and he became more alert and responsive, speech therapy was to be initiated to address feeding and communication impairments.

Tests and Measures

Impairments

T.W. exhibited severely impaired skin integrity with minimal closed skin areas; the majority of his skin was still open. He had significant burned areas, and his head/scalp was used as a donor site. His left anterior-lateral thigh had undergone a compartment release due to the development of a compartment syndrome and as a result had a "filleted" appearance. Range of motion throughout his trunk and all extremities was highly limited in all planes of movement, and he did not come with any splinting when transferred. Because of his medically induced coma, he was highly unresponsive, and no further examinations were completed at the time.

Once his medications were reduced and his alertness increased, complete functional motor skills assessment and testing would need to be completed.

Continued

CASE STUDY OF A CHILD WITH BURNS—cont'd

Functional Limitations and Disability

T.W. initially exhibited limited responsiveness due to a medically induced coma, but once sedative medications were decreased, standardized testing with the Peabody Developmental Motor Scales, Second Edition (PDMS-2) was completed. He displayed gross motor skills at a 2-month level for reflexes, a 2-month level for stationary skills, and a 3-month level for locomotion skills.

Diagnosis

Upon synthesis of the examination information, the following diagnoses were determined for T.W.: impaired arousal, attention, and cognition, most likely due to medically induced coma for pain management; impaired integumentary function; impaired range of motion; impaired motor functioning; impaired sensory integration; and impaired functional mobility. Because of the seriousness of his burn injuries, T.W. exhibited severe impairments in all of the areas listed above.

Prognosis

Given the extent of T.W.'s burn injuries, he will most likely exhibit lifelong integumentary, range of motion, and functional limitations, likely requiring surgical intervention to address these impairments as he grows. The psychologic implications for T.W. are currently unknown, but will likely need to be addressed as he ages and begins school and socialization with peers. With the excellent care he received both at the trauma center and now at the rehabilitation center, T.W. could make excellent progress with highly intensive services.

PLAN OF CARE

T.W.'s length of stay in the intensive rehabilitation program was estimated at the time of the examination to be approximately 24 to 28 weeks to best maximize his potential for integumentary, motor, sensory, psychologic, and cognitive recovery.

The following goals and outcomes for physical therapy were determined:

Goals

1. T.W. will tolerate passive, active, and active assistive range of motion for all affected joints.
2. T.W. will maintain independent sitting.
3. T.W. will tolerate prone play and creep independently.

4. T.W. will exhibit an intact integumentary system with no open areas.
5. T.W. will use all of his extremities in play.
6. T.W. will cruise on a supportive surface.

Outcomes

1. T.W. will tolerate all skin and burn care during daily hygiene activities.
2. Once identified, T.W.'s foster parents will increase their understanding of scald burns and their effects and the anticipated goals and expected outcomes.
3. T.W. will participate in age-appropriate social interactions with modifications, as required.
4. T.W. will tolerate wearing pressure garments to minimize scarring.
5. T.W. will play with toys and interact with other children and adults.

INTERVENTION

T.W. received extensive physical therapy services in an inpatient rehabilitation program for 26 weeks, with physical therapy services delivered twice to three times a day Monday through Friday, daily on Saturdays, and for the first 8 weeks of his rehabilitation admission, daily on Sundays as well. (T.W. was unable to maintain his range of motion without daily intervention, so Sunday treatment was initiated.) Intervention included weekly staffing/care conferences and multidisciplinary rounds, reintegration of T.W. into child life activities once or twice daily as he became more alert, and extensive caregiver training once a specialized foster placement was identified. A foster family was identified during week 20 of T.W.'s 26-week rehabilitation stay, and his foster parents became highly involved in his day-to-day care and therapy programs. His foster mother was a registered emergency room nurse, and his foster father was a pharmacist.

Treatment interventions focused on passive, active, and active assistive range of motion, splinting, positioning for edema control, and restoration of functional mobility. As T.W.'s pharmacologic management became more simplified and his narcotics began to be tapered, his alertness began to increase. Age-appropriate play activities were introduced in therapy to promote increased functional use of his hands and functional developmental mobility.

CASE STUDY OF A CHILD WITH BURNS—cont'd

The use of pressure garments was initiated once his skin no longer had open areas. Silicone gel sheets provided lubrication of his skin surfaces.

OUTCOME

At the time of discharge, T.W. was beginning to independently cruise along furniture approximately 5 to 6 feet. He was able to creep independently on a level surface and was able to creep up and down 4 stairs with supervision. At the time of readministration of the PDMS-2, T.W. was 16 months of age and functioning at a gross motor age equivalency of 10 months for reflexes, 12 months for stationary skills, 12 months for locomotion skills, and 12 months for object manipulation skills. This indicated a great improvement in his developmental mobility since admission, but also demonstrated the success of his range-of-motion and positioning programs as well. He had begun to talk and say single words. Although the use of his hands for fine-motor play was his greatest remaining impairment, he demonstrated amazing improvements during his inpatient rehabilitation stay. T.W. was discharged home with his foster parents, who lived in a suburban setting on a horse farm and inquired about the appropriateness of taking T.W. horseback riding. T.W. was also going to continue intensive rehabilitation services at a day rehabilitation program near his home 5 days per week for 4 hours per day. As of 3 years post-burn injury, T.W. is a very happy, ambulatory little boy who will always have integumentary impairments that require ongoing therapy services and future surgical interventions.

ANALYSIS OF CASE USING THE ICF MODEL (AT DISCHARGE)

Body functions: Healing burns on four extremities and trunk, decreased range of motion.

Activity limitations: Decreased fine and gross motor skills, decreased self-care, limited play and interactions.

Participation restrictions: Extended inpatient status secondary to guarded medical condition, cannot play, cannot participate in age-appropriate activities, living with a new family.

Environmental factors: Extended inpatient stay at hospital transitioning to rural home setting; involved with child protection agency.

Chapter Discussion Questions

1. Discuss why young children are more susceptible to scald burns than older children.
2. Identify the characteristics of first-, second-, and third-degree burns based on alternative labels for burn classification, physical characteristics, pain/sensation, and cause of burn.
3. Describe total burn surface area (TBSA) and the three ways to measure TBSA.
4. Compare and contrast acid and alkaloid burns.
5. Identify two possible complications from a burn injury.
6. How can healing tissue cause difficulties in the rehabilitation process?
7. What are the two main goals for someone who is recovering from a burn injury?
8. Why would a family be more accepting of a clear facemask versus a cloth facemask?

REFERENCES

1. Warden GD, Lang D, Housinger TA: Management of pediatric hand burns with tendon, joint and bone injury. Paper presented at the meeting of the American Burn Association, Cincinnati, March 1993.
2. Brigham P, data compiler: Burn Foundation, Allentown, Pa, 1999.
3. Lucchesi M: *Burns, thermal* (website): www.emedicine.com. January 2004.
4. Hostetler MA, *Burns, electrical* (website): www.emedicine.com. January 2004.
5. Hostetler MA: *Burns, chemical* (website): www.emedicine.com. January 2004.
6. Feller I: Burn epidemiology: focus on youngsters and the aged, *J Burn Care Rehabil* 3:285, 1982.
7. Bennett B, Gamelli R: Profile of an abused burned child, *J Burn Care Rehabil* 19(1):88, 1998.
8. Herndone DN, Rutan RL: Have we improved burn care? In Carlson RW, Reines HD, editors: *Critical care state of the art* 13:389, Anaheim, 1992, Society of Critical Care Medicine.

9. Bull JP, Squire JR: A study of mortality in a burn unit: standards for the evaluation of alternative methods of treatment, *Ann Surg* 130(2):160, 1949.

10. Carrougher GJ: *Burn care and therapy*, St Louis, 1998, Mosby.

11. Mikhail NJ: Acute burn care: an update, *J Emerg Nurs* 14:1, 1988.

12. Doane CB: Children with severe burns. In Pratt PN, Allen AS, editors: *Occupational therapy for children*, St Louis, 1989, Mosby.

13. Cassell OC, Hubble M, Milling MA, and others: Baby walkers—still a major cause of infant burns, *Burns* 23(5):451, 1997.

14. Monafo WW: Initial management of burns, *N Engl J Med* 335(21):1581, 1996.

15. Bennett GB, Helm P, Purdue GF, and others: Serial casting: a method for treating burn contractures, *J Burn Care Rehabil* 10:543, 1989.

16. Staley MJ, Richard RL: Use of pressure to treat hypertrophic burn scars, *Adv Wound Care* 10(3):44, 1997.

RESOURCES

Burn Recovery Center
877-640-3200
www.burn-recovery.org
About.com: Physical Therapy
www.physicaltherapy.about.com
Burn Survivors Online
www.burnsurvivorsonline.com
Severe Burns, by Andrew M. Munster
Coping Strategies for Burn Survivors and Their Families, by Norman R. Bernstein and others

Chapter 14

Roberta Kuchler O'Shea, PT, PhD

Limb Deficiencies

Guide Pattern 4J: Impaired Motor Function, Muscle Performance, Range of Motion, Gait, Locomotion, and Balance Associated with Amputation
Guide Pattern 7A: Primary Prevention/Risk Reduction for Integumentary Disorders
Guide Pattern 7E: Impaired Integumentary Integrity Associated with Skin Involvement Extending into Fascia, Muscle, or Bone and Scar Formation

key terms

Acquired limb deficiency

Amelia

Amniotic band syndrome
  (ABS)

Congenital limb deficiency

Hemimelias

Prosthesis

Residual limb

outline

learning objectives

At the end of the chapter the reader will be able to do the following:

1. Label the amputation levels using current appropriate terminology.

2. Compare and contrast congenital and acquired amputations/limb deficiencies.

3. Design an exercise program based on level of amputation.

DEFINITION

Limb deficiencies in children may affect the upper or lower extremities and may involve one limb or several limbs. Causes fall into one of two categories: **congenital limb deficiency** or **acquired limb deficiency** (amputation). Congenital deficiencies are further classified into transverse and longitudinal. Nomenclature of the acquired types has changed over the last several years, but both previously accepted labeling (above knee [AK], below knee [BK], above elbow [AE], and below elbow [BE]) and current labeling (transfemoral, transtibial, transhumeral, transradial) continue to be used.[1] For this chapter, when appropriate, the historical system is in parenthesis.

PATHOLOGY

CONGENITAL

Congenital amputations occur in utero. These include absence or deformities of limbs or loss of muscles and ligaments in the limbs. **Amelia** refers to the occasion where an entire bone/segment is missing, **hemimelias** refer to a longitudinal anomaly where all or part of one bone is missing, and *phocomelia* refers to the congenital absence of the proximal section of the limb.[2] Transverse amputations occur in the transverse plane of the extremity through the shaft of the involved bone. These amputations occur in the proximal, middle, or distal third of the involved limb. Longitudinal deficiencies may be unilateral or bilateral. One of the bones in the segment is missing or malformed along the long axis of the segment (e.g., the ulna or fibula may be missing). These deficiencies may cause the remaining bones in the segment to be malformed; in the case of a missing ulna, the radius may be bowed. Segments proximal or distal to the limb deficiency may be completely formed.

A common cause of congenital amputation is **amniotic band syndrome (ABS)**, which occurs in 1 out of 1200 live births; 80% involve anomalies of the fingers and hands.[2] The entrapment of fetal parts in a fibrous amniotic band while in utero is believed to cause ABS. The amnion ruptures early and entangles the fetus. This may in turn cause several varying birth defects, including amputation of the arms, legs, and digits.[2] Interestingly ABS is sporadic, not hereditary, and there is typically no risk of recurrence within families.[2]

ACQUIRED

Acquired amputations may be due to trauma, vascular disease, tumors, infections, or burn injuries. Amputations secondary to trauma occur twice as frequently as amputations due to disease. Partial or complete removal of the limb may be necessary following a traumatic incident.[3] Different types of amputations are described in Table 14-1.

INTERVENTION

The rehabilitation team typically includes the child and family; physicians; nurses; physical, occupational, and developmental therapists; social workers; and prosthetists. The rehabilitation team works closely to design a plan that includes **residual limb** shaping and desensitization, exercise and strengthening, improving endurance, and prosthetic tolerance. The child and the family play an important part in the child obtaining full independence. As the child grows and matures, he or she should be given a progressively larger role in making prosthetic decisions.

Children with congenital limb malformations or deficiencies may undergo surgery to adapt the residual limb for prosthetic wear. Surgery should be undertaken with the goal of restoring function. Typically a multidisciplinary team, including the child/family, makes a decision regarding surgery and follow-up rehabilitation. With a traumatic amputation or disease process, surgery may be the only option, and the medical team will lead that decision. Following surgery, however, the entire rehabilitation

TABLE **14-1** Types of Amputations

AMPUTATION	CHARACTERISTICS
UPPER EXTREMITY	
Shoulder disarticulation	Humerus and all distal structures are missing.
	Child will require prosthesis that includes a mechanical shoulder joint, elbow joint, and hand components.
Transhumeral (above elbow)	Amputation occurs through the shaft of the humerus.
	Child will require prosthesis with an elbow and hand components.
Transradial (below elbow)	Amputation occurs through the shaft of the radius and ulna.
	Elbow joint remains intact.
	Prosthesis includes a hand component.
Wrist disarticulation	Amputation occurs at wrist level.
	Prosthesis will include hand component.
Hand	Amputation includes all or part of the hand and all or part of the fingers.
	Prosthesis will include hand components.
LOWER EXTREMITY	
Hemipelvectomy	Amputation includes half of the pelvis and all anatomic structures of the ipsilateral lower extremity.
	Prosthesis will include a bucket socket to contain distal trunk structures; mechanical hip, knee, ankle, and foot components will be attached to this bucket socket.
Hip disarticulation	Amputation includes femur and all distal anatomic structures.
	Prosthesis will include hip, knee, ankle, and foot components.
Proximal femoral focal deficiency (PFFD)	A longitudinal deficiency in which the femur is malformed and shortened
	Typically the remaining femoral segment is held in flexion, abduction, and external rotation.
	This deformity is classified into four types: Class A, B, C, or D.
	• Class A: normal hip joint with intact and well-seated femoral head and acetabulum, shortened femoral segment with subtrochanteric varus angulation
	• Class B: femoral head present, acetabulum adequate but defective, capital fragment within acetabulum
	• Class C: femoral head and acetabulum absent, short femoral fragment, no articulation between femur and acetabulum
	• Class D: femoral head and acetabulum absent, no relation between femur and acetabulum
	Several surgical intervention strategies are available to the child with PFFD, depending on the length of the remaining limb. Prosthetic components may or may not include a knee joint, but will include ankle and foot components.[1]
Transfemoral (above knee)	Amputation occurs through the shaft of the femur.
	Prosthetic components include knee, ankle, and foot.
Knee disarticulation	Amputation occurs at the knee joint.
	Femur is intact; distal lower extremity is removed/missing.
	Prosthesis includes a knee joint, ankle, and foot components.
Transtibial (below knee)	Amputation occurs through the shaft of the tibia and fibula.
	Anatomic knee remains intact.
	Prosthesis includes ankle and foot components.
Syme amputation	Ankle disarticulation with intact heel pad
	Prosthesis includes foot component.
Foot	Amputation includes all or part of the foot and all or part of the toes.
	Prosthesis includes shoe filler.

team cooperatively creates a postsurgical rehabilitation and prosthetic plan.

In the case of a baby with a congenital amputation, the parents can be initially devastated by the defect. They may feel shame and anger and want to hide the child or the affected limb. The parents may try to blame themselves for an incident, real or perceived, that occurred during pregnancy. It is vital for the family to be connected with a rehabilitation team as soon as possible and a social network that includes individuals who have experienced what they are currently experiencing. These connections can help the family adjust to the child's missing limb and formulate a story to share with others. Families need time and peer assistance to put together the words that positively describe their child and acknowledge their child's disability as a secondary consideration. Other parents will share their experiences, triumphs, and pitfalls, thus easing the pain and journey.

Limb Deficiencies Interventions

- Shape and desensitize residual limb
- Plan a program for exercise and strengthening
- Improve endurance
- Improve tolerance of prosthetic

CONGENITAL UPPER EXTREMITY LIMB DEFICIENCY

For the child with a congenital amputation, prosthetic fittings and therapy begin when developmentally appropriate. Typically the child should be evaluated as soon as possible to determine a plan of action and introduce the family to the remedial medical systems. For a child with an upper extremity limb deficiency, prosthetic wear will occur as early as 3 months of age. This will enable the child to develop prone skills and bimanual skills age-appropriately. As the child grows, the components of the **prosthesis** should match the child's development. Decisions concerning passive versus dynamic hand, voluntary opening versus voluntary closing hand, and traditional versus myoelectric should be made in light of the child's development and

activity level. See Table 14-2 regarding appropriate outcomes by age for children with upper extremity amputations.

Myoelectric prosthetics use the body's power to open and close the terminal device. The child must have sufficient activation of muscle groups to be able to activate at least two directions of motion. Children can be fitted for a myoelectric prosthetic device when they can cognitively understand and motor plan a volitional muscle contraction on demand. Thus the muscle must generate a contraction when commanded to do so and not necessarily within the framework of a functional activity. Myoelectric devices have many pros and cons that must be considered prior to recommending them. These devices are heavier than their traditional body-powered prosthetics, they are battery operated, they require a higher level of maintenance and care, and they do not hold up well against sand, water, grime, or dirt. On the other hand, children perceive myoelectric devices as "cool." Additionally, myoelectric devices nicely mimic a biologic hand.

CONGENITAL LOWER EXTREMITY LIMB DEFICIENCY

As in the case of upper limb deficiency, the team should evaluate the child with a congenital lower extremity deficiency as soon as possible. Prosthetic wear typically occurs as the child begins to develop lower extremity weight-bearing skills. These skills include assuming and maintaining four point position, pulling to stand, cruising, and standing. Decisions concerning prosthetics will need to be made in light of the child's amputation level as well as developmental level.

TRAUMATIC OR SURGICAL AMPUTATION

For the child with a traumatic amputation, postsurgical rehabilitation should begin as soon as medically feasible. Particular care should be paid to range of motion, skin condition, and the strength and shape of the residual limb. The child may also have issues of phantom pain and hypersensitivity in the residual limb. Family

TABLE **14-2** Intervention Outcomes for Children with Upper Extremity Deficiencies and Their Parents

AGE OF CHILD	INTERVENTION OUTCOMES FOR CHILDREN	INTERVENTION OUTCOMES FOR THEIR PARENTS
Infant	Comfort with the prosthesis Tolerate wearing prosthesis Can clasp large objects using prosthesis Use the prosthesis to aid in sitting and crawling	Can apply and remove the prosthesis correctly Can care for child's skin and child's prosthesis Can recognize and report any problems with the prosthesis
Toddler	Child can control terminal device and elbow unit Child can perform bimanual prehension activities Child can use prosthesis as an assist in functional activities	Should provide toys that require bimanual prehension/manipulation Encourage child to think of the prosthesis as an assistive device Inspect skin regularly for signs of irritation Encourage child to be independent in all activities of daily living and play
School-aged	Child has an opinion about type and function of prosthesis Child can maintain proper prosthetic fit and recognize when repairs are needed Child can grasp firm or fragile objects without dropping or crushing them Child can successfully open and close the terminal device Child can don and doff prosthesis independently Child can dress self independently	

Data from Lusardi MM, Nielson CC: *Orthotics and prosthetics in rehabilitation*, ed 2, Philadelphia, 2006, Butterworth-Heinemann.

support is another integral part of the rehabilitation process.

Traumatic amputations or surgical amputations are equally traumatic for the family nexus. In the case of traumatic amputation, perhaps the incident that caused the child's injury may have been preventable. The parents may experience guilt and remorse, even if there is no way they could have prevented it. Similarly, families will grapple with issues surrounding surgery and limb salvage. It seems that most caregivers' and clients' initial response is to save the limb; however, as time progresses the family or child may decide that a revised limb with a prosthesis is more functional, stronger, and more cosmetically acceptable than the salvaged limb.

Families and children require peer support as well to help them journey through this process. Following amputation surgery, peers with the same level amputation can offer support, encouragement, and direction to the family and child. Professionals should be available to visit the child's school with the parents before the child returns from amputation surgery and recovery. This visit will allow the child's school peers to ask questions, touch and feel different prostheses and components of prostheses, and talk through some of their fears and concerns about their classmate. The hope is that these sessions will help ease the transition back to school and minimize any apprehension the children and school staff may be experiencing. The child with an amputation should be encouraged to resume his or her previous activities and routines as soon as possible. Table 14-3 details appropriate outcomes by age for children with lower extremity amputations.

PROSTHETIC COMPONENTS

Although prosthetic components change and are upgraded frequently, categories of components share commonalities. These generalizations will be discussed, keeping in mind that new technology is constantly evolving. It is crucial for the comprehensive rehabilitation

TABLE **14-3** Intervention Outcomes for Children with Lower Extremity Deficiencies and Their Parents

AGE OF CHILD	INTERVENTION OUTCOMES FOR CHILDREN	INTERVENTION OUTCOMES FOR THEIR PARENTS
Infant	Comfort and tolerance of prosthesis Child can stand by leaning against a table Child can cruise around furniture Child can walk with or without support of an age-appropriate push toy	Parents can apply and remove the prosthesis correctly Parents can care for child's skin and child's prosthesis Parents can recognize and report any problems with the prosthesis
Toddler	Child tolerates wearing prosthesis all day Child uses prosthesis when completing age-appropriate ambulatory activities	Encourage use of the prosthesis Provide toys and equipment that require age-appropriate activities and mobility Inspect skin regularly for signs of irritation
School-aged	Child has an opinion about type and function of prosthesis Child is able to independently monitor and maintain proper prosthetic fit, including skin inspection, and recognize when repairs are needed Child can independently don and doff prosthesis, as well as dress independently Child can complete all ambulatory activities and mobility activities independently	Encourage child to be independent in all activities of daily living and play Encourage child to be active in group sporting activities

Data from Lusardi MM, Nielson CC: *Orthotics and prosthetics in rehabilitation*, ed 2, Philadelphia, 2006, Butterworth-Heinemann.

team to include members who have up-to-date knowledge of prosthetic technology.

Transtibial prosthetic components include the following:

- Hard socket: The hard socket is made of a rigid laminate material. It can be reinforced with carbon fiber for strength. The socket is shaped to exactly fit the child's residual limb. The socket helps to maintain the soft tissues of the residual limb in a safe and efficient position.
- Prosthetic socks: Socks come in a variety of thicknesses, typically 1-, 3-, 5-, and 10-ply. They are made of cotton or wool and must be carefully cared for. As the residual limb shrinks in size, the sock offers a mechanism to take up some of the excess room, so that the residual limb will not experience shearing or friction from pistoning. A sock also acts as a shock absorber for the residual limb.
- Soft liner: A thin, soft liner can be used in lieu of socks. It acts as a shock absorber between the residual limb and prosthesis

socket. Care must be taken to ensure that the liner fits properly and is cleaned regularly.

- Suspension mechanics: When properly suspended, the prosthesis should not swivel or move on or about the residual limb. Similarly, the residual limb should not piston or move about within the prosthesis. If movement occurs or areas are not properly loaded for appropriate weightbearing, the child could be at risk for skin breakdown, development of sores or blisters, and inefficient and unsafe gait.
- Supracondylar suspension systems: Supracondylar suspension grips the child above the medial and lateral femoral condyles and is used with a transtibial prosthesis. The condyles provide an ideal surface area for suspension.
- Cuff: The suspension cuff is added to the distal part of the transtibial prosthesis. The cuff is tightened around the femur just proximal to the femoral condyles.

This arrangement secures the prosthesis to the residual limb and prevents pistoning or movement of the residual limb.

- Suction: With suction the air is milked out of the socket, forming a suction seal that secures the prosthesis to the residual limb. This seal should be strong enough to maintain the prosthesis securely in place during all normal activities. When the prosthesis is to be removed, the suction seal is broken.
- Sleeve: A roll-on sleeve can be used over the standard suspension mechanisms. The sleeve provides added suspension and helps minimize any remaining movement between the residual limb and the prosthesis. Some children use the sleeve when they participate in sports or activities requiring fast movements.

Transfemoral prosthetic components include the following:

- An ischial containment socket: This type of socket contains the ischium with the posterior prosthetic wall. The femur maintains normal adduction position, thus allowing the child to use a narrower base of support. The ischial containment design allows for more optimal force distribution along the residual femoral shaft. This socket is the design of choice for most children and adults with transfemoral amputations.
- A quadrilateral socket: This socket design was used successfully for years before the advent of the ischial containment socket. In this design, the socket has a quadrilateral shape, with each wall having a different purpose. Most notably the ischial tuberosity sits up on the posterior wall and acts as a weightbearing surface along with the gluteal musculature. The medial wall is relatively high to contain the adductor tissues and provide counterpressure to the lateral wall. The lateral wall provides a working support surface for the residual femur in midstance. The anterior wall blocks forward motion of the residual limb, and the medial corner of the anterior wall contains a channel for the adductor tendon.
- Prosthetic knee options: There are several pediatric knee options, ranging from a single hinge with a manual lock to those with hydraulic components. It is commonly thought that the ambulatory child should be fitted with a working knee as soon as possible. This allows the child to develop normal gait rhythm and cycle from the onset of ambulation. Infants may use a single-axis joint that when released has full flexion and when strapped or locked is maintained in extension.

Components used for both transfemoral and transtibial prosthetics include the following:

- Prosthetic foot options: The standard foot is still considered the solid ankle cushion heel (SACH foot). This design allows for a more normal gait pattern, but does not store energy generated as part of push-off and does not necessarily allow for inversion or eversion movements, which accommodate for uneven surfaces. The SACH foot, however, is a durable, reliable foot for children, especially young children. As growth progresses toward middle and late childhood age, the child may consider other options like an energy-storing foot or at least a dynamic foot. These are more accommodating and higher-performance prosthetic feet, allowing the child greater flexibility.

Prosthetic coverings include the following:

- Exoskeletal: The covering of the prosthesis is a hard laminate material. Once fabricated, it cannot be easily modified in color or shape.
- Endoskeletal: The covering of the prosthesis is a softer foam laminate with a nylon sheath covering. The shape and color of the cover can be modified if necessary. The downside is that the cover may be damaged or torn more easily than the exoskeletal cover.

CASE STUDY OF A CHILD WITH A LIMB DEFICIENCY

Jason was born a typically developing child. At 18 months, he contracted bacterial meningitis. By the time the devastation of the disease could be arrested, Jason's four extremities were severely affected. He lost his limbs at the following levels: bilateral transfemoral, a left upper extremity transradial, and a right wrist disarticulation. He was fitted with four prostheses. The lower extremity prostheses had solid sockets with hip joints and a waist belt for suspension. The knee joints were single-axis hinges that could be locked in extension or swing loose for flexion. He used bilateral SACH feet. Primary therapy and teaching entailed maintaining skin integrity, because his skin had rough scarring from the meningitis and multiple surgeries. Therapy also consisted of improving his strength, coordination, balance, and equilibrium reactions and helping him learn to fall safely.

As a toddler, Jason learned first to ambulate with a reverse wheeled walker. The handle grips needed to be modified so that he could grasp and control the walker easily. As he learned to balance and shift weight more easily, Jason began to ambulate around his home with bilateral Lofstrand crutches. Finally he learned to ambulate with a single Lofstrand when indoors. He preferred to use a walker when ambulating outside or longer distances. If traveling a far distance, he would be pushed in a stroller. Jason used bilateral Adept terminal devices, each with a single cable to operate the hand function. The terminal device rests in the opened position (this is the opposite of a traditional hook terminal device) and closes via the cable system, which is attached to a figure-eight harness worn over the shoulders. Jason needed to learn initially how to operate the devices so he could accomplish self-help skills such as feeding or dressing. After learning to use his prostheses as assists, he then moved on to master more delicate fine motor skills such as grasping and maintaining a hold on different objects, manipulating small objects, and performing self-help and self-care activities. He also learned rather quickly that he could cause pain without feeling pain by squeezing or pinching with his terminal devices.

At 3 years old, Jason attended a special education program to receive PT and OT in the school. He was transitioned into the state pre-kindergarten room at age 4. He did well in school and learned to adapt his environment to be as independent as possible. He propelled a manual wheelchair for long-distance outings. At school he carried his supplies in a backpack and used bilateral Lofstrand crutches for mobility around the school building. After 3 years of preschool and kindergarten, he left the special education system to attend regular public school first grade. He was independent in all his school skills, and he and his family were self-sufficient in caring for his skin and recognizing when he needed prosthetic adjustments or replacement equipment. Jason typically had growth adjustments made over the summer so that his sudden change in height would not be as obvious to school peers. Before growth adjustments, Jason was commonly shorter in stature than his classmates. After summer break, he would return with 2 years worth of estimated growth built into his new prostheses, making him one of the taller students in his group.

As he grew and became a more skilled prosthetic wearer, Jason considered more technically advanced prosthetic components. He preferred to use hydraulic knee joints, energy-storing feet, and suction sockets in his lower prostheses. He tried a myoelectric upper extremity device, but ultimately preferred the performance and durability of manual terminal devices. He learned to ride a bike with great determination and some modifications. He credits his ability to overcome his impairments and grow into an independent young man to self-determination and a supportive family.

ANALYSIS OF CASE USING THE ICF MODEL:

Health conditions: Status post bacterial meningitis

Body functions: Quadrimembral amputee, scar tissue on distal residual limbs, four prostheses

Activity limitations: None, as long as prostheses are functioning

Participation restrictions: None, as long as prostheses are functioning

Environmental limitations: Requires prostheses to be independent and functional

Chapter Discussion Questions

1. What body parts are most commonly affected by amniotic band syndrome (ABS)?
2. If a baby is born with ABS, what is the risk that future children in the family will have it?
3. What are the two categories of limb deficiency?
4. What is the current nomenclature for the following previously accepted terms for levels of amputation: above knee, below elbow?
5. What is the difference between an amelia, a hemimelia, and a phocomelia?
6. Describe a proximal femoral focal deficiency.
7. At what age would a baby be fitted with an upper extremity prosthesis?
8. At what age would a child be fitted with a lower extremity prosthetic device?
9. What design of knee joint would you recommend for a child just beginning to stand and take steps?
10. What are two desired intervention outcomes for a young child with a lower limb deficiency?

REFERENCES

1. Lusardi MM, Nielson CC: *Orthotics and prosthetics in rehabilitation*, ed 2, Philadelphia, 2006, Butterworth-Heinemann.
2. Amniotic Band Syndrome: *Amniotic band syndrome* (website): www.amnioticbandsyndrome.com. Accessed August 15, 2005.
3. Seymour R: *Prosthetics and orthotics: lower limb and spinal*, Philadelphia, 2002, Saunders.

RESOURCES

National Limb Loss Information Center

900 East Hill Ave
Suite 288
Knoxville, TN 37905
888-267-5669
www.amputee-coalition.org

National Rehabilitation Information Center (NARIC)

4200 Forbes Blvd., Suite 202
Lanham, MD 20706
800-346-2742
www.naric.com

Association of Children's Prosthetic and Orthotics Clinics (ACPOC)

6300 N. River Rd., Suite 727
Rosemont, IL 60018-4226
847-384-4226
www.acpoc.org

Chapter 15

Jeanne Kelly, RN, BSN
Roberta Kuchler O'Shea, PT, PhD

Asthma

learning objectives

At the end of the chapter the reader will be able to do the following:

1. Identify the warning signs of asthma.

2. Respond to a child in respiratory distress secondary to asthmatic conditions.

3. Design an appropriate exercise regimen for a child with asthma.

DEFINITION

Asthma is a chronic respiratory condition with inflammation of the airways; its symptoms include breathing problems such as coughing, wheezing, shortness of breath, and chest tightness.

PATHOLOGY

Asthma episodes are classified as mild, moderate, and severe, because the degree to which a person reacts to a trigger varies (Figure 15-1). Often there are triggers that cause an asthma sufferer's airways to react by swelling, closing down, and producing excess mucus. Triggers include physical activity, allergens such as pollen or pet dander, irritants such as chemicals or smoke, and respiratory coughs or colds.

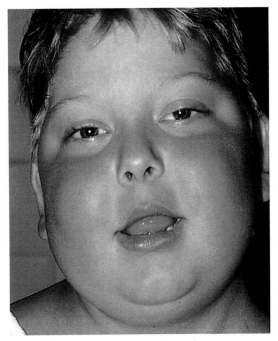

Fig. 15-1 A child with steroid-dependent asthma.
(From Zitelli BJ, Davis HW: *Atlas of pediatric physical diagnosis*, ed 5, Philadelphia, 2007, Mosby.)

Asthma rates continue to increase all over the world and have nearly doubled in the United States during the past decade. According to the Centers for Disease Control and Prevention (CDC), more than 4 million children under age 18 in the United States have asthma, making it one of the most common chronic health conditions of childhood.[1,2]

Racial and economic disparities are apparent in both the number of hospital and emergency room visits attributable to asthma and deaths from asthma. Children of color in low-income neighborhoods have shown the highest increase in rates of asthma in recent years, perhaps related to both indoor and outdoor air pollution.[3]

A study by Mount Sinai Medical Center in New York City showed that emergency room visits for asthma varied dramatically by zip code, with the number of visits much higher in poor areas having large minority populations. Spanish Harlem had 223 visits for every 10,000 residents, while some parts of more affluent lower Manhattan did not record any emergency room visits.[3]

The CDC reports that emergency room and hospitalization rates for asthma are higher for black children than for white children, particularly for those under age 5. Among non-Hispanic black and white children aged 5 to 14, black children are five times more likely to die from asthma than white children.[2]

CLINICAL SIGNS

Signs and symptoms of asthma vary from person to person. As stated previously, symptoms include wheezing, shortness of breath, chest tightness, and coughing. An increased respiratory rate (tachypnea) and difficulty breathing (dyspnea) may accompany an asthma attack. A child may also be using accessory muscles in the ribcage to breathe; in this instance, the child may appear winded. Asthma attacks are generally recurring episodes, and by definition airway obstruction is reversible.

Asthma Clinical Signs
Wheezing
Shortness of breath
Chest tightness
Sputum production
Coughing
Airway inflammation, obstruction, or hypersensitivity to extrinsic and intrinsic stimuli
Episodic in onset

INTERVENTION

PHYSICAL THERAPY ASSESSMENT

After a review of the child's medical history, physical therapy evaluation should focus on identifying any areas of impairment, functional limitations, and activity and participation limitations.[4] Table 15-1 describes some of asthma's secondary impairments that can interfere with functional activity.

PHYSICAL THERAPY INTERVENTION

Physical therapy intervention of asthma comprises both short- and long-term goals. Short-term goals include addressing medical needs and musculoskeletal restrictions. Long-term goals are focused on reducing secondary impairments, usually through an established exercise regimen.[5]

In caring for children with asthma, it is imperative to have their diagnosis and **asthma management plan** in the charted history. Anyone involved with the child's care should be well instructed on signs and symptoms of asthma, as well as how and when to administer asthma medications or call for emergency help if needed. An individualized asthma management plan includes the child's asthma history, triggers and symptoms, ways to contact the parent/guardian and healthcare provider, physician and

TABLE **15-1** Assessing Functional Limitations Associated with Asthma

FUNCTIONAL ACTIVITY	SECONDARY PROBLEMS
Breathing	Inadequate breath support and inefficient trunk muscle recruitment at rest or with activities, such that breathing or postural control are compromised
	Asthmatic triggers such as rapid air flow caused by sudden increase in physical activity, dry air, extreme temperatures, or other triggers that trip an asthmatic reaction
Coughing	Ineffective mobilization and expectoration strategies
Sleeping	Breathing difficulties, signs of obstructive or central sleep disorders
	Nocturnal reflux (GERD)
Eating	Swallowing dysfunction
	Reflux (GERD)
	Dehydration
	Poor nutrition
Talking	Inadequate lung volume and/or inadequate motor control for eccentric and concentric expiratory patterns of speech
	Poor coordination between talking (refined breath support) and moving (postural control)
Moving	Inadequate balance between ventilation and postural demands
	Breath holding with more demanding postures: use of the diaphragm as a primary postural muscle for trunk stabilization
	Inadequate lung volume to support movement
	Inadequate and/or inefficient muscle recruitment patterns for trunk/respiratory muscles, causing endurance problems or poor motor performance
	Ineffective pairing of breathing with movement, especially with higher-level activities

GERD, gastroesophageal reflux disease.
NOTE: These activities require adequate lung volumes and coordination of breathing with movement for optimal performance. Typical secondary problems associated with asthma should be screened for to determine their possible contribution to the child's motor impairment or motor dysfunction.
From Campbell SK, Vander Linden DW, Palisano RJ: *Physical therapy for children*, ed 3, Philadelphia, 2006, Saunders.

parent/guardian signatures, the child's target peak flow reading, and a list of current asthma medications. The plan will also include the child's treatment plan for medications, based on symptoms and peak flow readings.

Peak flow monitoring can be effectively used in children age 5 and older. There are many different peak flow meters available on the market. The simple device measures how well air is moving out of a person's airways. To use the device, one takes a deep breath in, places the mouth on the peak flow meter, and exhales as fast and completely as possible. A reading will appear on the meter. Usually the steps are repeated a few times to ensure accuracy. Each person who uses peak flow monitoring has a personal best or target reading. Lower numbers may call for attention with medications and additional monitoring. Very low numbers demand emergency attention. Peak flow numbers or zones should be included in the asthma management plan. Though quite effective, peak flow monitoring is only one indicator of asthma stability or problems. Other symptoms such as coughing, wheezing, complaints of shortness of breath, and chest tightness should also be considered.

Asthma may be treated and controlled with a variety of pharmacologic interventions. Many patients have at least two types of medications (Table 15-2). The first type is used as a preventive or maintenance medication. **Preventive medications** can be oral or inhaled and are used to help decrease the inflammation of the airways or decrease the response to triggers such as allergens. The second is a **rescue medication**. Rescue medications are usually supplied in the form of an inhaler that contains a bronchodilator such as albuterol. Albuterol quickly helps to open the airways, enabling an asthmatic to breathe easier. It is important to distinguish between the two types of medications. A preventive inhaler will be of no help during an acute asthma attack. People with asthma should carry their rescue inhaler with them. Children with asthma should also keep extra rescue inhalers at school and at any caregivers' homes.

A **spacer** is a large chamber that is fitted to an inhaler and is useful in dispensing a dose of medication more effectively. Spacers serve to increase the amount of medication that actually reaches the lungs, instead of being deposited in the mouth and throat. For children

TABLE **15-2** Current Medications for the Quick Relief and Long-Term Management of Asthma

TYPE OF DRUG	DRUG NAMES	FUNCTION
Bronchodilators	Albuterol	Preventive (long-acting)
	Levalbuterol	Rescue (short-acting)
	Salmeterol	
	Ipratropium	
	Theophylline	
Combined beta-agonist/corticosteroid	Salmeterol/Fluticasone (Advair Diskus)	Preventive
Corticosteroids	Fluticasone (Flovent)	Preventive (inhaled)
	Triamcinolone (Azmacort)	Rescue (systemic)
	Beclomethasone (Vanceril, Beclovent, Qvar)	
	Prednisone (Deltasone, Orasone, Meticorten)	
	Budesonide (Pulmicort Turbuhaler, Rhinocort)	
Leukotriene receptor antagonists	Montelukast (Singulair)	Preventive
	Zafirlukast (Accolate)	
Mast cell stabilizers	Cromolyn (Intal)	Preventive
5-Lipoxygenase inhibitors	Zileuton (Zyflo)	Preventive

Data from Morris MJ: *Asthma*, e-Medicine (website): http://www.emedicine.com/med/topic177.htm. Accessed 2/13/07.

there is the added advantage of not having to coordinate the inhalation of medication, as they must with a multi-dose inhaler. The medication dose is released into the spacer and then can be inhaled at will by the child. In the event that the lung tidal volume is low and inhalation is difficult, he or she can breathe in and out several times with the chamber and still get an effective dose. Caution must be used to avoid spraying more than one puff at a time into the spacer. If the child's dose is two puffs, spray one and have the child inhale from the spacer, then repeat with the second puff after waiting 1 full minute.

It is vital for caregivers to be able to identify when a child is having difficulty breathing or having an acute episode. Activity should be stopped when these symptoms are noticed. If a child has an asthma management plan, instructions with regard to medications should be closely followed. If the child does not respond to medications or fails to improve, emergency help should be sought. Furthermore, if a child is hunched over, straining to breathe, has difficulty completing a sentence, looks ashen or has blue lips and fingernails, immediate emergency help (i.e., a 9-1-1 call) is warranted.

Exercise-induced asthma is a special consideration. Children and caregivers can try to reduce triggers like allergens and irritants, but exercise should not be avoided to avert an asthma attack. Rather, with medications and possibly some modifications to physical activity, the symptoms can be controlled. Often a physician will recommend giving a dose of rescue medication prior to exercise to decrease the child's chances of having an acute asthma episode. This can be very effective. In addition, a child who has had a recent asthma episode is more likely to have additional episodes, and therefore the level of exertion should be modified. The physical therapist assistant can create an individualized exercise regimen that will improve muscle function while minimizing the risk of an asthma attack.

Exercising indoors or in a warm, humid environment rather than outdoors or in a cold, dry environment can reduce the frequency of asthma attacks.[4]

Recent research[6,7] has determined that weather factors, pollen, and the different seasons have an effect on the severity of asthma symptoms. High temperature and barometric pressure were the most highly correlated weather factors with severity of asthma symptoms.[7] Additionally, airborne irritants such as pollen and mold also correlated with asthma symptoms.[7] Finally, in most of the subjects, summer was the least difficult season for asthmatics, followed by spring; fall was the worst, followed by winter.[7] This research is important to the PT and PTA when designing exercise protocols for asthmatics or for the PT and PTA who work in schools. Warm days with high barometric pressure, allergy-alert days when the airborne irritant count is high, and the fall season are specific times when healthcare providers must be keenly aware of the status of children with asthma.

Asthma Interventions

Design an exercise protocol
Implement low-cost measures for indoor allergen avoidance
Restore, maintain, and promote optimal physical functioning

Chapter Discussion Questions

1. Describe two triggers that may affect an asthmatic child's ability to breathe.
2. What racial and economic groups demonstrate the highest rate of childhood asthma?
3. What are the components of an asthma management plan?
4. What is the purpose of the peak flow meter?
5. Is it better to have a high reading or a low reading on the peak flow meter?
6. What is the difference between preventive medication and rescue medication?

7. What are two accommodations that children with asthma may make in order to participate in an exercise routine/activity?
8. What are three common signs or symptoms of an asthma attack?
9. What is the appropriate action to take if a child begins to have an asthma attack while exercising?
10. What weather-related factors and season seem to correlate with the severity of asthma symptoms?

REFERENCES

1. Centers for Disease Control and Prevention: *Asthma* (website): http://www.cdc.gov/asthma/default. htm. Accessed September 1, 2004.
2. Children's Defense Fund: *Asthma* (website): www. CDF.org/Asthma. Accessed September 1, 2004.
3. Mitchell H, Senturia Y, Gergen P, and others: Design and methods of the National Cooperative Inner-City Asthma Study, *Pediatr Pulmonol* 24:237, 1997.
4. Morris MJ: *Asthma*, e-Medicine (website): http:// www.emedicine.com/med/topic177.htm. Last updated 2/13/07.
5. Campbell SK, Vander Linden DW, Palisano RJ: *Physical therapy for children*, ed 3, Philadelphia, 2006, Saunders.
6. Altintaş DU, Karakoç GB, Yilmaz M, and others: Relationship between pollen counts and weather variables in east-Mediterranean coast of Turkey. Does it affect allergic symptoms in pollen allergic children? *Clin Dev Immunol* 11(1):87, 2004.
7. Weber G: *Asthma and weather: a mathematical model (electronic version online)*: http://www.hcs.harvard. edu/~weber/HomePage/Papers/Asthma AndWeather/. Accessed January 15, 2005.

RESOURCES

Childhood Asthma Foundation
1-800-373-5696
www.childasthma.com
American Academy of Allergy, Asthma, and Immunology
555 East Wells Street
Suite 1100
Milwaukee, WI 53202-3823
414-272-6071
www.aaaai.org
U. S. National Library of Medicine
www.nlm.nih.gov

Pediatric Sports Injuries

learning objectives

At the end of the chapter the reader will be able to do the following:

1. Identify the variances of children's sports-related injuries.

2. Describe appropriate exercise regimens for the child athlete.

3. Identify the differences in children's anatomy as compared to adults.

4. Recognize common childhood sports injuries and their etiologies.

As the number of children who participate in organized sports increases, the number of children injured increases as well (Figure 16-1). Child athletes are not smaller versions of adult athletes.[1] They have different physiologic responses to exercise, different musculoskeletal structures, and thus are susceptible to different injuries.

INJURY CONSIDERATIONS

There are many physiologic differences between the adult and the child during exercise. The child has a smaller heart than the adult; thus there is a smaller stroke volume, or in simple terms, a smaller heart pushes less blood. A child has a higher heart rate during submaximal and maximal exercise. This increased heart rate offsets some of the decreased stroke volume, but not enough to compensate for the size difference.[2] Because of these factors, the child cannot exercise as efficiently as an adult can and must be watched very closely.

Another difference in the response to exercise is the effect on muscle mass. It has been shown that a limited amount of weightlifting improves strength in the child muscle; however, there is little gain in muscle mass. The strength increase is due to improved coordination and neuromuscular recruitment. **Strength training** can assist the normal muscle development occurring throughout puberty. Because of their decreased muscle mass, the recommended weightlifting program for adolescents is low weight–high repetition activity. This is especially true in the beginning stages of

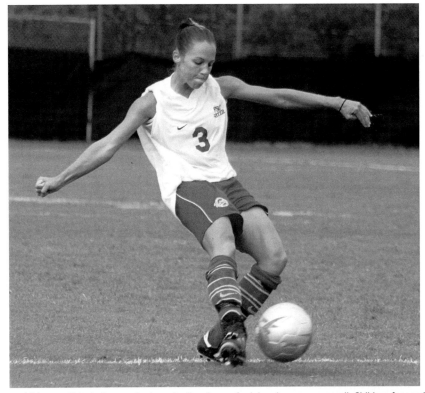

Fig. 16-1 As more children participate in organized sports, the chance for injury increases as well. Children face unique considerations with sports injuries. (From Cummings NH, Stanley-Green S, Higgs P: *Perspectives in athletic training*, St Louis, 2009, Mosby.)

weightlifting. Proper lifting technique is the key to avoiding injuries in the adolescent population. Once the technique has been perfected, 8 to 15 repetitions should be performed. The weight should not be increased until 8 to 15 repetitions can be performed with good technique, and then it should be increased in small increments. This is why supervision is essential for adolescent strength training. Strength training should be done 2 to 3 times per week. There is evidence showing that there is no benefit to strength training more than 4 times per week.[3] Recommendations by the American Academy of Pediatrics Committee on Sports Medicine and Fitness are listed in Box 16-1.

A common question among parents is when a child can safely begin strength training. There is no exact chronological age when this can begin. Instead, strength training can begin when the child is able to understand and follow detailed instructions on proper technique and progression of the program.[4]

There are two general classifications of musculoskeletal differences between children and adults: bone and muscle. The differences in these structures at varying maturation stages leads to a separate set of common injury patterns. The osteology of a child varies from the adult in many ways. The bone is more porous and more susceptible to compression fractures. A greenstick fracture can also occur when there is a perpendicular force placed upon a bone and the bone begins to bend. The fracture occurs on the convex side of the curve. Stress fractures are common in females with delayed menarche or amenorrhea due to hormonal imbalances prior to and during puberty.[5] The general rehabilitation of these types of injuries involves rest, biomechanical examination, orthotic bracing, and strengthening and stretching of the surrounding soft tissue structures. Surgery may be involved if the fracture requires more support.

Another injury unique to the child is a physeal or **growth plate fracture**. There are many areas in the body where this can occur, and the most common ones will be discussed later in the chapter under the headings of each anatomic region. A growth plate in a long bone is most commonly found near a joint. These growth plates provide for axial and circumferential growth of bones. These areas are the weakest point around joints, thus injuries usually occur in the growth plate, not the joint.[6] Salter and Harris described the most common way to classify the extent of the fracture. This classification separates these fractures into five categories (Table 16-1).[7] The general rehabilitation for these types of injuries involves rest, biomechanical examination, orthotic bracing, and strengthening and stretching of the surrounding soft tissue structures. Surgery may be needed to stabilize the fracture if the fracture is too extensive or unstable.

Another common injury to the bone is a fracture to an apophysis, which is growth cartilage connecting bone to tendon. In adults this junction is ossified and is not as easily injured. These injuries in children can be the result of a traumatic incident or from an overuse type of injury with an insidious onset.[8]

Box **16-1**	Strength-Training Recommendations for Children

A thorough medical examination should be completed before a strength-training program begins.

If general health benefits are the goal, aerobic exercise should be included.

Warm-up and cool-down periods are an essential part of the strength-training regimen.

Specific strength-training exercise should be learned with no weight to perfect the technique. Small increments of weight should be added in 8- to 15-repetition sets.

All muscle groups should be included, and the activities should include full range of motion.

If any sign of injury occurs, all activity should stop, and a thorough medical examination should be completed.

From American Academy of Pediatrics: Strength training by children and adolescents, *Pediatrics* 107(6):1470, 2001.

TABLE **16-1** Salter-Harris Fracture Classification

CLASSIFICATION	DESCRIPTION
I	A fracture along the entire length of the growth plate that does not involve the surrounding osteology
II	A fracture of part of the growth plate and part of the osteology away from the joint
III	A fracture involving part of the growth plate and part of the osteology nearest to the joint
IV	A fracture through the growth plate and both sides of the osteology
V	A compression fracture in the mid-substance of the growth plate

From Salter R, Harris W: Injuries involving epiphyseal plate, *J Bone Joint Surg* 45A:587, 1963.

The more common injury sites are the knee, hip, and shoulder. Apophyseal fractures will be addressed later in the chapter under the headings for each anatomic region.

The general rehabilitation for fractures to growth plates, either a physis or an apophysis, should be conservative before surgical. Conservative intervention involves rest, biomechanical corrections, orthotic bracing, and strengthening and stretching of the surrounding soft tissue structures. Surgery may be involved to fixate the apophysis or physis if it becomes unstable. Surgical intervention is the last resort and rarely needs to occur. Caution is always the rule when treating these injuries.[8] Growth plate injuries may lead to an alteration in normal bone growth and subsequent biomechanical problems with injuries later in life. The regional anatomy sections will detail a rehabilitation program for specific injuries.

Osteochondritis dissecans is an injury to the articular cartilage and the corresponding bone. The bone and cartilage may split from the rest of the bone and can in some instances separate from the bone and become loose in the joint. These injuries may be asymptomatic if no displacement occurs. The elbow, knee, and ankle are common sites for this type of injury.[9]

The general rehabilitation for these injuries is similar to the rehabilitation for physeal or apophyseal injuries: conservative before surgical. Conservative intervention should involve rest, biomechanical corrections, orthotic bracing, and strengthening and stretching of the surrounding soft tissue structures. Surgery may be necessary to fixate a partially separated injury or to remove a loose body if it is interfering with normal joint function.[5]

Muscle tissue injury causes different problems for the child. As bone growth occurs, especially during growth spurts, the muscle must adapt and lengthen. This process may take some time to occur, and during this adaptation period the joints and growth plates have increased stress placed upon them. This excess stress can lead to numerous types of injuries in any of the musculoskeletal structures.[3] General rehabilitation for these problems entails increasing the flexibility of the involved muscles and appropriate action for any of the other involved musculoskeletal structures.

COMMON INJURY SITES

CERVICAL SPINE

Cervical injuries in children need to be treated with great caution. Studies have shown that a large portion of cervical injuries in this age group are sports-related. Any injury to the cervical spine, or any injury that causes neurologic symptoms in the upper extremity, needs thorough examination because of the possibility of long-lasting complications for the child. A three-view radiographic series consisting of lateral, anteroposterior, and oblique views is the most effective approach to diagnosing any significant problems in the cervical spine. One study found this process to be 94% sensitive to all cervical spine injuries that can lead to long-lasting deficits.[10] Once the radiographs determine the spine is stable with no osteologic, ligamentous, or neurologic deficits, examination and intervention for the musculature can continue.

The general intervention protocol will consist of a soft collar for rest, with heat or ice for analgesic effect. Once the pain subsides, a progressive strengthening and stretching program should be initiated. The stretching program should begin with gentle stretching in the lateral, anterior, and posterior directions, as well as the diagonals of anterior-lateral and posterior-lateral bilaterally. The stretching program should address unilateral and bilateral rotation as well. The stretching should be pain-free with no residual soreness. The strengthening program should begin with isometrics in the cardinal planes of motion and rotation and progress to the diagonals. The program should advance to active strengthening in the pain-free range of motion once the isometric exercises are no longer difficult and exhibit no residual effects. The active exercises should begin in the cardinal planes of motion and rotation, then progress to the diagonal planes. Active resistance using manual resistance by the child is a common exercise. The most important aspect of the rehabilitation program is technique. To prevent injuries, detailed instructions are very important. The child should not progress to a more difficult exercise until he or she practices the next exercise and the therapist is certain he or she can do it properly.

THORACIC SPINE

Thoracic spine injuries mostly consist of osteologic injuries. The most significant difference between the mature and immature spine, as with all other bones, is the presence of growth plates. There are growth plates at each end of the vertebral body. These appear between the ages of 8 and 12 and begin to fuse at age 15. Injuries are most common at age 14 to 16 around the time these growth plates begin to fuse and are susceptible to fractures. The most common problem associated with these fractures is the wedging of the vertebral body. If this occurs, it will cause an increase in the kyphosis of the thoracic spine and lead to many biomechanical problems later in life.[11] The most common

mechanisms of injury are hyperflexion with or without compression, shear forces, or distraction forces.[12]

If these fractures are stable, conservative intervention is the norm. Bed rest or a thoracolumbosacral orthosis (TLSO) allows the fracture to heal. Once the fracture has sufficiently healed, the recommended rehabilitation is a progressive stretching and strengthening program focusing on extension of the thoracic spine and scapular strengthening. A postural rehabilitation program will assist in decreasing the possibility of a habitual hyperkyphosis forming. If surgical intervention is required, the therapist should follow a physician's protocol as to when to begin the stretching and strengthening progression.[5]

Another common problem in the thoracic spine is **Scheuermann's disease**. This is similar to the wedge-shaped fracture discussed previously, but it has an overuse, postural etiology.[13] The rehabilitation for this problem is similar to that for acute fractures, focusing on thoracic extension stretching and strengthening and postural education to decrease the kyphosis. Scapular strengthening may help; the biomechanics of this area can be affected by increased kyphosis.

LUMBAR SPINE

Injuries to the lumbar spine are more common than either thoracic or cervical spine injuries. Posture plays a significant role in the incidence of most injuries in this area. During periods of rapid growth, muscle and fascia may become tight and cause postural changes. These dysfunctions are common in the dorsal lumbar fascia and hamstrings.[5]

The child with an increased lumbar lordosis posture is more susceptible to an injury to the pars interarticularis. The pars interarticularis prevents the vertebral body from gliding anteriorly on the vertebral body inferior to it. A fracture to this area with no subsequent vertebral movement is a *spondylolysis*. If the vertebral body glides anteriorly due to this injury, it is a *spondylolisthesis*. Spondylolisthesis is classified by the distance the vertebral body translates anteriorly as confirmed by radiographs.[14] The most common sites for this injury are L5-S1 and L4-L5, respectively. This injury is common in sports where forced hyperextension occurs—gymnastics or football, for example. The rehabilitation for this injury is usually conservative. The intervention consists of trunk stabilization exercises avoiding lumbar extension. These exercises may include back stretching and abdominal strengthening. In severe cases surgery may be required to stabilize the unstable vertebral segment.[15]

The child with a decreased lumbar lordosis posture is susceptible to a flexion injury of the intervertebral body or intervertebral disc. The injury to the intervertebral body is in the growth plate near the superior and inferior borders of the vertebral body. If the injury is severe enough, it can cause the wedging described earlier for the thoracic spine. In children fractures are more common in the lumbar region than intervertebral disc injuries. The reason is because in the immature skeleton the disc is hydrophilic and stronger than the growth plates in the vertebral body. Overuse repetitive trauma or acute trauma can cause either of these injuries.[12] Intervention for both injuries should include postural retraining and lumbar stabilization exercises.

Sciatica is a problem not commonly seen in children, but it can occur. Many problems can cause it, including those listed above. Tight piriformis muscles can cause sciatica. Symptoms are similar to those associated with other lumbar spine problems.[5] Intervention consists of general lumbar stabilization and flexibility if the cause arises from the lumbar spine or piriformis flexibility exercises if the piriformis muscles are the cause.

SHOULDER

The most common type of shoulder injury in the young athlete is an overuse injury. These occur most often in sports involving use of the arm overhead in activities such as throwing, racket sports, or swimming. The most common injuries are growth plate fractures and impingement.

For the athlete who does a great deal of throwing, prevention is the best medicine for all injuries. The primary factor responsible for the injury is the technique or biomechanics of the throwing motion. A detailed analysis of the throwing motion, with corrections and proper coaching afterwards, is essential to preventing problems in the shoulder. For pitchers, the athletes who throw the most, a detailed pitch count and frequency of pitching performance is also important. Another factor for pitchers is the type of pitch thrown. Pitchers under the age of 12 should not throw breaking pitches.[6]

For racket sport athletes and swimmers, biomechanics and coaching are also important. Repetitive use of the arm overhead creates a great deal of force, and only with proper form and training can most of these problems be avoided.

One of the common overuse injuries is the proximal humeral growth plate fracture. This may be referred to as *little league shoulder*. Poor technique and underdeveloped musculature are primary causes for this injury. Rehabilitation often consists of rest until the fracture has healed, usually 6 to 8 weeks, followed by a progression of rotator cuff strengthening exercises. The exercises consist of external rotation, internal rotation, abduction, extension, and diagonal patterns to increase the strength and stabilization of the shoulder.[5]

Another common injury is an impingement in the subacromial area of the shoulder. With this injury the rotator cuff musculature is underdeveloped and is not capable of generating enough force to maintain the stability of the glenohumeral joint. The humeral head begins to glide superiorly in the glenoid fossa and impinge upon the subacromial structures against the undersurface of the acromion. These structures include the rotator cuff muscles, the subacromial bursa, the glenoid labrum, and the attachment for the long head of the biceps brachii.[11]

Rehabilitation for this injury consists of a period of rest followed by progressive strengthening of the rotator cuff muscles to increase the stability of the joint and general strengthening of the entire shoulder complex. The strengthening progression starts with isometrics in the cardinal planes and the rotator cuff muscles and progresses to active strengthening in the diagonal planes, including the rotator cuff muscles. The final phase of the progression is strengthening during functional activities in the respective sport (e.g., throwing). During the functional training phase, a large part of the focus should be on technique and the importance of supervised training.

Children and adolescents may also sustain acute injuries to the shoulder area. Dislocations at the glenohumeral joint can occur but are rare. Acute injuries are more common in the joints surrounding the shoulder. An acromioclavicular joint separation occurs in contact sports such as football or wrestling as a consequence of falling on the lateral aspect of the shoulder.[5]

Rehabilitation for this injury consists of a period of rest to allow healing and then a progressive strengthening program for stability. Since there is very little musculature that crosses the joint, surrounding muscles such as the deltoid and scapular stabilizers will be the focus of the strengthening program.

A fracture of the clavicle is a common injury in children. As with acromioclavicular separation, a fall on the lateral aspect of the shoulder is usually responsible. The intervention for this injury is rest and immobilization, possibly in a figure-eight sling, to facilitate the healing of the bone in a normal alignment.

ELBOW

Like shoulder problems, overuse injuries of the elbow occur more frequently in children than acute injuries. Most elbow problems are associated with throwing and racket sports. Proper technique and biomechanics are essential for preventing injuries to the elbow. The same guidelines that apply to the shoulder as related to throwing apply to the elbow.

Little league elbow is a term used for pain around the medial aspect of the elbow. A variety of injuries can cause medial elbow pain. All of these injuries are overuse injuries and most commonly seen in throwers.[6]

One of the more common injuries implicated in little league elbow is medial epicondylitis. This is an inflammation of the origin of the wrist flexor tendons. It is an overuse injury that occurs with "dropping the arm too low" during throwing, throwing too many pitches or too often, or throwing breaking pitches at an early age (Figure 16-2). Rehabilitation consists of rest and gentle massage until the pain subsides, progressing to friction massage and progressive strengthening of the wrist, finger flexors, and forearm pronators.

Another injury to the elbow is a partial or complete avulsion of the medial epicondyle from the humerus through the growth plate. The cause can be a progression from medial epicondylitis or spontaneous separation. This injury is an overuse injury that occurs when the growth plate begins to widen under repetitive stress from excessive valgus forces placed upon the elbow. Rehabilitation consists of rest followed by progressive strengthening exercises, always strictly supervised by a qualified professional. Correction of a biomechanical flaw in the throwing motion, if one exists, is also necessary. If the avulsion progresses too far, surgery to stabilize the medial epicondyle is necessary for adequate healing. Primary concerns in any elbow rehabilitation are elbow stiffness and decreased range of motion. Thus active assistive movement or active range of motion should begin as soon as possible.

Ulnar nerve irritation is a problem caused by any instability on the medial side of the elbow. The ulnar nerve stretches during an

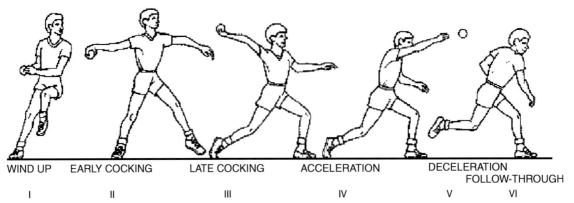

WIND UP   EARLY COCKING   LATE COCKING   ACCELERATION   DECELERATION
FOLLOW-THROUGH
I   II   III   IV   V   VI

Fig. 16-2 Little league elbow is an overuse injury that is common in pitchers. Late cocking, acceleration, deceleration, and follow-through are the phases most associated with elbow injury. (From Gerbino PG, Waters PM: Elbow injuries in the young athlete, *Oper Tech Sports Med* 6[4]:259, 1998.)

excessive valgus movement at the elbow, and this causes a "tingling" or "shooting" pain from the elbow to the little finger. Rehabilitation depends on the cause of the instability.

Osteochondritis dissecans of the radial capitellum can cause lateral elbow pain. This is a condition where there is pain, swelling, and possibly locking or catching in the elbow. A portion of the articular cartilage from the capitellum can be disassociated or attached. Either way, it changes the mechanics in the elbow. Rehabilitation generally consists of rest followed by progressive strengthening of the elbow musculature. If the problem is severe enough or persists long enough, surgery may be required to remove the loose body.[5]

Many elbow problems in children can cause or be caused by accelerated or delayed growth of the medial supracondylar growth plate or the superior radial growth plate. The primary cause of most of these injuries is throwing; however, upper extremity weightbearing sports such as gymnastics or wrestling can also cause these injuries in either acute or overuse variations. Medial (ulnar) collateral ligament injuries are common in adult athletes but rare in children, because at this stage of skeletal maturation the ligament is stronger than the growth plate and is not injured.

WRIST

Fractures are common injuries to the distal radius and wrist. Greenstick fractures are acute injuries usually sustained from a fall on an outstretched hand. These fractures typically occur in the middle to distal portion of the radius. Many of these can be treated with closed reduction and a short arm cast for approximately 4 weeks followed by flexibility and range-of-motion exercises to regain full motion.[9]

Growth plate fractures can occur in the distal radial growth plate. The causes of these injuries can be either acute or secondary to overuse. Acute injuries commonly result from a fall on an outstretched hand. Overuse injuries are often associated with upper extremity weightbearing sports such as gymnastics and wrestling. The rehabilitation is rest with immobilization if necessary. These injuries are commonly seen in athletes in contact sports.[6]

HAND

Fractures of the hand are less common than those of the wrist, but they are similar in origin. In adults dislocation or sprains of the fingers are common. In the child these injuries are often mistaken for phalanx growth plate injuries. These injuries may necessitate reduction and splinting for proper rest and healing. Active range of motion needs to begin as soon as possible to regain full function. Ligament avulsion injuries can also occur in the fingers but are more common in the thumb. Avulsions of the ulnar collateral ligament occur at the proximal phalanx of the thumb.[5] This injury is normally treated with a cast and rest, with range-of-motion exercises beginning as soon as possible to regain flexibility. Rehabilitation also includes strengthening in all planes of motion for the thumb.

PELVIS

There are a number of muscle attachment sites throughout the pelvis where growth plate avulsion fractures commonly occur. Sites include the iliac crest, anterior superior iliac spine, anterior inferior iliac spine, the ischial tuberosity, and the pubic symphysis. Avulsions at these sites are usually the result of quick and abrupt muscle contractions. Such injuries are common in sports where sprinting, stopping and starting, and an abrupt change of direction occurs. Rehabilitation of these injuries includes rest during the early stages of recovery until the avulsion has healed. The key to a full recovery from the injury and return to full function is stretching of the muscle attached at the site of the avulsion. As with most other growth plate injuries, conservative intervention is usually effective; however, for severe or displaced cases, surgery may be required.[8,9]

HIP

In children, assessing any and all hip pain should start with ruling out a growth plate injury in the femoral head. This condition is a slipped capital femoral epiphysis and can result from trauma or overuse. Intervention for this condition nearly always requires surgery followed by extensive range of motion, stretching, and progressive strengthening.[5]

Fractures and dislocations of the hip in children are rare. The bone, capsule, and ligaments are stronger than the growth plates in children, so the growth plate is usually the structure that fails first under stress.[6]

KNEE

The knee is one of the most common regions for overuse injuries in children. The sites where growth plate injuries occur in the knee are at each end of the patellar tendon. The injury when an avulsion or split of the bone occurs at the proximal end of the patellar tendon at the junction of the tendon and the patella is called *Sinding-Larsen-Johansson disease*. *Osgood-Schlatter disease* is an avulsion or split of the bone where the patellar tendon attaches to the tibia. Both problems can arise from a period of growth in which the bones have grown faster than the tendon. Children who participate in sports that involve jumping (e.g., basketball) are more vulnerable to this type of injury.[6] Rehabilitation consists of ice for acute pain and inflammation and rest until the split has healed. The next step is an aggressive stretching program to minimize the stress on each end of the patellar tendon. After the stretching program reaches a satisfactory point, the progressive strengthening program should begin concentrating on eccentric exercises. The functional portion of the progression may include plyometrics to coordination of jumping activities.

Jumper's knee is a term used to describe a number of different injuries that cause pain in the extensor mechanism of the knee. Two of the injuries that may be implicated in this category are Sinding-Larsen-Johansson disease and Osgood-Schlatter disease, but another common injury in this category is patellar tendonitis. This is an inflammation in the tendon generally caused by jumping or squatting, common activities in all sports. Rehabilitation for tendonitis is a gentle stretching program with ice for pain, followed by a progressive strengthening program focusing on eccentric activities.

Growth plate injuries of the long bones also occur in the knee region. The distal femoral epiphysis is a common site for injuries. This injury can have important consequences. If the growth plate does not heal properly, growth of the involved limb can be altered, and surgery may be required to fixate the fracture if it is unstable. Rehabilitation is rest until the growth plate fracture heals, then a general stretching and strengthening progression.

One of the most common regions for osteochondritis ossificans is the knee. This is a condition where the articular cartilage and associated bone may split or detach from the rest of the bone. The injury can range from a slightly split portion of cartilage to a loose body floating in the knee joint. The problem may be asymptomatic in the mildest cases. If the cartilage detaches, surgery may be necessary to remove it.[5] Rehabilitation should begin with ice to control pain and edema, then rest until the radiographs show the split has healed. A general stretching progression follows to ensure full motion returns.

Another musculoskeletal problem of the knee is patellofemoral pain syndrome. The precise cause of this syndrome is not certain, but there are a few theories. One theory is that there is a malalignment between the patella and distal femur. Another theory is that the vastus medialis obliquus (VMO) may be weak and allow excess lateral movement of the patella on the femur. Excess genu valgus is another possibility for the cause of patellofemoral pain. This condition changes the mechanics of the extensor mechanism and may force the patella to slide more laterally. Rehabilitation for patellofemoral pain syndrome includes strengthening of the quadriceps muscles, particularly the VMO, and stretching of the tensor fascia lata and iliotibial band. A biomechanical examination may be needed to rule out any mechanical problem arising from the hip or ankle. The strengthening program should consist of basic strengthening and progress to functional activities, including closed kinetic chain and eccentric exercises.[6]

Shin splints, or medial tibial stress syndrome, is a common injury in child athletes, especially runners. This is another syndrome that may have many different causes. The primary symptom is medial tibial pain. One injury may be an inflammation of the connection between the posterior tibialis and soles interposes membrane and the periosteum of the tibia. Another possibility is medial tibial stress fracture.[3] There are a few possible causes for these problems. One is a biomechanical problem in the foot, usually excessive pronation. Another common cause is repetitive eccentric contraction of the ankle dorsiflexors during gait. Rehabilitation begins with corrections in the gait pattern deficiencies during walking and running. Landing more toward the midfoot instead of the heel will reduce the stress in the medial tibia. Aquatic exercises work very well for low-impact activities. The intervention should progress from ice for pain and inflammation, along with strengthening and stretching of the pretibial muscles, to functional low-impact activities. The strengthening should include eccentric activities.

ANKLE

Sever's disease is a growth plate injury to the posterior portion of the calcaneus near the attachment of the Achilles tendon. Decreased flexibility of the Achilles tendon contributes to the cause of this injury. The decreased flexibility of the Achilles tendon can be from the bone growing faster than the muscles. As the traction force increases, the calcaneal growth plate can separate. This very rarely becomes displaced.[5] Interventions include temporary heel lifts to decrease pressure on the injury site, along with ice massage to decrease the pain and inflammation. After the injury heals, stretching of the Achilles tendon is the priority. After flexibility improves, strengthening of the calf muscles is next, including functional activities.

Ankle sprains are very common injuries in adults. However, in children this injury is not as common. In children the ligament structure is stronger than the bone structure, especially near growth plates. The growth plate near the distal end of the fibula can be easily injured with inversion injuries of the ankle. This injury can have serious ramifications later in life for the child. Alterations of normal growth of the bone can occur. This may result in any number of biomechanical problems, from the lower extremity to the lumbar spine. The ankle can also become unstable, causing frequent lateral ankle injuries with only mild inversion forces in adulthood.

Rehabilitation for this injury is general rest until the fracture heals, followed by a strengthening and proprioceptive progression. The strengthening program should consist of cardinal plane exercises for plantar flexion, dorsiflexion, inversion, and eversion, followed by diagonal plane strengthening. The focus of the strengthening program should be on eversion activities to strengthen the peroneal (fibularis) muscles to prevent further inversion injuries. The proprioceptive progression should include activities that begin with a good base of support and progress to minimal support. A typical progression may begin with double-leg-stance activities, progress to single-leg-stance activities, and end with activities using double- and single support on balance boards or mini-trampolines.

Osteochondritis dissecans can occur on the talus and cause pain, swelling or locking of the ankle. Intervention is conservative, with rest and bracing until the bone heals. A general stretching and strengthening progression follows. If the articular cartilage becomes disassociated, surgery may be necessary to remove the loose body.

FOOT

For the child athlete, stress fractures are the most common injuries seen in the foot. These are overuse injuries where the force is enough to cause injury to the bone but not enough to cause it to fully fracture. These may be difficult to diagnose on normal radiographs, and bone scan may be needed. Stress fractures are

more common in girls, especially as they near puberty.[6]

Rehabilitation for these injuries will include rest until they heal and biomechanical corrections of the foot and ankle. The use of soft foot orthoses to decrease stress in the injured area is a common intervention.

Sports Injuries Interventions

Conservative rehabilitation
Rest (which is the primary factor in allowing the bone to heal) before initiating a rehabilitation program
General progressive rehabilitation program that consists of strengthening and flexibility exercises for the respective area, focusing on functional activities
Surgery only when there is a loose body interfering with normal joint motion or when a displaced fracture may interfere with normal bone growth

Summary

As more and more children participate in organized athletics, more injuries will occur. The therapist must remember that a child is not a small adult. There are many physical, mental, and emotional differences between the age groups. The child cannot exercise in the same manner as an adult because of physiologic and hormonal differences. Physiologic differences include heart size, volume of blood, and decreased stroke volume among others. Prepubertal hormonal differences do not allow the muscles to increase in size or strength. Children can participate in weightlifting and strengthening exercises; however, the strength gains are due more to neuromuscular improvements in coordination and muscle recruitment than to pure strength gains. Children should not begin strengthening exercises and weight training programs until they can fully understand and follow detailed instructions to prevent injuries.

Injuries that are common in children who participate in athletics are physeal (growth plates in the long bones) fractures, greenstick fractures, stress fractures, apophyseal (growth plates in the bone-tendon junctions) injuries, and muscle stress injuries resulting from bone growing at a more rapid rate than the attached muscles.

Chapter Discussion Questions

1. Why is a child's heart rate higher than an adult's during exercise?
2. How does strength improve in children without an increase in muscle mass?
3. Describe two skeletal injuries unique to children.
4. Describe Salter-Harris categories I and V of growth plate fractures.
5. What is Osgood-Schlatter disease? Who is more susceptible to getting this disease?
6. Describe general rehabilitation guidelines for childhood athletic injuries.
7. Why are foot stress fractures common in children?
8. Describe *little league elbow* injury.
9. Describe *little league shoulder* injury.
10. When can a child safely begin to participate in a strength-training program?

REFERENCES

1. American Academy of Pediatrics: Strength training by children and adolescents, *Pediatrics* 107(6):1470, 2001.
2. Wilmore J, Costill D: Children and adolescents in sports. In Wilmore J, Costill D, Kenney WL, editors: *Physiology of sport and exercise*, ed 3, Champaign, Ill, 2004, Human Kinetics.
3. Faigenbaum A, Millikin L, Burak R, and others: Comparison of 1 and 2 days per week of strength training in children, *Res Q Exerc Sport* 73(4):416, 2002.
4. Faigenbaum A, Westcott W: The effects of different resistance training protocols on muscular strength and endurance development in children, *Pediatrics* 104(1):e5, 1999.
5. Trepman E, Micheli L, Backe L: Children and adolescents. In Kolt G, Snyder-Mackler L, editors: *Physical therapies in sports and exercise*, London, 2003, Churchill-Livingstone.
6. Koutures C: An overview of overuse injuries, *Contemp Pediatr* 18(11):44, 2001.
7. Salter R, Harris W: Injuries involving epiphyseal plate, *J Bone Joint Surg* 45A:587, 1963.
8. Aksoy B, Ozturk K, Ensenyel C, and others: Avulsion of the iliac crest apophysis, *Int J Sports Med* 19(1):76, 1998.
9. Kaeding C, Whitehead R: Musculoskeletal injuries in adolescents, *Prim Care* 25(1):211, 1998.
10. Faigenbaum A: Strength training for children and adolescents, *Clin Sports Med* 19(4):593, 2000.
11. Widhe T: Spine: posture mobility and pain. A longitudinal study from childhood to adolescence, *Eur Spine J* 10(2):118, 2001.
12. Baker C, Kadish H, Schunk J: Evaluation of pediatric cervical spine injuries, *Am J Emerg Med* 17(3):230, 1999.
13. Katz D, Screpella T: Anterior and middle column thoracolumbar spine injuries in young female gymnasts. Report of seven cases and review of the literature, *Am J Sports Med* 31(4):611, 2003.
14. Ikata T, Miyake R, Katoh S, and others: Pathogenesis of sports-related spondylolisthesis in adolescents. Radiographic and magnetic resonance imaging study, *Am J Sports Med* 24(1):94, 1996.
15. Clark P, Letts M: Trauma to the thoracic and lumbar spine in the adolescent, *Can J Surg* 44(5):337, 2001.

Part FIVE

Special Considerations
for Pediatric Practice

Chapter 17

Cheryl A. Mercado, OTR/L

Therapeutic Intervention in the Neonatal Intensive Care Unit Environment

key terms

Adjusted age (AA)
Chronological age (CA)

Developmentally supportive care
Gestational age (GA)

Neonatology
Postconceptual age (PCA)

outline

learning objectives

At the end of the chapter the reader will be able to do the following:

1. Understand the perinatal complications that result in a neonatal intensive care unit (NICU) stay.

2. Be familiar with terminology used in the NICU environment.

3. Know the therapeutic interventions appropriate for babies in the NICU.

Care of the neonate (the first 4 weeks of life) and provision of therapy services in the neonatal intensive care unit (NICU) require specialized knowledge and skills beyond basic physical therapy education and general pediatric practice. Given the advanced knowledge and skill NICU practice requires, it is typically not considered an appropriate practice area for the physical therapist assistant. However, infants discharged from the NICU often require continued therapy services (Figure 17-1) in settings where physical therapist assistants do provide care (e.g., early intervention programs, family homes, preschools, and day care centers). Providing comprehensive care for NICU graduates and their families requires the treating therapist to understand the family dynamics and stressors that accompany the birth of a premature or special needs infant, as well as knowledge of the infant's complex medical history (Box 17-1). This chapter will serve as an overview of therapeutic principles,

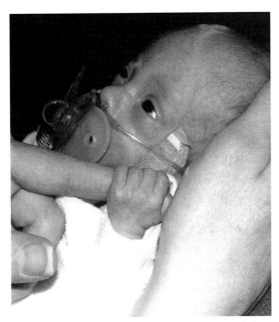

Fig. 17-1 Infants discharged from the NICU can benefit from continued physical therapy services. (Courtesy NICU, Medical Center of Plano, Plano, Texas; photography by Vicky Leland.)

Box **17-1**	Commonly Used Abbreviations

Preparing to provide treatment for a NICU graduate will involve review of the medical record and/or NICU discharge summary. The following list of abbreviations will help the PTA to discern some of the terminology:[1]

A's & B's	Apnea and bradycardia
AGA	Appropriate for gestational age
BAER	Brainstem auditory evoked responses
BPD	Bronchopulmonary dysplasia
BPM	Beats per minute (heart rate)
BW	Birth weight
CHF	Congestive heart failure
CMV	Cytomegalovirus
CPAP	Continuous positive airway pressure (type of ventilation)
CS	Cesarean section delivery
CSF	Cerebrospinal fluid
GT	Gastric tube
KCAL	Kilocalories
MCA	Multiple congenital anomalies
NG	Nasogastric feeding tube (also known as *gavage*)
NJ	Nasojejunal feeding tube
NNS/NS	Nonnutritive suck, nutritive suck
PO	Per os ("by mouth"—usually indicates feeding taken from a nipple)
PROM	Premature rupture of membranes
PTL	Preterm labor
RDS	Respiratory distress syndrome
Sats	Oxygen saturation levels
SVD	Spontaneous vaginal delivery
TORCHS	Screening for toxoplasmosis fetalis, rubella, cytomegalovirus, herpes simplex, and syphilis
TPN	Total parenteral nutrition

commonly seen problems, interventions, equipment, and terminology associated with the NICU environment.

OVERVIEW OF THE NICU

Neonatal intensive care nurseries have existed since the 1950s. Regional NICUs were established and have been in existence since the late 1960s. With subsequent advances in technology and care, physicians were able to improve outcomes for the very-low-birth-weight infant. With this increase in the number of surviving infants, the necessity of providing specialized care also grew. The complex needs of these very young infants necessitated involvement from multiple healthcare professionals. Physical therapists, occupational therapists, and speech-language pathologists began to expand their knowledge and scope of practice to provide care for the premature and/or ill neonate. Therapists have been providing care in the NICU for decades. **Neonatology** is now a technologically sophisticated area of pediatric medicine, and infants as premature as 24 weeks gestation (16 weeks early) and less than 500 grams (less than 1 pound) at birth have a good chance of survival.[2]

The philosophies guiding NICU care have evolved over the decades as well. Theories guiding care in the late 1960s and early 1970s suggested that the preterm or ill infant in the NICU experienced a kind of sensory deprivation. Intervention at that time was guided by the belief that infants required supplemental sensory stimulation in an effort to mimic the intrauterine environment. However, after further research indicated that these sick and preterm infants appeared to experience more stress from this imposed sensory stimulation, practice shifted to a model of reduced stimulation.[3,4]

The current standard of care in NICUs, **developmentally supportive care**, first emerged in the 1980s after parents and medical staff noted a variety of negative physiologic, motor, state, and attentional responses. The developmentally supportive care approach is based on the belief that infants are vulnerable to sensory overload and overstimulation. Optimal developmental care is based on minimizing this stress and increasing the infant's ability to self-organize through very careful monitoring of the infant's behavioral and physiologic cues.

More recent perspectives in care also recognize the family as the constant in the infant's life. Treatment is now directed toward facilitating parent/professional collaboration at all levels of care. One of the most important concepts of family-centered care recognizes the importance of an accessible healthcare system that is flexible, culturally competent, and responsive to family-identified needs.[5] Developmentally supportive care has now shifted to encompass optimizing the infant's long-term outcomes and development. This can be accomplished through the delivery of relationship-based individualized care geared to enhance the strengths of each infant and infant's family. This approach requires a high degree of interpersonal and intrapersonal collaboration between infants and families, as well as among infants, families, and professional caregivers.[5]

NEWBORN NURSERY LEVEL DESIGNATIONS

Hospital units specialized for neonatal care are designated as Level I, Level II, or Level III nurseries on the basis of their responsibilities and the availability of special services. The Level I nursery, essentially a *healthy newborn nursery*, can provide care for infants of routine, uncomplicated deliveries. Unexpected complications must be medically managed until transfer can be arranged to a more sophisticated facility. Level II nurseries, commonly referred to as *special care nurseries*, have the personnel and equipment available to manage neonatal care after uncomplicated deliveries, as well as many common problems of high-risk mothers and neonates. Level III nurseries, or *NICUs*, have specialized personnel and high technology equipment available to provide appropriate care to infants all along the risk and pathology spectrum, from term infants with increased care requirements like ventilatory support to preterm, critically ill, and malformed infants in need of the full range of intensive care interventions.[6]

CLASSIFICATION OF NEWBORN INFANTS

Newborn infants are typically classified by **gestational age (GA)** (number of weeks postconception). Gestational age or estimated gestational age (EGA) is expressed in weeks. The terms *postconceptual age, adjusted age,* and *chronological age* are also used. Classifications by GA are listed in Table 17-1.

TABLE **17-1** Gestational Age Classifications

CLASSIFICATION	AGE
Extremely preterm	Under 28 weeks
Preterm	28-37 weeks
Full term	37-42 weeks
Postterm	Above 42 weeks

Chronological age (CA) refers to the age of the child in days, weeks, or months from the time of birth. It is the actual amount of time since the child's birth. **Adjusted age (AA)** refers to the child's age after adjusting for prematurity. It is the age the child should be if they had been born full term, or the CA minus the weeks premature. For example, a child who is 16 weeks old (CA) but was 10 weeks premature has an AA of 6 weeks. Age is adjusted for prematurity until the child's second birthday. **Postconceptual age (PCA)** is the CA plus the GA. Thus a 4-week-old infant (CA) born at 28 weeks gestation (GA) has a PCA of 32 weeks.

Infants are also classified by birth weights. Birth weights in the NICU environment are typically expressed in grams, as opposed to pounds/ounces. One pound is equal to 454 grams. The most common birth weight classifications are listed in Table 17-2.[7]

Newborns are further classified in terms of how adequate their weight is in relation to their postconception age. The most common age-weight classifications are *appropriate for gestational age (AGA)*, which encompasses the 10th through 90th percentiles; *small for gestational age (SGA)*, for those infants who fall below the 10th percentile; and *large for gestational age (LGA)*, for those who fall above the 90th percentile.

NICU PERSONNEL

Neonatology is a technologically sophisticated area of pediatric medicine. The therapist working in the NICU is surrounded by a multitude of other professionals, all striving to meet one goal: optimizing the infant's potential for development. All of these therapists will work in a highly collaborative manner with one another, as well as with the NICU personnel, with the neonatologist (physician) as the leader of the team. Each specialist is equipped with unique knowledge to enhance the quality of life for infants and their families.

Most regional and Level III nurseries utilize multiple therapy services personnel, including physical and occupational therapists and speech-language pathologists. Physical and occupational therapists work in collaboration with NICU staff and families to help infants avoid unwanted or atypical movement patterns. In an effort to promote the overall development of the baby, physical and occupational therapists use facilitation and inhibition techniques and positioning to promote desired movement patterns and enhance function.

Speech-language pathologists are often consulted to address oral-motor and feeding/swallowing function. They also work with older infants to facilitate prelinguistic skills. As stated previously, all therapists work in a highly collaborative manner with one another, as well as with the NICU personnel. Each infant will be cared for by a neonatal nurse with advanced training. Because of the intensity of patient intervention and length of stay in most NICUs, patients are assigned a primary and secondary nurse who follow the infant throughout the weeks or months of hospitalization to provide continuity of care, support, and teaching for the family.

Other team members may include a neonatal nurse practitioner (NNP), who may direct care for infants in the intermediate care setting/

TABLE **17-2** Birth Weight Classifications

CLASSIFICATION	WEIGHT
Extremely low birth weight (ELBW)	Under 1000 grams
Very low birth weight (VLBW)	1000 to <1500 grams
Low birth weight (LBW)	1500 to 2500 grams
Average birth weight	Above 2500 grams

step-down nursery or for those infants retained only to feed and grow. These nurse practitioners undergo intensive training and testing and are supervised by the neonatologist. Also included in the NICU team is a respiratory therapist, usually assigned one to each room in a NICU, who monitors ventilator equipment. A pharmacist is typically on staff and assigned exclusively to the NICU to assist doctors and nurses with the complex balance of pharmacology. A nutritionist assists doctors, nurses, and families in providing the appropriate number and type of calories to help these tiny patients grow. A lactation consultant is available to help mothers in pumping breast milk, and when the infant's health and development permit, bringing infants to breast to initiate breastfeeding. Social workers and parent liaisons are typically available to assist families with the emotional responses to their infant's complex care. Many hospitals will also employ the services of child life personnel or developmental therapy professionals to provide additional stimulation and developmental activities and toys for the long-term but stable infant patient.

COMMON NICU EQUIPMENT

The NICU environment is filled with technology. Therapists working in the NICU require basic knowledge of the equipment for safe and effective delivery of service. Following is an introduction to some of the most commonly used equipment in the NICU:

- A *radiant warmer* is a bed with mattress on an adjustable tabletop covered by a radiant heat source. This type of bed is used for the gravely ill or newly admitted neonate to allow open space for tubes and equipment and rapid access for personnel to assess and care for the infant.
- A self-contained *isolette*, formerly known as an *incubator*, is an enclosed unit of transparent material; it provides a heated and humidified environment with a "servo" system of temperature monitoring. Caregivers can gain access to the infant through

portholes or by opening a door on the face of the unit. Most stable preterm infants will be placed in an isolette for the first several weeks of admission until they can maintain appropriate body temperature.
- An *oxygen hood* is a plastic or Plexiglas hood that typically covers the infant's head and provides a closed environment for controlled oxygen or humidification delivery.
- *Mechanical ventilators*: A *pressure ventilator* delivers positive-pressure ventilation. Pressures are limited, with the breath volume delivered dependent on the stiffness of the lung. A *volume ventilator* delivers positive-pressure ventilation, delivering the same tidal volume with each breath. A *negative-pressure ventilator* creates a relative negative pressure around the thorax and abdomen, thereby assisting ventilation without an endotracheal tube.
- *Nasal and nasopharyngeal prongs* are used to provide continuous positive airway pressure (CPAP); the apparatus consists of nasal prongs of varying lengths and an adapter for pressure source tubing.
- *Monitor*: Usually one unit will display one or more vital signs on a digital display. Electrodes are placed on the infant's chest or abdomen, and the same monitor will typically display heart and respiration rates, as well as oxygen saturations. High and low limits are typically set, and an alarm will sound if the limits are exceeded. The following are recommended safe limits:
  - Heart rate (HR) between 100 and 200 beats per minute (BPM). The ideal HR is between 120 and 160 BPM.
  - Respiration rate (RR) between 20 and 60 breaths per minute.
    Therapists working in the NICU should be aware that many false alarms are set off when the infant is moving. However, the nurse should always be consulted for all real alarms. Clinical observation of the infant's behaviors and skin color will help to discern real from false alarms.

- An *oxygen saturation monitor (pulse oximeter)* measures the amount of oxygen carried in the blood. Normal oxygen concentration ranges between 90% and 100%, and the alarm is usually set to trigger if the concentration falls under 85%. The sensor for this monitor is usually attached to one of the infant's toes.
- *Infusion pumps* are electric pumps that control the flow and rate of intravenous fluids, medications, fat emulsions, and transpyloric feedings. When an infusion pump alarm sounds, therapists should not alter the settings, but notify the nurse.
- *Extracorporeal membrane oxygenator (ECMO)* is a lifesaving therapy for infants with severe neonatal respiratory failure who, despite intensive therapy, fail to recover from hypoxemia or respiratory acidosis. The procedure involves passing the infant's blood through a filter and supplementing it with oxygen outside the infant's body. Infants undergoing ECMO are critically ill and usually are not candidates for therapy until they are stabilized and off the ECMO. Infants on ECMO are typically immobilized with their heads turned to one side. They are almost always in need of therapeutic intervention following ECMO treatment to help facilitate typical movement patterns and symmetry of posture.[2]

REASONS FOR THERAPY REFERRAL

The goal of therapeutic intervention in the NICU is to optimize the infant's potential for development. NICU physicians and nurses recognize the valuable role therapists can play in optimizing outcomes for premature and ill newborns. While referral criteria will vary between institutions, common reasons for referral include the following:
- Caregiver observations of increased tone with stiffness and arching
- Decreased range of motion or joint contractures

- Persistent asymmetric postures
- Known diagnosis or syndromes (e.g., spina bifida, Down syndrome)
- Poor state control or limited calming
- Disorganized feeding

Referrals are also frequently made to obtain a baseline evaluation for infants with questionable neurologic status. Commonly observed neuromotor profiles are listed in Table 17-3.

COMMON MEDICAL DISORDERS

The majority of the many medical problems experienced by newborn infants are directly related to their premature birth and the immaturity of various systems. However, other problems can arise as a result of iatrogenic complications resulting from the medical management of life-threatening situations. Following is a list of the most prevalent neonatal medical problems, causes, and the effects on neonatal development.

RESPIRATORY DISORDERS

Transient tachypnea of the newborn (TTN) occurs when an infant experiences minor respiratory difficulty soon after delivery. This condition is

TABLE **17-3** Common Neuromotor Profiles

PROFILE	CHARACTERISTICS
Typical preterm profile	Hypotonia Decreased antigravity actions Neck hyperextension Elevated/retracted shoulders Decreased UE/LE midline Excessive trunk extension Limited pelvic mobility
Hypotonic profile	Low arousal Decreased antigravity action Fixing at hips/shoulders Weak suck Poorly coordinated feeding
Hypertonic profile	Irritable Diminished handling tolerance Disorganized/tremulous actions Extensor posturing

Data from Toby M. Long, Dynamic Therapy Services, Inc., Clifton, New Jersey.

characterized by fast breathing (>80 breaths per minute). Other clinical signs are nasal flaring, intercostal retractions, and cyanosis. For the majority of neonates TTN generally resolves in 2 to 3 days. It is most commonly seen in term or near-term infants and infants born by cesarean section (in whom TTN may be attributed to lack of vaginal squeeze on the infant's thorax). This condition is treated with oxygen, typically administered in an oxygen hood or via "blow by" (oxygen tubing placed near the infant's face). Occasional short-term endotracheal intubation may be required in severe cases.

Perinatal asphyxia occurs when a newborn does not breathe spontaneously. The asphyxia may develop before or during labor or occur immediately after delivery. Intervention consists of maintaining adequate ventilation and oxygenation. Neurologic involvement is common in severely asphyxiated infants (Apgar scores below 5). Apgar scores are an evaluation of an infant's physical condition, usually performed at 1 minute of life and again at 5 minutes after birth. Scores are based on the sums of five factors that reflect an infant's ability to adjust to extrauterine life. The infant's heart rate, respiratory effort, muscle tone, reflex irritability, and color are scored from a low value of 0 to a normal value of 2. The five scores are combined, and the totals at 1 and 5 minutes are noted. Asphyxiated infants often experience neurologic problems. Associated conditions are hypoxic seizures or hypoxic ischemic encephalopathy (HIE).

Respiratory distress syndrome (RDS), also known as *hyaline membrane disease*, is a specific respiratory disorder common in premature infants and attributed to inadequate pulmonary surfactant. It is caused by collapse of lung tissue due to lack of pulmonary surfactant and an overly flexible chest wall. As the air sacs collapse, the surface tension of the lungs increases, making ventilation very difficult. Medical management requires ventilatory support, typically via endotracheal intubation.

Bronchopulmonary dysplasia (BPD), or chronic lung disease (CLD), is the most common form of chronic lung disease in premature infants; it is a consequence of continued damage and abnormal healing of the lungs after a severe respiratory distress disorder. Infants born at <32 weeks EGA who need supplemental oxygen after 36 weeks GA and infants born at ≥32 weeks GA who need additional oxygen after 28 days CA are defined as having BPD or CLD.

Apnea and bradycardia ("A's & B's") is another common problem in the NICU. Apnea is an absence of spontaneous respiration lasting longer than 20 seconds; it is commonly seen in premature infants. Apnea is frequently accompanied by bradycardia, a slowing in the heart rate to less than 100 BPM. Apnea of the newborn frequently requires physical stimulation of the infant. Bradycardia, if not directly related to apneic episodes, may be treated pharmacologically with caffeine. Infants cared for in the NICU are typically monitored, and alarms are set to track and alert staff to the occurrence of A's & B's. Some infants are discharged home with apnea monitors as well.

CARDIOVASCULAR/CARDIOPULMONARY DISORDERS

Patent ductus arteriosus (PDA) occurs when the fetal ductus arteriosus fails to close spontaneously at birth. When this happens, blood from the left side of the heart is able to pass to the right side, decreasing oxygenation and potentially causing cardiovascular overload. A PDA is more common in premature infants. The main diagnostic criterion is a characteristic heart murmur heard on auscultation and confirmed by echocardiogram. Those PDAs that do not resolve spontaneously are treated pharmacologically with indomethacin or through surgical ligation.

Persistent pulmonary hypertension of the newborn (PPHN) is characterized by an increase in vascular tension in the lungs that causes a right-to-left shunt through the ductus arteriosus and foramen ovale; it generally resolves spontaneously. Infants with persistent PPHN are treated with medication or mechanical ventilation.

Ventricular septal defect (VSD) is an abnormal opening in the septum separating the heart ventricles, permitting blood to flow from the left ventricle to the right ventricle and recirculate through the pulmonary artery and lungs, compromising peripheral oxygenation. It is the most common congenital heart defect and in many cases requires surgical correction.

CNS DISORDERS

Intraventricular hemorrhage (IVH) describes bleeding into the ventricular system of the brain and occurs almost exclusively in premature infants. Fifteen percent of infants with weights of <1500 grams and 80% of preterm infants <1000 grams will develop some degree of IVH. Diagnosis is typically made by cranial ultrasound or CT scan. Common symptoms include a bulging fontanel, sudden anemia, apnea, bradycardia, acidosis, high blood pressure, hydrocephalus, and changes in muscle tone and/or level of consciousness. The severity of IVH is classified according the extent of the lesion:

- Grade I: Subependymal, germinal matrix hemorrhage
- Grade II: Intraventricular bleeding without ventricular dilation
- Grade III: Intraventricular bleeding with ventricular dilation
- Grade IV: Intraventricular and intraparenchymal bleeding

The prognosis for infants with IVH is variable. Outcomes depend upon the severity of IVH, the presence or absence of other complications, and birth weight/GA. Infants with Grade I and Grade II bleeds typically recuperate with little or no deficits. Infants with Grade III and Grade IV IVH are at increased risk for long-term neurologic impairments, cerebral palsy, and cognitive impairment. Recent studies show that MRI is superior to cranial ultrasound in improved detection, classification, and thereby prognosis of IVH.

Periventricular leukomalacia (PVL) can occur as a severe form of IVH or as an independent diagnosis. This condition is characterized by ischemic white matter tissue surrounding the ventricles as a result of hypoxia associated with perinatal asphyxia. Diagnosis is established if paleness of the white matter is evident on cranial ultrasound or CT scan. Infants with PVL are at exceptionally high risk for CNS damage and cerebral palsy.

MISCELLANEOUS DISORDERS

Retinopathy of prematurity (ROP) results from an alteration in the normal development of retinal blood capillaries. Found exclusively in premature infants, especially those with very low birth weights, ROP affects approximately 65% of infants with a birth weight <1250 grams, and 80% of those <1000 grams will develop some degree of ROP. The incidence of ROP is most consistently associated with early GA, LBW, and duration of mechanical ventilation. The following classification system is a simplified version of the International Classification of ROP:

- Stage I: Thin demarcation line between the vascular and nonvascular regions of the retina
- Stage II: Demarcation line develops into a ridge that protrudes into the vitreous
- Stage III: Extraretinal fibrovascular proliferation occurs
- Stage IV: Fibrosis and scarring occurs, with traction on the retina resulting in retinal detachment
- Plus disease: Occurs when vessels posterior to the ridge become dilated and tortuous

Routine ophthalmoscopic examinations are now performed in NICUs for all infants with a birth weight <1500 grams or GA <32 weeks. Screening typically begins at 4 to 6 weeks CA, and reevaluations are conducted every 2 weeks until the retinas become fully mature. Laser surgery may be indicated if ROP is detected.

Necrotizing enterocolitis (NEC) is a serious disease in which the immature intestinal tissue, usually the intestinal wall, dies and sloughs off. The exact cause of NEC is unknown, but it may be related to intestinal ischemia. Infants may develop intestinal hemorrhage, gangrene, submucosal gas, and in severe cases perforation of the intestine. Typically seen in premature infants, NEC often first becomes evident around the third to tenth day of life as abdominal distention. The diagnosis of NEC is confirmed by x-ray. Medical management can be complex, and surgical intervention is indicated when perforation of the intestines has occurred. In severe cases a colostomy may be required. Oral or nasogastric feeding will be suspended and reintroduced very gradually.

Intrauterine growth restriction (IUGR) occurs when the development and maturation of the fetus is impeded or delayed by genetic factors, maternal disease, or fetal malnutrition caused by placental insufficiency. Infants weighing less than the 10th percentile for GA or less than 2 standard deviations below the mean for GA are classified as IUGR.[2]

INTERVENTION

PHYSICAL THERAPY ASSESSMENT

There are relatively few assessment tools available to physical, occupational, and speech-language therapists for assessing the baby in the NICU. The most valid and reliable tool is the Test of Infant Motor Performance (TIMP). Physical therapists might also evaluate the baby's emergence/dominance of primitive reflexes, tone, and range of motion. Most NICUs have adapted to the shortage of assessment tools by borrowing a variety of clinical observations from standardized tools to create their own OT/PT/SLP evaluation tools. Some formal tools commonly used and modified are the following:

- Neurological Assessment of the Preterm and Full-Term Newborn Infant (NAPFI): Used to document status of the nervous system in infants, document neurologic maturation and/or change in infants, and detect deviations in neurologic signs.[8]

- Neonatal Neurobehavioral Examination (NNE): A quantitative analysis of neonatal and neurologic status.[9]
- Neurobehavioral Assessment of the Preterm Infant (NAPI): Used to assess neurobehavioral status of prematurely born infants, monitor effects of intervention, and document individual differences.[10]
- Newborn Individualized Developmental Care and Assessment Program (NIDCAP): Used to develop a profile of the infants' physiologic and behavioral responses to environmental demands and caregiving.[11]

PHYSICAL THERAPY INTERVENTION

Therapists working in the NICU assist families and NICU staff in enhancing infant outcomes. The range of possible interventions includes fostering caregiver-infant interactions; positioning, feeding, sensory stimulation, or sensory/environmental modification; motor development intervention; splinting; and preparation for discharge.

Fostering Parent Interaction/Caregiving

Optimizing the infant's potential is the thrust of all NICU intervention. Therapists work as a part of a collaborative team to enhance the infant's outcome. Parents, as the constant in the baby's life, should be their first and foremost consideration. The birth of an infant with special needs or a premature birth creates profound stress on the family. Awaiting the birth of a baby is an emotionally charged time in the best of circumstances, but when problems occur, families experience emotional responses like fear, apprehension, shock, guilt, anger, depression, frustration, helplessness, and denial. Such emotions will affect the family's perception of how their newborn is being cared for and how they are able to participate in that care. Therapists working in the NICU and those working with NICU graduates must recognize these emotions and empower families to participate in providing care for their premature and ill infants. Parent education is fundamental in the NICU.[1]

Neonatal Interventions
Providing information about the infant's condition and management
Recognizing, monitoring, and appropriately responding to the infant's cues, particularly to stress indicators
Decreasing the infant's stress responses
Facilitating alertness and enhancing attentional stability
Optimizing the infant's interactive abilities through environmental modulation and appropriate timing of caregiving interventions, according to the infant's signals

Neonatal Interventions
Careful observation to assess baseline level of stress and readiness intervention
Gradual changes in lighting
Taking the infant gently into your arms
Recognizing and inhibiting stress indicators
Gentle but firm stroking or deep pressure
Gentle vertical vestibular stimulation while holding the infant in an upright position
Unswaddling an infant who is swaddled
Presenting stimuli from one sensory modality at a time
Quiet talking or singing/humming
Infant massage

Sensory/Environmental Modulation

Neonatal therapists must be able to accurately assess an infant's state or neurobehavioral readiness for intervention. Brazelton's state classification is the most commonly recognized indicator, with six defined states: deep sleep, light sleep, drowsy, quiet alert, active awake, and crying.[12] Current best practice in the NICU recognizes the quiet alert state as most appropriate for therapeutic intervention and incorporates the concept of *clustered care*. Most infants are fed at regular 3-hour intervals. Nursing procedures such as checking of vital signs, administration of medications, and diaper changing are "clustered" to also occur on this 3-hour schedule. Therapeutic interventions should ideally be timed with this same philosophy in mind. Therapy sessions should be scheduled immediately before or after a feeding to take advantage of periods of greater wakefulness and to minimize disrupting the infant's rest.

Helping an infant to achieve a quiet alert state is accomplished by a graded approach to modifying the infant's environment. Intervention strategies must be employed with a very gradual progression and with careful attention to physiologic responses and stress indicators, including gaze aversion, grimace, motor agitation, hand/arm salutes, hand/arm on face maneuver, finger/toe splays, changes in vital signs, vomiting, bowel movements, yawning, sneezing or hiccups, gape face, arching or extension, and crying.

Positioning

Premature and very ill neonates have a number of positioning problems that if not managed appropriately may lead to the development of postural abnormalities and a variety of developmental and movement problems. Common position-induced deformities include the following:[1]

- Neck and trunk hyperextension with shoulder retraction and elevation
- "W" posturing of the upper extremities (shoulder abduction with external rotation and elbow flexion)
- "Frog-leg" positioning of the lower extremities (hip abduction and external rotation with knee flexion)
- Out-toeing posturing (hip external rotation with ankle eversion and external tibial torsion)

The most common indicator for positioning intervention in the NICU is hypotonia. Hypotonia and hyperextension are common in premature infants, due in part to the lack of physiologic flexion and the immaturity of the nervous system. When the preterm infant is placed supine, he will typically assume a fully extended or hyperextended position as a result of his in ability to move or flex against gravity. Extension is further reinforced by the infant's tendency to fix against the supporting surface in efforts to move, to seek boundaries, or to avoid noxious stimuli.

When placed prone, these infants will typically be unable to maintain prone flexion due to low tone and lack of strength and balance between flexors and extensors. The aforementioned "W" and "frog-leg" postures are common in the preterm infant lacking physiologic flexion and antigravity movement/ strength to maintain prone flexion. These postures may also be observed in the very ill term neonate who has been sedated with paralytic drugs to control pain or reduce motor activity.

Care must also be taken to observe the infant's head shape. Head flattening, a common deformity, is the result of prolonged sidelying or supine positioning. The infant skull assumes the shape of the surface on which it is lying, so children positioned in sidelying positions for extended periods of time will have flattening of the sides of the skull. Children who are positioned supine for long periods of time will experience flattening on the posterior skull. This skull deformity may also be accompanied and/or exacerbated by torticollis or increased tone, both of which will assert asymmetric forces on the skull. A torticollis occurs when there is spasm or shortening of unilateral cervical muscles, rotating the head and neck to one side. Regular position changes or commercially available gel cushions can be used to prevent head flattening. Even the gravely ill infant will require position changes at regular intervals.

Caring for the very ill neonate or premature infant takes place in a high-technology environment alongside many invasive procedures. Physicians and nurses are the lead personnel in providing lifesaving care. Therapists can, however, make great contributions in enhancing outcomes for these infants. Positioning is one of the least intrusive neonatal interventions and can be implemented even with the medically unstable infant. Nurses in the NICU are now quite knowledgeable about appropriate positioning, but therapy staff can further assist them

in promoting normal postural development and preventing positioning-induced disorders.[13] When placed prone, infants are said to sleep more, expend less energy and oxygen, breathe slower, and remain calmer.[1] Infants will require support to maintain the prone position. The stable infant can be swaddled in flexion and placed prone. However, this limits access to the infant for caregiving and necessitates disruption when unswaddling. Boundaries can be formed around the infant using blanket rolls or commercially available bumpers. The same techniques can be employed if an infant must be positioned supine.

Motor agitation or disorganized movements are commonly seen in NICU infants. Limiting this type of movement is desirable and can also be accomplished with appropriate positioning and containment/boundaries.[13]

Motor Development Intervention

Motor development intervention or handling is based on the concepts of neurodevelopmental therapy. Like positioning, handling techniques are employed in an effort to prevent the development of abnormal postural or movement patterns and facilitate normal development. A sequence of normal development is followed. Efforts are directed toward handling or positioning the infant to decrease neck and trunk hyperextension, shoulder retraction, and total body extension while facilitating active work in all the flexor muscle groups. As with all interventions, handling should be conducted in a gentle, graded manner with careful attention to the infant's responses.

Feeding

Therapists working in the NICU are often consulted by nursing staff to assist in the progression of oral feeding. While feeding intervention is more often addressed by the occupational therapist or speech-language pathologist, in some settings physical therapists are also involved. Absent direct feeding intervention, all

NICU therapists do in fact address the underlying physical support required for efficient oral feeding.

Full-term infants begin feeding shortly after birth. They are fully equipped with the appropriate reflexes, muscle strength, and oral motor coordination to participate in feeding. They also have a biomechanical advantage. Physiologic flexion with shoulder elevation and protraction provide a stable base of support for the oral structure. Cheek stability and a large tongue give the term infant the oral posture to compress, suck, and extract milk from a nipple. In contrast, preterm and ill infants lack all of these fundamental components, as well as the physical strength and neurologic maturity to participate in oral feeding. Positioning, handling, and motor development strategies employed and taught by therapy staff most certainly contribute to the infant's readiness to participate in oral feeding. Even after discharge from the NICU, infants may continue to experience feeding difficulties, so all treating therapists should understand the role of posture and regulation of physiologic state in facilitating efficient feeding.

Splinting

Therapists are frequently consulted by NICU staff when an infant is believed to require splinting of the upper or lower extremities. Neonatal splinting should be considered in an effort to provide immobilization and support, to prevent contractures, or for maintaining or increasing range of motion. Therapists must also take into very careful consideration the very fragile skin of the newborn or premature infant. The role of the therapist is to fabricate the splint and educate the nursing staff and family about its use, wearing schedule, and precautions.

Preparing for Discharge

While parents may look forward to the day they can finally bring their infant home, discharge from the NICU can also be a frightening and anxious time. Parents face the reality of having sole responsibility for the care of their baby absent the security of medical professionals. The transition is further complicated when an infant goes home still in need of medical supports such as oxygen or monitors or even requires continued in-home nursing care. Therapists must ensure that parents feel comfortable with the carryover of therapeutic positioning and handling and the use of any equipment or splints that are recommended. The NICU team will likely also call upon the services of a discharge planner or medical social worker to assist families in moving on to the next level of care. Referrals and recommendations for additional therapies through a home care agency or early intervention program are vital in helping families adjust to caring for the NICU graduate.

Families typically return to the hospital NICU follow-up clinic at regular intervals, where therapists take an active role in assessing the infant's progress and functional level or limitations and providing recommendations for continued therapy or access to early intervention services. It is imperative that parents keep their child's appointments with the follow-up team. In some instances doulas provide continuity between the hospital and home. Likewise, some states have funded parents-as-teachers programs that send trained community workers or parenting peers into the homes of recently discharged infants. These individuals are trained to help parents acclimate their child to the home environment. They can also help parents organize appointments and offer age-appropriate child development suggestions.

CASE STUDY OF A CHILD IN THE NEONATAL INTENSIVE CARE UNIT

G.M. is a 33-week PCA infant girl referred for therapy services. G.M.'s primary NICU nurse reports G.M. is very floppy, has trouble moving her arms against gravity, and does not bring her hands together at midline. She tends to arch and is not able to lift her legs from the bed. She recently began to feed orally, but has frequent A's & B's during and after feeding. The infant's history is significant for premature birth at 27 weeks EGA following a pregnancy complicated by breech positioning, premature rupture of membranes (PROM), and preterm labor (PTL). Delivery was by emergency cesarean section due to fetal heart rate decelerations. Birth weight was 1315 grams. G.M. required resuscitation and intubation and was then transferred to a Level III NICU 1 hour from home. Apgars were 1 and 8 at 1 and 5 minutes, respectively. She was placed on mechanical ventilation and remained on the vent for 7 days, at which time she was transitioned to nasal CPAP. She is now on 1 liter of oxygen via nasal cannula.

Problems identified upon review of the chart include Grade III IVH, PDA treated with Indocin, anemia, and apnea. G.M.'s parents are often at her bedside, even though they must travel a great distance to be with her. She is their first child. The nurse reports they have frequent questions about her movements and facial expressions when they hold her. They are also concerned that she does not feed well and that her head is flat on the left side. They are very concerned about providing care for her after her discharge. The doctors have projected she will go home in 3 to 4 weeks. Answer the following questions based on this information.

Chapter Discussion Questions

1. What is G.M.'s newborn classification based on her gestational age and birth weight?
2. The concerns expressed by the primary nurse indicate a profile consistent with what neuromotor profile?
3. Review of the medical record indicates what complications during the pregnancy/delivery?
4. Further review revealed what other problems and risk factors that may impact outcomes?
5. After evaluating the infant, meeting the parents, and consulting with the primary nurse, the physical therapist provided information for all caregivers regarding positioning. The parents also had many questions regarding feeding, and her mother stated she is interested in breastfeeding. What could the PT suggest to assist the family further?

REFERENCES

1. Greneir IR, Bigsby R, Vergara ER, and others: Comparison of motor self-regulatory and stress behaviors of preterm infants across body positions, *Am J Occup Ther* 57(3):289, 2003.
2. Cloherty JP, Eichenwald EC, Star AR, editors: *Manual of neonatal care*, Philadelphia, 2004, Lippincott Williams & Wilkins.
3. Als H: Towards a synactive theory of development: promise for the assessment of infant individuality, *Infant Ment Health J* 3:229, 1982.
4. Als H: A synactive model of neonatal behavioral organization: framework for the assessment of neurobehavioral development in the premature infant and for the support of infants and parents in the neonatal intensive care environment, *Phys Occup Ther Pediatr* 6(3/4):3, 1986.
5. Als H, Gilkerson L: The role of relationship-based developmentally supportive newborn intensive care in strengthening outcome of preterm infants, *Semin Perinatol* 21:178, 1997.
6. Hautch JC, Merenstein GB, editors: *Guidelines for perinatal care*, ed 4, Grove Village, Ill, 1997, American Academy of Pediatrics.
7. Vergera E: *Foundations for practice in the neonatal intensive care unit and early intervention*, vol 1, Rockville, Md, 1993, American Occupational Therapy Association.
8. Dubowitz L, Dubowitz V: The neurological assessment of the preterm and full-term infant. In *Clinics in developmental medicine*, No. 79, London, 1981, Heinemann.
9. Morgan AM, Koch V, Lee V, and others: Neonatal neurobehavioral examination. A new instrument for quantitative analysis of neonatal neurological status, *Phys Ther* 68(9):1352, 1988.

10. Korner AF, Thom VA: *Neurobehavioral assessment of the preterm infant*, New York, 1990, The Psychological Corporation.
11. Als H, Lawhon G, Duffy FH, and others: Individualized developmental care for the very low birthweight infant: medical and neurofunctional effects, *J Am Med Assoc* 272:853, 1994.
12. Brazelton TB: *Neonatal behavioral assessment scale*, ed 2, Philadelphia, 1984, Lippincott.
13. Sweeney JK, Gutierrez T: Musculoskeletal implications of preterm infant positioning in the neonatal intensive care unit, *J Perinat Neonatal Nurs* 16(1):58, 2002.

RESOURCES

When Your Baby's in the Neonatal Intensive Care Unit

www.kidshealth.org/parent/system/ill/nicu_caring.html

A Mothers Diary: How to Survive the Neonatal Intensive Care Unit, by Menetra Hathron

Seating and Wheeled Mobility

Roberta Kuchler O'Shea, PT, PhD

key terms

Assistive technology device   **Contoured system**   **Planar system**
Assistive technology service   **Custom-molded system**   **Wheeled mobility**

outline

learning objectives

At the end of the chapter the reader will be able to do the following:

1. Identify the three categories of seating components.

2. Identify the similarities and differences between manual and power mobility.

3. Advocate for appropriate seating and mobility equipment for a child.

4. Recognize laws that impact assistive technology.

Assistive technology (AT) is an integral part of modern living and varies from low-level non-mechanical picture books to complicated robotic machinery that allows an individual with a severe disability to live independently. Availability of AT services and equipment spans the rehabilitation spectrum. In this chapter, seating and mobility will be the focus. (This text will not address the widespread availability of AT for computers, communication, home, and worksite modifications. Please refer to other resources for these topics.) Prior to delving into descriptions of the equipment, it behooves one to understand the historical and legal developments of the AT field.

Attempts at integrating therapy goals in home and classroom settings often included homemade adaptive equipment for positioning, mobility, and communication. An **assistive technology device** is defined by legislation to include any item, piece of equipment, or product system that increases, maintains, or improves an individual's functional status.[1] In contrast an **assistive technology service** is legally defined as any service, such as physical therapy, occupational therapy, or speech therapy, that directly assists someone with a disability in the selection, acquisition, or training of AT.[1] Over the recent years, AT has come to encompass a vast range of materials, designs, and applications. It is used to promote the development and acquisition of skills that a client lacks as a result of disease or injury. It can also provide compromises or adaptations in motor function when the attainment of certain skills is unrealistic or impossible.[2] Also referred to as *enabling technology*, AT can often generate new opportunities and open new doors for individuals with physical impairments or overall developmental delays.

Seating and **wheeled mobility** are just a small segment of the AT available to individuals with disabilities. Activity limitations, such as the inability to sit unsupported, the inability to walk or move from one place to another, the inability to effectively use the hands because of a weak, unstable trunk, or the inability to produce speech are often primary reasons for prescribing ATs and AT services. Assistive technology that is correctly prescribed and used, especially in therapeutic positioning (adaptive seating), may help prevent secondary impairments such as skin breakdown, cardiopulmonary compromise due to scoliosis or slouched posture, and contractures or deformities due to inadequately supported body segments. Other potential benefits at this level are the reduction of tone or excessive muscle activity and a decrease in pathologic movements.

HISTORICAL OVERVIEW

In the past three decades, an explosion in the number and type of assistive devices has occurred. In 1972 the creation of several federally funded rehabilitation engineering centers focused efforts on research and development of new products, as well as on the delivery of services to the consumer.[3] This process brought together professionals from many fields: biomedical and rehabilitation engineering, physical therapy, occupational therapy, speech and language pathology, and special education. The Rehabilitation Engineering and Assistive Technology Society of North America (RESNA), an outgrowth of this shared interest, is an interdisciplinary association of professionals who bring applied technology to persons with disabilities. Assistive seating technology in particular has been evolving rapidly in many different regions of North America, creating a confusion of locally adopted language and terminology, so RESNA has published a list of standardized seating terminology that is helpful in improving communication among research and service centers, clients, and funding sources.[4]

Since 1975 many laws have been passed to ensure that the rights of people with disabilities are included in all education and work environments. These laws include PL 101-476: Education of All Handicapped Children Act; 1986-2004 Amendments to the individuals with Disabilities Educational Act (IDEA);

PL 105-394: Technology-Related Assistance for Individuals with Disabilities Act of 1988 (TRAIDA [Tech Act]); PL 93-112: Rehabilitation Act; and PL 101-336: Americans with Disabilities Act (ADA). These laws have helped focus attention on, and create a growing market for, new technologies and products. Consumer demands for increased durability and performance have prompted manufacturers to apply technologies created by the aerospace, medical, and information industries to their own products. The field of AT represents a well-established cross-disciplinary specialty.

The 1988 federal legislation known as *TRAIDA*, or the Tech Act, defined ATs and services and recognized the importance of technology in the lives of individuals with disabilities.[2,5] The Assistive Technology Act of 1998 has extended funding to develop permanent comprehensive technology-related programs. All states and territories are eligible for 10 years, and states that have completed the 10 years are eligible for an additional 3 years of federal funding. IDEA funds programs that promote research and technology while the 1998 Amendment states that assistive technology devices and services be considered on all individualized educational plans (IEPs). In 2000, Quality Indicators for Assistive Technology Services became available to provide practitioners with a description of the essential elements of assessing, ordering, and implementing AT services under the auspices of IDEA.[6] It is the intent of these Indicators to assist therapists in providing appropriate and quality ATDs and services to children, especially young children. The Rehabilitation Act and the ADA protect individuals with disabilities against civil rights violations.

ASSISTIVE TECHNOLOGY TEAM

Interestingly, team relationships entwine and define pediatric service provision. It is rare that an individual works in isolation with a child without input from the family, other professionals, or the child himself. Assistive technology implementation defines the importance and essence of team collaboration.

As in any rehab team, the client/family must play an active role in the selection and procurement of the equipment. The makeup of the team and the setting in which it functions can vary greatly. For example, in many hospitals and rehabilitation centers with comprehensive technology service delivery programs, physicians (especially physiatrists and orthopedic surgeons) may be an integral part of the core team. In schools and residential centers, one or more of the client's primary therapists, along with an equipment supplier, may function as the core team.

A successful team recognizes that each of its members, even a minor player, contributes important information and perspective; communication must be multidirectional. The core team takes the responsibility of imparting information and training to the patient and caregivers to ensure proper use, maintenance, responsibility, and safety of the prescribed devices.

ASSISTIVE TECHNOLOGY FOR MOBILITY

A large portion of this chapter is dedicated to seating and mobility, as it is the most complex system of AT for the physical therapist and physical therapist assistant. However, there are several pieces of adaptive mobility equipment that bear discussion.

In order to gain independent mobility, a child may require an ambulation aid. These include canes, axillary crutches, Lofstrand crutches, forward walkers, and reverse walkers. Canes provide minimal balance support to a child. They offer effective assistance if the child has good static and dynamic balance. Canes give the child a stability boost. Some children prefer to use bilateral canes to gain stability. Many children prefer Lofstrand crutches over axillary crutches, because they can use their hands for a task and allow the crutch to be suspended from the forearm, thus preventing the crutch from falling to the ground. There is some debate about the use of a forward walker versus a reverse walker. The forward walker may get away from the child as it rolls if the child is slow to pick up his or her feet. The reverse walker may pitch the child posteriorly and does not allow the child to ambulate in a typical alignment with the weight forward. Both seem to be successful in assisting children with ambulation and should be regarded equally.

SEATING SYSTEMS

The purpose of the seating system is to provide external postural sitting support for the child who has functional limitations due to impairments in musculoskeletal alignment, postural control, muscle tone, or strength. Seating is the interface between the child and the mobility device.[7] The goal is to enable the child to compensate for functional limitations and thereby maximize participation levels (Box 18-1). Letts stated that to achieve stable sitting, biomechanical forces and moments in all planes must be balanced.[8] "Good positioning" usually consists of an upright midline orientation of the entire body with a near-vertical alignment of the trunk and head. In children the "90-90-90" rule often is used to maintain the hips, knees, and ankles at 90 degrees. As the child grows, it may not be reasonable (due to leg length) to maintain the knees at 90 degrees. In this case the decision to go with a different angled front rigging must be made. Additionally, if the child has significant contractures of the lower extremities or trunk, it may not be possible to position them in 90 degrees of hip, knee, and ankle flexion. Kangas has seriously challenged the idea of static positioning, stating that it is unnatural and impedes function.[9] In the next section, studies that have examined the effectiveness of seating systems are reviewed, and considerations in prescribing seating systems are discussed.

MEASURING THE CLIENT

It is imperative to record accurate body segment measurements when fitting a child for a seating system and mobility device. Final cushion measurements should account for 2 or 3 years of potential growth. Figure 18-1 offers a template to assess body measurements. The measurements should be taken with the child seated.

MATCHING THE INTERVENTION TO THE CLIENT'S LEVEL OF NEED

Postural support systems typically are classified in three levels: planar or linear, contoured, and custom molded. The first and least intensive level of intervention is the **planar system**; it consists of a flat seat and back (Figure 18-2). Children with good postural stability, sitting balance, and a minimum of deformities are the most appropriate candidates for this level of intervention. The seat and back are constructed of a solid base (plywood or plastic) covered by foam and upholstered with vinyl or knit fabric. Linear trunk or pelvic supports may be added laterally. Many commercial variations are available, or they can be constructed in the clinic. This system is easily changed and adapted and typically the least expensive for the client.

Box **18-1**	Potential Outcomes of Proper Seating and Positioning

Facilitation of optimal postural control to enable engagement in functional activities
Provision of an optimal balance between stability and mobility in the seated position
Maintenance of neutral skeletal alignment
Prevention of skeletal deformities
Maintenance of tissue integrity
Maintenance of a position of comfort
Decreased fatigue
Enhanced respiratory and circulatory function
Facilitation of caregiver activities

From Cook A, Polgar J: *Cook and Hussey's assistive technologies: principles and practice*, ed 3, St Louis, 2008, Mosby.

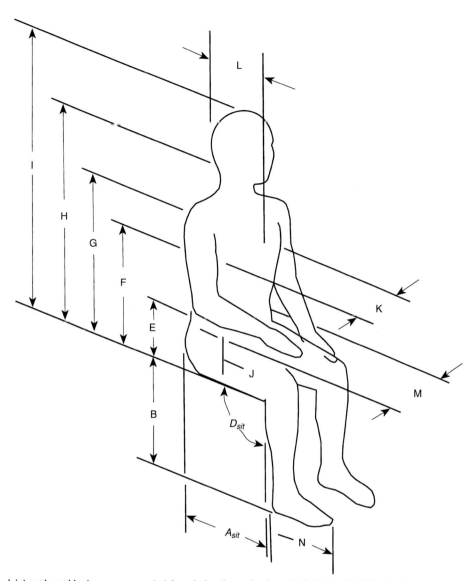

Fig. 18-1 Joint angle and body measurements taken during the evaluation. A_{sit} (R & L), behind hips/popliteal fossa; B (R & L), popliteal fossa/heel; D_{sit}, knee flexion angle; E, sitting surface/pelvic crest; F, sitting surface/axilla; G, sitting surface/shoulder; H, sitting surface/occiput; I, sitting surface/crown of head; J, sitting surface/hanging elbow; K, width across trunk; L, depth of trunk; M, width across hips; N, heel/toe. (From Bergen AF, Presperin J, Tallman T: *Positioning for function: wheelchairs and other assistive technologies*, Valhalla, NY, 1990, Valhalla Rehabilitation.)

The second level of intervention is the **contoured system**, which provides external postural control by increasing the points of contact, especially laterally. The seat and back surfaces are rounded by shaping layers of firm foam, air, or gel to correspond to the curves of the body (Figure 18-3). Contours also help distribute pressures more evenly. Contouring can range from simple to aggressive. Simple contouring can improve comfort and stability

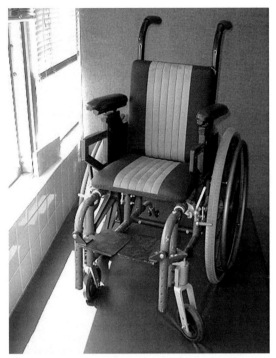

Fig. 18-2 Planar/linear seating system. (From Campbell SK, Vander Linden DW, Palisano RJ: *Physical therapy for children*, ed 3, Philadelphia, 2006, Saunders.)

for many clients, and aggressive contouring may provide enough support for some clients with severe impairments. Table 18-1 lists the varieties of seating that can be fabricated in the clinic from solid bases with varying densities and configurations of foam, air, or gel materials to create the contours. This level of system can accommodate for growth with modifications or adjustments to the positioning materials.

The third level of intervention is the **custom-molded system**. It provides an intimate fit by closely conforming to the shape of the client's body, thereby giving the most postural support. When carefully molded, it theoretically provides the greatest amount of pressure relief as well. The time and expense involved in the fabrication of these systems is considerable, and the molding process requires a great deal of skill. Production of the mold usually involves either a vacuum consolidation method or a chemical reaction of liquid foams injected into a special bag. Several varieties of custom-molded systems are available, including those that can be completed on site and those that

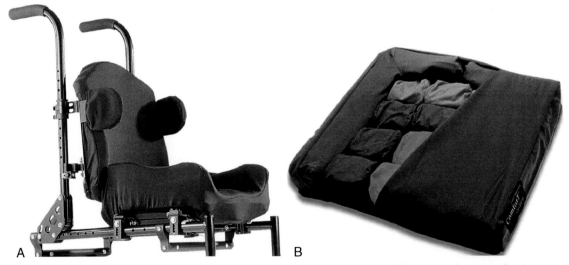

A   B

Fig. 18-3 Generic contour seating systems. **A,** Jay-fit adjustable contour system. **B,** ComforT cushion. (**A** courtesy Sunrise Medical; **B** courtesy Otto Bock Health Care.)

TABLE **18-1** Various Types of Seating Fabrication Materials

CUSHION TYPE	ADVANTAGES	DISADVANTAGES
Foam	Inexpensive	Affected by light and air, which cause
	Lightweight	degradation of the foam
	Nothing leaks	Loses shape
Gel/viscous fluid	Good pressure relief	Heavy
	Easier than air to maintain	Chance of leakage
		May bottom out
Air without foam	Lightweight	Less stable
	Waterproof	Chance of puncture/damage
	Good pressure distribution over entire seated surface	High maintenance
	Adjustable via valves to relieve sores or provide postural support	
Thermoplastic elastomer/ Urethane honeycomb	Lightweight	Can produce unwanted shear force if used without a cover
	Good support	
	No risk of leakage	
	Machine washable/dryable	
Custom-molded cushions	Designed to meet individual pressure and positioning needs	Expensive
		No ability to modify once fabricated

are sent to a central fabrication center. Computer-aided design technology allows the clinician to bypass the construction of molds by mapping and digitizing body shape data directly using an instrumented simulator. The information is then transferred via computer disk, fax, or modem to a computer-driven carving machine that produces the cushion. Custom-molded systems do not allow for growth and cannot be modified. Additionally, if a child is not positioned properly within the molded cushion, high-pressure spots can develop and result in trauma to the underlying soft tissues.

PRESCRIPTION AND APPLICATION OF SEATING SYSTEMS

The scope of this chapter and the rapidly evolving nature of technology preclude a thorough discussion of all options and features of postural support systems. Many excellent resources that describe these in more detail and provide problem-solving lists and charts exist.[7,8,10-13] In this section attention is focused on some of the most salient points in the decision-making process (Figure 18-4).

SEAT CUSHIONS

In most cases the seat cushion is the most critical element of the seating system. The use of true planar seats is becoming more rare, because most clinicians have found that a small amount of lateral contouring for even the highest-level sitter adds comfort and stability.[10,14] The benefit of adding contours to help relieve pressure problems is evidenced by the number of commercially available air and gel pressure cushions that have foam blocks and wedges to allow customization of cushion shape. On the other hand, strategically placing commercial gel pads in a custom-made, contoured foam cushion can also supply that extra critical amount of pressure relief needed by some clients. Antithrust seats have a block of high-density foam placed just anterior to the ischial tuberosities; the foam block keeps the pelvis from sliding forward

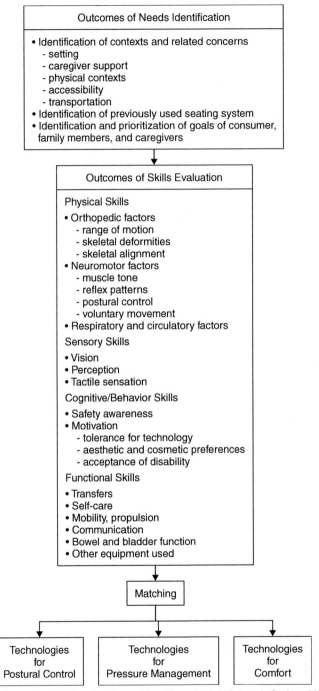

Fig. 18-4 Framework for seating and positioning decision making. (From Cook A, Polgar J: *Cook and Hussey's assistive technologies: principles and practice*, ed 3, St Louis, 2008, Mosby.)

and equalizes pressure distribution along the thighs.[15] Antithrust seats can be added to planar as well as contoured systems, but they are thought to work best with deep lateral contours of the pelvis and lateral thigh supports (adductor pads).

Seat placement within the wheelchair frame is an important consideration. A thick cushion or inappropriate mounting hardware can place the seat too high, causing loss of independent transfers or wheeling. Poor seat placement can also change the center of gravity to an unsafe position. Forward or backward placement, especially in very small children, can affect the knee angle required for foot placement on the footrests and can change the ease of wheeling by affecting access to the wheel rims or loading or unloading the front casters. For individuals who propel with their lower extremities, it is important to maintain a lower seat-to-floor height and a flat front edge of the seat cushion. Often these individuals find it helpful to relieve the front edge of the seat to allow full knee flexion without irritating the hamstrings.

BACK CUSHIONS

A back support with a gently curved surface can improve lateral trunk stability, posture, and comfort. Simple contouring and lateral support can often be achieved by shaping the back cushion. Many back cushions are available with accompanying customized support options. More aggressive contouring can be achieved using high-density foam blocks/wedges. A custom-molded back should be used for clients with severely fixed spinal deformities. Some children who need specific contact and support along the paraspinals but are still growing can benefit from a hybrid back cushion. This type of back cushion is custom-molded and only contours along the paraspinal region and flattens laterally. Linear lateral trunk supports are then added to the contoured back. This allows for growth and maintains significant proprioceptive input along the spine.

Sagittal plane alignment of the spine has traditionally been adjusted using lumbar rolls; however, control of sagittal curves begins with the pelvis and sacrum rather than the lumbar spine.[16,17] A "biangular back" has a vertical section behind the pelvis, with the section above the pelvis angled back a few degrees to encourage lumbar extension or sacral disks or pads that can be added to the back surface. The client must have sufficient range of motion and flexibility for these items to work. Over the long term, this back cushion may cause increased lordosis in the child, so it is imperative to monitor spinal alignment.

PELVIC STABILIZATION

The most effective technique for pelvic stabilization control continues to remain largely a matter of clinical opinion and user preference.[18] A seat belt placed at a 45-degree angle at the seat-back junction is the most typical form of pelvic stabilization. For high-functioning individuals, placement of the belt across the anterior thighs, just in front of the hips, allows more natural active trunk and pelvic mobility.[10] The pelvic positioning belt can use a 2-point or 4-point attachment system. The 4-point system allows for more comprehensive control of the pelvis and greater distribution of the pressures maintaining postural control.

The subASIS bar is a form of rigid pelvic stabilization consisting of a padded bar attached to plates lateral to the pelvis.[17] The pelvis must be maintained in a vertical orientation or the client will slide under the bar. A less rigid variation is the semirigid pelvic stabilizer (SRPS),[19] which is constructed of high-density foam mounted on a reinforcing strip of thermoplastic splinting material. It incorporates wedges that fit under the anterior superior iliac spine while providing relief across the lower abdomen. Like the subASIS bar, the SRPS provides direct control of the pelvis for stabilization, yet the angle of placement can be varied, as with a seat belt, making it an option for clients with a mild fixed posterior pelvic tilt.

The flexibility of the SRPS may result in fewer pressure problems than the subASIS bar, and it works especially well for clients who demonstrate a strong asymmetric thrusting pattern.

Dynamic pelvic stabilization uses individually contoured pads that fit around the pelvis, with a pivot mechanism allowing anterior-posterior tilting of the pelvis without loss of stability.[20] Adjustments allow deformity accommodation, control of the amount and direction of tilting, and a dynamic force to return the pelvis to a neutral position. Anterior knee blocks, another form of pelvic stabilization, direct a long axis force up the length of the femurs to counter sliding of the pelvis.[10,19]

ANGLES

There is no consensus about the effects of seat and spatial angles on alignment and function. Factors that must be considered in determining fixed angles include severity and nature of postural tone abnormalities, contractures and deformities, level of motor control for sitting, and design and purpose of the mobility base. Although the concept of upright 90-90-90 sitting is theoretically sound, it may not be a biomechanically possible option for many clients. Slight anterior wedging of the seat may improve head alignment or keep very young children from sliding. Opening the hip angle (tipping the front seat edge) may be necessary when hip extension contractures are present. Allowing the knees to flex brings the feet back under the seat and reduces the rotary force on the pelvis, thus minimizing the effect of tight hamstrings.

The anteriorly tipped seat has potential benefits for clients with hypoextensible lower extremity musculature, but fair to good upper body control, who "sacral sit" on a flat surface. It is also used for the more severely involved child in a forward-lean position with a solid anterior chest support. Good pelvic stabilization must be achieved to prevent sliding. Unfortunately, when anteriorly tipped seating is used in wheelchairs, the client often lacks enough knee extension to keep the heels from interfering with caster movement.

Variable seat-to-back angles allow adjustments of tilt and recline throughout the day. Tilt is useful for relief of pressure or relief of trunk or neck fatigue, and it provides a combination of active sitting and rest positions. When in a tilt system, the seat-to-back angle does not change. Recline is useful for relief of fatigue, for hip or back pain, and for catheterizations or other hygiene procedures that must be performed in the chair. In a reclining seating system, the seat-to-back angle changes as the reclining position changes.

Some clinics have engineered dynamic or compliant seating systems for clients with severe and abrupt extensor spasms.[21,22] Often the severity of tone or spasm is exacerbated by the rigidity of a conventional system. These devices use hinges, pivot points, and springs to allow movement of the seat or back with the child and provide a gentle returning force. Clients who use these systems exhibit a decrease in the severity of spasms or fluctuating tone over a period of weeks, as well as improved comfort and ease of transfers.

UPHOLSTERY

Upholstery for seat and back cushions can be made out of a variety of materials. When choosing a covering, consideration must be given to whether the child is incontinent, whether the child is typically hot, and who will care for the coverings. Vinyl is a durable cushion covering; however, it can be hot and slippery and typically cannot be removed from the seating system. Synthetic knit fabrics with waterproof backing are also a popular choice of covering. They are less slippery, thus decreasing shear, and they can be removed for easy cleaning. Ideally a child should have at least two sets of cushion covers so that one can be laundered while the other is in use.

FRONT RIGGINGS

Front riggings, or leg supports, which are considered a component of the mobility base, are discussed here because of their direct influence on the entire seating system. Elevated legrests are set farther forward of the seat than fixed legrests and can contribute to forward sliding on the seat or poor positioning of the feet for weightbearing. They should never be ordered unless they are specifically required.

Choice of footrests on small pediatric chairs can be especially difficult, because they may interfere with caster action. Footplates that extend backward under the seat are helpful when clients have tight hamstrings. Footplates can be positioned parallel to the floor or angled to match a client's foot/ankle deformity. Shoe holders and foot straps hold the feet in the desired location to assist with lower body stability and weightbearing. For clients with deformities or limited joint movement, forcing the foot into neutral alignment on the footrest may impose undesirable stresses at the knees or hips.[10] Other clients who exhibit natural postural adjustments and placement of the feet during weight shifting and active movement should have their feet left free. If the child is learning to transfer independently, can already transfer independently, or is using a sit-to-stand transfer, the front riggings and footplates should be able to swing out of the way. An exception to this rule must be made for the client who uses tapered front riggings and fixed footplates for performance. These users will transfer out of their mobility base with the front riggings in a forward position.

LATERAL AND MEDIAL SUPPORTS

Lateral trunk supports (or scoliosis pads) range from simple, flat, padded blocks to contoured, wraparound supports. Swivel or swing-away mounting hardware allows the wraparound supports to fit properly and enables the child to transfer into and out of the seating system easily.

Contoured seats usually provide the most effective lateral thigh and pelvic support, as well as good pressure relief. Square or rectangular pads such as lateral thigh supports can maintain position of the lower extremities and allow for growth. Medial thigh supports (abductor wedges or pommels) maintain hip

alignment in neutral or slight abduction and should not function to stretch tight adductors or prevent forward sliding of the pelvis. Removable or swing-away pommels facilitate transfers and urinal or catheter use.

ANTERIOR SUPPORTS

Anterior trunk supports maintain the spine erect and upright over the pelvis. Butterfly-shaped straps should not be used, because they present extreme safety hazards. Instead, anterior support can be gained via an H or Y harness or anterior chest strap. Rigid shoulder retractors that project over the top of the backrest provide significant anterior shoulder control but may be poorly tolerated. Padded axillary straps, sometimes known as *Bobath straps* or *backpack design straps,* also help maintain the trunk in an upright posture. They attach to the underside of the lateral thoracic support, are directed superiorly and medially over the front of the axilla, and attach at the top of the backrest, controlling shoulder protraction without crossing the chest. Trefler and Angelo reported no significant clinical differences in performance for children with cerebral palsy after completing a switch activation task while using different anterior chest supports.[23] They concluded that style of anterior chest support should be based on client preference.

HEADREST

Facilitating good head position can be one of the most difficult tasks. In the almost totally immobile client, the head is the one body part that is likely to move, and poor head positioning can make an otherwise effective postural support system fail. On the other hand, barium-swallow studies suggest that some clients with the most severe physical and mental impairments may need to adopt a forward-hanging head position to cope with increased oral secretions or reflux.[24] Correcting these clients' heads to a position that "looks good" may increase their risk of aspiration or choking.[24]

Support under the occiput provides better head support than a flat contact on the back of the head. Neck rings, two-step head supports, and contoured head supports are available in several options. Halos encircle the forehead and should always be used with caution, particularly during vehicular transport, because of the potential for neck injury. Static and dynamic forehead straps position and maintain the head securely on the headrest. Collars with soft anterior chin support (which are not attached to the wheelchair) may be effective for clients who have constant neck flexion, regardless of seating angles. Care must be taken that the head support does not unduly block the child's peripheral visual fields. Additionally, head supports can be the ideal mounting location for switches that control the AT or augmentative communication systems.

UPPER EXTREMITY SUPPORTS

Cutout trays are the most typical form of upper extremity support and can be designed for a multitude of special purposes. Posterior elbow blocks help reduce the tendency to retract the arms and maintain the upper extremities in a forward position. Clients with severe dystonia often prefer wrist or arm cuffs to reduce unwanted movement of one or both arms.

WHEELED MOBILITY

The purpose of the mobility base is dependent on the child's level of function. For some the primary purpose will be independent mobility, and the therapist must determine how best to achieve this. For others the purpose of the base is to provide a means of being transported by a companion, and this must be accomplished in a comfortable and efficient manner. In either case the base serves the additional role of supporting the seating system. Selection of a mobility base requires consideration of the seating system it will support, the environments in which it will function, and the client's lifestyle (Box 18-2). Assessment for a new mobility base should ideally be done at

Box **18-2**	Factors to Consider when Selecting a Wheelchair

Consumer profile: Disability, date of onset, prognosis, size, and weight
Consumer needs: Activities, contexts of use (e.g., accessibility, indoor/outdoor), preferences, transportation, reliability, durability, cost
Physical and sensory skills: Range of motion, motor control, strength, vision, perception
Functional skills: Transfers and ability to propel (manual or powered)

From Cook A, Polgar J: *Cook and Hussey's assistive technologies: principles and practice*, ed 3, St Louis, 2008, Mosby.

the same time as assessment and simulation for the postural support system, because much of the same information regarding the client and the environment must be gathered.

Many factors affect performance and mobility in users of manual wheelchairs, including human physiologic capacities such as strength and endurance, which are dependent on the user's diagnosis, age, sex, lifestyle, and build.[25] The position of the individual within the wheelchair, particularly in relation to the handrims or other propulsion method, determines the mechanical advantage of the user to act on the chair. Wheelchair factors that affect mobility are rolling resistance, control, maneuverability, stability, and dynamic behavior. These depend on the quality and construction of the wheelchair and factors such as weight, rigidity of the frame, wheel alignment, mass distribution, and suspension. Wheelchair propulsion in children with spinal cord injury is similar to that in a neurologically matched group of adults.[26] The adults wheeled faster, but the children spent a similar proportion of the wheeling cycle in propulsion, and the angular changes in the kinematics of the elbow and shoulder over time were the same for both groups. Therefore applications intended to improve wheeling efficiency in adults may be appropriate for children as well.

The developmental consequences of impaired movement are another area of functional limitation and disability. The typical developing infant's experience with independent forward progression has a profound impact on perceptual, cognitive, emotional, and social processes.[27] For the immobile child, early provision of artificial forms of locomotion has the potential to minimize deficits in spatial, cognitive, affective, and social functions. Prone scooters, caster carts, and walkers are alternatives for some young children with functional upper extremities. For the child with more severe involvement, however, early power mobility offers the best choice and allows the child to increase his or her self-initiated movements during play.[28]

Historically, prescription of power wheelchairs was put off until children reached their teens, after all attempts at effective ambulation were exhausted. Power wheelchairs were considered too expensive and too difficult for young children to learn to drive, and walking was too important a goal to give up. Studies indicate that children as young as 24 months can successfully learn independent power mobility within a few weeks.[29,30] Benefits attributed to the use of power mobility include increases in self-initiated behaviors, including change in location, rate of interaction with objects, and frequency of communication.[29,31] Others concluded that social participation of wheelchair users is a complex phenomenon. However, the benefits frequently reported are increased peer interaction, increased interest in other forms of locomotion, including walking, increased family integration such as inclusion in outings, and decreased perception of helplessness by family members.[32-35] Field concluded that the major issues affecting powered mobility performance are ability, technology features, environment, driving as an activity, and the interactions between these variables.[36]

Training is always an important facet of ordering power mobility devices for children. Hasdai, Jessel, and Weiss used simulator programs to provide training to children ages 7 to 22.[37] They determined that inexperienced drivers improved their overall driving performance after simulator training. The Internet is becoming a training site as well. The Oregon Research Institute has a public domain training program that is networked. A child can log on to the site, choose their virtual reality device and environment, and race with other children on the network. The program records performance measures related to the child's driving ability. The virtual environment responds to the child's improving skills, and the child is required to take interval skills assessment quizzes in order to continue using the program. The therapist and/or caregiver receive feedback about the child's performance.

SELECTION OF A MOBILITY BASE

The goal in selecting a mobility base is to provide an appropriate means of efficiently getting from one location to another. It is inappropriate to require someone to rely on his or her everyday mobility for exercise. Prohibiting a child with marginal ambulation to use a manual wheelchair or prohibiting a child with marginal manual wheelchair skills to use a power wheelchair places both at risk for poor functional and academic performance due to excessive energy expenditure. A creative and structured fitness program is a more appropriate way of addressing strength and cardiovascular endurance goals.

It is generally agreed that positioning needs take precedence over the issuance of a mobility device. At the same time, the design of the seating system should maximize potential for independent function in the wheelchair whenever possible. This in turn influences chair modifications and the interface hardware needed. For example, if a 3-inch modular composite foam cushion is necessary for pressure relief, but the client has short extremities (as in myelodysplasia), both independent transfers and wheeling will be more difficult. A possible solution is to order a chair frame with a lower seat height and without upholstery so that drop brackets can be used to lower the cushion between the seat rails.

To assess driving skills and controller placement once the desired seating position has been obtained, some seating simulators can be mounted on a power base. A remote, attendant-held control can override the user's control, ensuring safety and appropriate feedback during assessment and training. The client should be offered test drives in a variety of bases, using appropriately simulated postural support wherever possible.

The first step in selecting a mobility base is to determine what type of functional mobility is desired. Three general types of mobility bases are (1) companion chairs for dependent wheeling, (2) standard manual wheelchairs, and (3) power wheelchairs. Ideally the selection should be based on the potential level of independent mobility, but other factors often come into play, including methods of transportation, type of housing, availability of training or supervision, and availability of funding.

The second step is choosing the style of the base. Within each type, there are several styles with different features and performance characteristics. Factors that influence this choice are the level and type of seating system required, the level of independence in other skills such as transfers and activities of daily living, the specific environments in which the chair will be used, the method of transportation, and the needs of caregivers.

Selection of size may influence both the style and type chosen and is based on client size, expected growth rate, growth capabilities of the chair itself, and the size and style of the seating system. Mobility bases designed specifically for pediatric clients are available in a variety of sizes and designs. Growth capabilities have been greatly improved as funding sources have demanded longer life from purchased items.

The final step is choosing the model and manufacturer of the chair. Often the finer details of construction are important at this stage, for example, the proportions of the chair; angles; orientations; adjustability of parts such as footrests and armrests; and swing-away, detachment, or folding mechanisms. Other important influencing factors are performance characteristics, styling, comfort, rate of breakdown, availability of parts, service record, and cost. Regional preferences for various models and manufacturers are evident across North America.

DEPENDENT PROPULSION WHEELCHAIRS

Dependent propulsion wheelchairs, transporter chairs, and dependent mobility bases are intended for individuals who will not need to access the wheels for independent mobility, including those with the most severe impairments and very young children (Figure 18-5). In other cases this type of chair may be used as backup transportation for a child who ambulates or

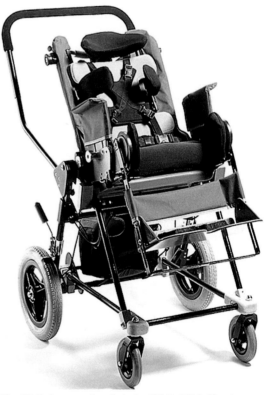

Fig. 18-5 A companion chair, the Kid Kart TLC. (Courtesy Sunrise Medical.)

uses a power wheelchair. Many styles of companion wheelchairs exist, and occasionally manual wheelchairs are used as companion chairs. Companion chairs often include firm seats and backs and have a wide variety of positioning components as options. Alternatively, contoured or custom-molded seating systems can be fabricated and mounted on these frames. Some of these chairs can be used as vehicular transport seats and comply with federal safety standards. Others are designed for very young children and look and perform like a stroller.

When choosing a dependent mobility base, the primary caregiver must be considered a user as well. Attention should be given to his or her comfort and ease of use, including push handle height, rolling resistance, maneuverability, and ease of disassembly and transport. Parents of young children who are receiving their first mobility base and seating system may be very sensitive to the need for a wheelchair. Mobility bases that look like a stroller are popular and are often much less threatening. Some funding sources deny stroller bases because of their limitations in growth and adaptability if the child's independent capabilities progress.

Manual tilt and recline features are incorporated into many companion chairs. A fixed angle of tilt or recline can be useful when designing the seating system for some clients. For others the ability to vary the amount of tilt or recline throughout the day is critical for prevention of pressure sores, fatigue, and discomfort.

MANUAL WHEELCHAIRS

The standard manual wheelchair has two large wheels, usually in back, for independent propulsion, and two small swiveling casters in front (Figure 18-6). Manual wheelchairs are often chosen as dependent mobility bases as well because of their ability to accept custom-designed seating systems, their ease of use, and their tilt and recline options. For independent propellers the 1980s were the "new age" of manual wheelchairs, when lightweight chairs

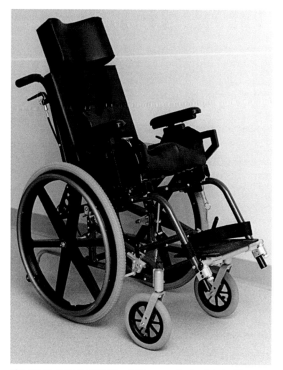

Fig. 18-6 Standard lightweight manual wheelchair. (From Campbell SK, Vander Linden DW, Palisano RJ: *Physical therapy for children*, ed 3, Philadelphia, 2006, Saunders.)

and chairs designed for recreational use and athletic competition became widely available. Lightweight and durable metals and fabrics, alternative wheel placement, improved frame proportions and designs, adjustability, and adaptability to custom seating have all helped streamline the manual wheelchair to improve its efficiency and control, ease of transfers, portability, and appearance. Lightweight chairs with the large wheels in front are much easier for young children to propel for short distances indoors. For the very active person, ultra-lightweight, high-performance chairs incorporate rigid frames and high-quality bearings for optimal performance. The serious athlete can find specialized designs dedicated to specific performance needs; these chairs barely resemble the traditional concept of a wheelchair.

One-arm-drive wheelchairs are designed for individuals with significant asymmetry of upper extremity strength and function that prevents bimanual propulsion. The classic style is the double-handrim on one side, with a linkage system to the other wheel. Styles that use a pumping action with a lever and ratchet system, although rarely used now, are generally easier and more efficient for both wheeling and steering, but they create more problems in dependent wheeling by caregivers. Operation of a one-arm-drive chair may exacerbate existing asymmetry in clients with tonal disorders such as CP.

POWER MOBILITY

Hays described four functional categories of children using power mobility.[38] The first group includes children who will never ambulate and who experience no independent mobility without the use of a power device. The second group includes children with inefficient mobility; that is, they ambulate or use a manual wheelchair but with unacceptable functional speed or endurance. The third group consists of children who have lost independent mobility through disease, brain injury, or spinal cord trauma. For this group, the developmental implications of independent mobility may be less important, but the acceptance of assisted mobility is a more significant issue. The fourth group includes children who require assisted mobility temporarily, either because they gain new ambulation skills through surgery or maturation or they recover lost function.

Advances in technology over the past decade have brought independent power mobility to a greater number of individuals with severe disabilities than ever before. A wide variety of power bases and options are available, with more reliable and precise controls than ever before possible (Figure 18-7).

The three main types of power wheelchairs are (1) the conventional design with integral seat and chassis (evolved from the traditional

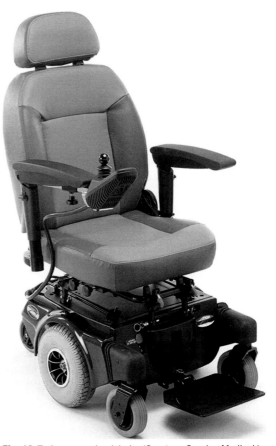

Fig. 18-7 A power wheelchair. (Courtesy Sunrise Medical.)

tubular manual wheelchair frame), (2) the powerbase or modular design with separate seat and chassis (often called an *all-terrain wheelchair*), and (3) scooters with either three- or four-wheeled platforms. Power chairs may be ordered with seats that tilt, backs that recline, units that recline and tilt, leg rests that elevate, and headrests that adjust, all with the touch of a switch. Manufacturers have responded to an increased demand for pediatric-sized power wheelchairs by producing wheelchairs that are lighter in weight, correctly proportioned for children, and have growth capabilities. Major advances in electronics have produced a greater variety of controls that are easier to access, more durable, and easier to adjust and customize. Power chairs are available in rear-wheel-, midwheel-, or front-wheel-drive options. The rear-wheel drive is the most common and longstanding traditional style. The front-wheel and midwheel drives allow the user a tighter turning radius.

The style of power mobility base chosen will depend in part on the client's upper body control. Scooters are steered using a tiller that requires a significant amount of upper extremity active range of motion and sitting balance. The control functions are usually mounted on the tiller and require a grip-type action of the thumb or fingers. Jones described a range of scooters from "light duty mall crawlers to heavy-duty barnyard rut jumpers."[39] Scooters are easier to dismantle and transport in the trunk of a car and look least like a wheelchair. Although they remain popular among adults, funding is often denied because of their limited indoor mobility and poor vehicle tiedown capabilities. Manufacturers have responded by making them more rugged and suited to outdoor use. Whereas wheelchair bases are generally easy to adapt to a seating system, scooter-seating systems have little room for adjustability and adaptability.

The conventional and powerbase designs offer the greatest range of seating and control options. The entire seating unit can be removed from the pedestal mount of the modular base. The traditional belt-driven chair is obsolete; the direct-drive motors of the powerbase improve power and control in turning. Front-wheel, midwheel, and rear-wheel drives offer different advantages and disadvantages in stability while driving and stopping, stability during recline or tilt, maneuverability in tight spaces, and ability to climb curbs. The type of drive system chosen for any given client must be as carefully considered as any other component of the wheelchair and seating system.

Power recline and power tilt capabilities offer excellent alternatives to individuals who need position changes throughout a long day of sitting to enable them to perform different functions or because of pain, fatigue, or pressure concerns associated with sitting too long. The act of reclining, however, causes shearing of tissues due to the disproportionate movement between the client and the seating system. On returning to the upright position, most clients will have shifted position in the system, and the more complex the seating system, the more significant the effects. Power recliners are available in low-shear and zero-shear models to help address these problems. Power tilt-in-space models work well for the client who has severe hypertonia or contractures and cannot tolerate having the seat-to-back angle opened up or who, once having done so, cannot return to an upright position without significant sliding.

Controls for power wheelchairs are available in two basic types: proportional and latched. The former has a proportional relationship between movement of the joystick and speed of the chair or sharpness of turning, whereas the latter has an on/off relationship to chair movement. The proportional control is the standard joystick found on most power wheelchairs. It is customarily mounted on either armrest and will move in a 360-degree arc. The movement of the joystick controls the speed and the direction of the wheelchair. An alternative to the standard joystick is a remote proportional joystick that is smaller and more compact. This feature allows a great deal of flexibility for joystick placement, provided sturdy mounting hardware is used. Proportional joysticks are also available in short-throw models that require less movement and force for activation and in heavy-duty models that can withstand a great deal of force. Head control joysticks are available for some wheelchairs.

A latched microswitch control system may consists of four separate switches, with each switch controlling one direction—forward, reverse, left, and right. All four switches might be in one control box (resembling a standard proportional control) or assembled into a smaller, more compact, remote control. Microswitches are also available in heavy-duty and short-throw models, as are the proportional controls. Microswitches are somewhat more flexible for assessment purposes. For example, they may be separated and set up in arrays to evaluate head control, or each of the four switches may be positioned at different body sites. The *wafer board* and *arm-slot* control are examples of microswitch technology. Microswitch-driven chairs tend to be less precise and smooth while turning and changing directions because a separate switch controls each direction.

With the recognition that age is no longer the determining factor in successful use of power mobility has come the need to define appropriate selection criteria. Schiaffino and Laux reported that children needed a cognitive level of at least 2 years of age, although these children would take longer to train than children with cognitive skills at the 3-year-old level or above.[34] More recently, transitional mobility programs are being developed for children as young as 12 to 14 months.[35] Barnes described a "motoric language" needed to learn to drive a powered chair that includes relational vocabulary (in, on, under), substantive vocabulary (nouns), directionality (forward, backward, right, left), perceptual concepts (visual and auditory feedback with switch activation), spatial concepts (depth perception, location of self in an environment, and problem solving to avoid obstacles), and serial or sequential concepts (first, second; before, after).[40]

It is possible that many of these concepts could actually be taught through training in a power device. Kangas provides a compelling argument for an experiential power mobility assessment for very young children that is based not on "readiness for driving" skills, but on the need for assistive mobility in any or all environments.[41] She suggests that the child be allowed to explore movement in the device over a period of many sessions by first being restricted to a single turning direction in a small, safe environment. Only after the child

has experienced going and stopping for the sake of being able to go again has he or she experienced mobility without regard for direction or purpose. This parallels the development of independent walking in toddlers. The child is never praised for "good driving," because this is meaningless. As the child's control over mobility expands and verbal labels for what is being accomplished are provided, the concepts described previously will develop. Power toys available at local toy stores make an excellent inexpensive alternative for power training of young children when the devices can be suitably adapted for seating and control.

Simulators have proven to be successful training tools. Hasdai, Jessel, and Weiss found that inexperienced drivers given simulator driving experience improved their accuracy and performance.[37] Newer virtual reality technology has allowed videogaming experiences to become wheelchair driver-training experiences.[42,43]

Oregon Research Institute/Applied Computer Simulation Labs has developed a virtual wheelchair mobility training course.[42] The intentionally designed training environments help children learn to drive a powered wheelchair safely, and 3-D computer gaming technology provides virtual reality environments in which students can practice driving with the use of an appropriately chosen joystick/input method. Additionally, software collects data regarding the student's driving performance. As the child's ability improves, the training environments become progressively more challenging. Internet connectivity allows the student to share training environments with others signed into the system.[42]

Galka and Lombard described functional criteria for safe driving, including the ability to turn the chair on and off, follow a straight course, turn both left and right, back the chair up, maneuver around objects and persons, and stop quickly.[44] The "marginal driver" is one of any age who may show borderline cognitive or physical skills or whose visuoperceptual problems significantly interfere with driving ability. With supervision these children may do well driving in a very specific setting, such as their school, but are not successful in novel or unpredictable community settings. The value of a power chair in increasing self-esteem and promoting independence in specific skills must be carefully weighed against the expense and amount of training and supervision required.

Besides the client criteria, there are several practical considerations that are unique to selection of power mobility. Building accessibility and space will affect where and how the device is used. Often it is kept and maintained at school, and a manual base is used at home. Care and maintenance of the power chair is more complex than that for manual systems. Transportation is also a more complicated issue. Some school districts refuse to transport certain types of power wheelchairs, such as scooters. The family may need a van for transporting the chair, and a ramp or a lift may be required for loading and unloading. Funding options for more expensive power wheelchairs may be more restrictive. Usually a backup manual chair is also required, especially during maintenance or repair of the power system. Responsibility for supervision, training, and routine wheelchair care should be determined prior to ordering the system.

TRANSPORTATION SAFETY

The U.S. society is generally mobile and on the go. This includes children and adults who use wheeled mobility. In recent years RESNA and the American National Standards Institute (ANSI) have set federal standards for using wheelchairs within vehicle transportation. Best practice dictates that when at all possible, wheelchair users should transfer out of their wheelchair and into an age- or weight-appropriate vehicle seat and occupant restraint systems that meet all the federal safety standards. The wheelchair should be stored and secured within the vehicle to prevent it from becoming a harmful projectile.

If the occupant cannot transfer, a seating system is required that can be attached to a transit wheelchair frame. Transport wheelchairs must meet ANSI/RESNA/WC19 standards, must have been frontal crash tested, and must have several advantageous features for use in vehicular transport, compared with standard wheelchairs. A WC19 transport wheelchair can be secured at four identifiable and crash-tested sites located on the floor of the vehicle, in less than 10 seconds per site, from an area accessible from one side of the wheelchair in enclosed space. Transit wheelchairs have crashworthy frames, smooth hardware edges, improved battery retention, better accommodation of vehicle-anchored belts, and proper instructions for use as a seat in a motor vehicle. It is imperative to face the wheelchair and occupant toward the front of the vehicle.

WC19 also set standards for lateral stability of a wheelchair within a forward-moving vehicle, because wheelchair users are often injured when the wheelchair tips after a quick stop or sharp turn in non-crash conditions. Effective May 2002, regulations allowed that a wheelchair occupant can use a crashworthy pelvic belt secured to the wheelchair frame, provided a separate vehicle-mounted shoulder belt could be inserted. This configuration may allow for restraint systems that fit more securely.

If the occupant cannot transfer and cannot use the transport wheelchair, a wheelchair with a metal frame should be used with a wheelchair tiedown and occupant restraint system (WTORS). Restraint systems that meet WTORS standards will be labeled as *SAE J2249*. Four tiedown straps are attached to strong places on the wheelchair frame, such as the welded frame joints. Attachment points should be as high as possible but below the seat surface. Rear tiedown straps should maintain a 30- to 45-degree angle with the vehicle floor.

Wheelchair occupants should ride in an upright position with the back reclined less than 30 degrees. The headrest should be positioned to support the head and neck, and trays should be removed and secured.

The 4-point tiedown system is considered the universal system. When used properly, the four-point system is effective and affordable. Tiedown straps should meet SAE J2249 standards.

Just as the wheelchair frame needs to be secured to the vehicle, the occupant needs to be secured with crashworthy lap and shoulder safety belts. Standard positioning belts and harnesses are not meant to restrain an occupant in a vehicle crash. Currently most lap and shoulder belts anchor to the vehicle independent of the wheelchair user. Newer models of WC19 wheelchairs have brackets for the occupant restraints mounted directly to the frame and allow the vehicle-mounted shoulder belts to attach directly to the lap belt.

EFFECTS OF MANAGED CARE ON ACQUISITION OF ASSISTIVE TECHNOLOGY

State-funded Medicaid programs, traditionally a major source of funding for children with disabilities, have contracted out much of their coverage to private managed care insurance organizations. In many cases this has affected accessibility to durable medical equipment and specialized devices.[24] Denials for requested items may increase, either because a narrower interpretation is used in determining medical necessity, or because nonstandard or customized items do not fit the billing codes. The time between the initial request and approval may be prolonged if the reviewers are less experienced in this specialized population and ask for more explanation, making repeated requests and justification necessary.

Choice of products may be restricted, because the amount that will be paid for a given item is often based on simpler adult equipment designs and does not cover the full cost of more expensive or more customized pediatric designs. The capitation rate paid to medical equipment suppliers is often inadequate to cover actual expenses, cutting their profit margins and making it difficult to provide and service sophisticated or customized equipment. In addition, many private insurance companies, as well as state-funded programs, have contracted with specific manufacturers to provide bulk orders of wheelchairs or other durable medical equipment, further restricting choice. Medical and equipment needs of individuals with disabilities are much higher than what many private companies anticipate. Some managed care companies have dropped contracts for state Medicaid patients, leaving those individuals with little or no choice of coverage and often requiring a change of provider. In the next decade the physical therapy profession will face the dilemma of reconciling knowledge of the huge variety of devices that can be designed and tailored for achieving independent function with the increasing restrictions in funding, choice, and accessibility of those devices.

ALTERNATIVE MOBILITY EQUIPMENT

Not all children with impaired mobility choose to use or require a wheelchair and seating system. *Mobility equipment* can be thought of as any devices that assist a child with mobility. Included in this group are canes, axillary crutches, Lofstrand crutches, forward walkers, reverse walkers, parapodiums, and harnessing systems.

Throughout the text, different mobility equipment is discussed in detail, particularly if a child with a certain diagnosis commonly uses a specific type of equipment. Children should attain mobility with the least number of devices; however, functional mobility across all environments relevant to the child must be considered. Some children ambulate at home using Lofstrand crutches but choose to use walkers for school mobility and wheelchairs for community mobility.

CASE STUDY OF A CHILD WITH SEATING AND MOBILITY DEVICES

EXAMINATION

History

General demographics: Anthony is an 11-year-old white male, and English is his primary language.

Social: Anthony attends fifth grade in an included classroom at his local public school. He is in Boy Scouts, on the school bowling team, and is involved in his church.

Growth and development: Anthony is left-hand dominant. He was born 8 weeks prematurely and contracted meningitis shortly after birth.

Living environment: Anthony lives with his two parents and his younger brother in an accessible single-family home. His father is a physical therapist.

History of current condition: Anthony needs a new seating and mobility system.

Functional status and activity level: Anthony requires minimum to moderate assistance with dressing and toileting. He can independently feed himself. He transfers with min-mod assist of 1. Anthony is independent in driving his power wheelchair indoors, within his community, and at school.

Medications: Anthony takes oral baclofen to decrease his spasticity.

Past history of current condition: Anthony received his first wheelchair at age 3. He initially used a linear seat and hybrid custom-molded back cushion with linear laterals on a power mobility system controlled by a joystick. It took him 6 months of driver training and practice to learn to drive the power chair independently.

Systems Review

Cardiopulmonary: There are no known pathologies or impairments.

Integumentary: There are no known pathologies or impairments. He has no history of pressure sores, and bilateral lower extremity scars are well healed.

Musculoskeletal: Bilateral de-rotation osteotomies 2 years ago.

Neuromuscular: See Test and Measures.

Tests and Measures

Endurance: Anthony is able to perform all activities required of him without difficulty. He does not become short of breath or fatigued.

Anthropometric characteristics: Anthony is a slender adolescent of average height and weight for his age.

Arousal/attention/cognition: Within normal limits (WNL).

Assistive and adaptive devices: Anthony uses bilateral solid ankle AFOs. He uses utensil modifications so that he can independently feed himself. He uses a wheel-in shower with water sprayer and a raised toilet seat in the bathroom. He uses an adapted computer at school and home for educational purposes.

Community integration: Anthony is fully integrated into his community and school.

Cranial nerve integrity: Intact. Anthony wears glasses for visual acuity.

Environmental barriers: Anthony's school is a single-level structure with an accessible playground. He rides a wheelchair-accessible school bus to and from school. Anthony's home has recently been structurally modified to allow for wheelchair-accessible common areas (kitchen, living room, bathroom, den) and an accessible bedroom suite. An elevator was installed to allow Anthony access to the basement area. Both front and rear home entrances are wheelchair accessible.

Gait/locomotion/balance: Anthony has excellent sitting balance. He requires upper extremity support to maintain standing. Anthony can ambulate with both hands supported by another person, but gains independent locomotion via his power wheelchair. Anthony uses a manual beach wheelchair (constructed of PVC tubing, mesh seat and back, and large inflated rubber wheels) when at the beach.

Integumentary integrity: All lower extremity scars are well healed.

Motor function: Anthony has spastic quadriplegia. He has increased spasticity in all four limbs that fluctuates with his activity level. He can roll and sit independently and transfer sit ↔ stand with min-mod assist of 1. When moving he tends to be influenced by upper extremity flexion synergies and lower extremity extension synergies. Gross Motor Function Classification System level 4: self-mobility with limitations. Child uses power mobility outdoors and in community.

Continued

CASE STUDY OF A CHILD WITH SEATING AND MOBILITY DEVICES—cont'd

Muscle performance: Modified Ashworth Spasticity Scale grade of 3; considerable increase in muscle tone, passive movement difficult.

Neuromotor development: Anthony's overall development is significantly influenced by his cerebral palsy, and he has a dominant startle reflex. He can volitionally move all extremities with effort. Anthony is left-handed and can easily move his left upper extremity and use his left hand to type and drive his power wheelchair. Anthony wears bilateral AFOs that fit him well. His current seating system and mobility devices no longer meet his needs. He has outgrown the customized seating system, and his mobility device is well worn and in need of repair. Anthony uses an adaptive computer with a modified keyboard for his schoolwork.

Pain: Anthony has no complaints of pain.

Posture: Anthony is relatively symmetric when in his seating system. He tends to laterally flex to the left when sitting unsupported.

All ROM measurements are WNL except:

LEFT (DEGREES)	MOTION	RIGHT (DEGREES)
0	Ankle dorsiflexion	0
0	Ankle inversion	0
−5	Knee extension	−5
0	Hip extension	0
25	Hip abduction	20
0	Hip internal rotation	0
WNL	Wrist extension	0
WNL	Wrist pronation	To neutral
−10	Elbow extension	−10
100	Shoulder abduction	100
110	Shoulder flexion	110

Reflex integrity: Anthony has a positive Babinski bilaterally.

Self-care: Anthony requires minimum assistance for dressing and toileting. He can independently feed himself, but requires assistance for food preparation. Anthony can independently manage his hygiene and oral care.

EVALUATION

Diagnosis
Guide to PT Practice Pattern: 5A

Prognosis
Anthony currently requires a new seating and mobility system. He needs a contoured seating system to maintain his musculoskeletal system in neutral and minimize deformities. He will continue to be independent and maintain good musculoskeletal alignment with a new system.

DIRECT INTERVENTION

Coordination/Communication/Documentation
To obtain new seating and mobility equipment, Anthony will require a medical prescription, as well as a medical need form from his physician and therapists.

Following delivery of the new system, Anthony will receive training on maintenance and care of his seating and mobility system.

Prescription of Device
Seating system: Anthony's seating system should include a generically contoured seat with moderate pressure relief. Bilateral hip blocks and an adductor pommel will maintain his lower extremity in neutral alignment. He will require a pelvic positioning device to maintain good positioning of his pelvis within the seating system. Anthony requires a low-maintenance pressure relief cushion. A fluid-filled cushion will provide appropriate pressure relief and sensory and kinesthetic feedback for his pelvis. A generically contoured back cushion with bilateral trunk lateral supports is recommended. The cushion contour should maintain Anthony's trunk in neutral alignment. Anthony requires a low-profile head support to protect against acceleration/deceleration injuries while in a motor vehicle.

Power mobility system: Anthony further requires a high-performance power mobility system that will integrate with his customized seating system. A rear-wheel-drive mobility system will allow him to achieve precise maneuverability at home, at school, and within the community. He should drive his system via a standard joystick input device placed on his left side. He will require 70-degree front riggings and footplates with shoe straps to maintain lower extremity positioning.

Reexamination
Anthony will need to be reassessed when the system is delivered. Anthony's seat/back may require slight modifications to ensure the most precise fit possible. Anthony should then be reassessed yearly.

CASE STUDY OF A CHILD WITH SEATING AND MOBILITY DEVICES—cont'd

Goals

1. Anthony will receive a new customized seating system to maintain good musculoskeletal alignment.
2. Anthony will receive a power wheelchair that interfaces with the recommended seating system, and the driver controls will be modified for his specifications.
3. Anthony will be independently mobile in his new seating and mobility system.

ANALYSIS OF CASE USING THE ICF MODEL:

Body functions: Severe spastic quadriplegia, musculoskeletal malalignment and imbalances.

Activity limitations: Requires a power wheelchair for mobility around home and community, requires assistance to complete motor tasks.

Participation restrictions: Requires modified computer equipment at home and school, requires assistance to participate in most nonverbal activities.

Environmental limitations: Requires accessible environments, requires assistance for ADLs, requires specialized transportation.

Chapter Discussion Questions

1. What are the three categories of seating systems?
2. What are the two categories of wheeled mobility?
3. If a child can ambulate but requires assistance for balance, what are appropriate devices to consider to assist the child with ambulation at home and at school?
4. A child with diplegia, who can ambulate but uses a wheelchair for long distances, would be most appropriate for what kind of seating system and mobility system?
5. What is the difference between a midwheel-drive power wheelchair and a rear-wheel-drive power wheelchair?
6. What laws influenced the availability of assistive technology for individuals with disabilities?
7. Why is the seating system an important component of a wheeled mobility or positioning system?
8. Your client is an 18-year-old girl with severe spastic quadriplegia. She attends a community college and lives at home. She has severe skeletal deformities, including scoliosis, hip dislocation, and leg-length discrepancy. Why would a custom-molded seating system and a midwheel-drive power chair be appropriate for her?

9. What is the difference between a tilt-in-space seating system and a reclining seating system? Give an example of when you would use each system.
10. If a child transitions from a manual mobility system to a power mobility system, what issues does the therapist need to be aware of?

REFERENCES

1. Parette P, McMahon GA: What should we expect of assistive technology? *Teaching Exceptional Children* 35(1):56, 2002.
2. Dorman SM: Assistive technology benefits for students with disabilities, *J Sch Health* 68(3):120, 1998.
3. Hedman G: Overview of rehabilitation technology, *Phys Occup Ther Pediatr* 10(2):1, 1990.
4. Medhat MA, Hobson DA: *Standardization of terminology and descriptive methods for specialized seating: a reference manual*, Arlington, Va, 1992, RESNA.
5. Langone J, Malone DM, Kinsley T: Technology solutions for young children with developmental concerns, *Infants Young Child* 4(11):65, 1999.
6. Long T, Tuscano K: *Handbook of pediatric physical therapy*, ed 2, Philadelphia, 2002, Lippincott Williams & Wilkins.
7. Galvin JC, Scherer MJ: *Evaluating, selecting, and using appropriate assistive technology*, Gaithersburg, Md, 1996, Aspen.
8. Letts RM, editor: *Principles of seating the disabled*, Boca Raton, Fla, 1991, CRC.
9. Kangas KM: Seating, positioning, and physical access, *Developmental Disabilities Special Interest Section Newsletter* 14(2):4, 1991.

10. Bergen AF, Presperin J, Tallman T: *Positioning for function: wheelchairs and other assistive technologies,* Valhalla, NY, 1990, Valhalla Rehabilitation.

11. Cook A, Hussey SM: *Assistive technologies: principles and practice,* St Louis, 1995, Mosby.

12. Cook A, Polgar JM: *Cook & Hussey's assistive technologies: principles and practice,* ed 3, St Louis, 2008, Mosby.

13. O'Sullivan SB, Schmitz T: *Physical rehabilitation: assessment and treatment,* ed 4, Philadelphia, 2001, FA Davis.

14. Bergen AF: Seating and positioning principles for the neurologically involved client, Presented at the American Physical Therapy Association Combined Sections Meeting, San Francisco, February 1992.

15. Siekman AR, Flanagan K: The anti-thrust seat: a wheelchair insert for individuals with abnormal reflex patterns or other specialized problems. In *Proceedings of the 8th annual conference on rehabilitation engineering,* Washington, DC, 1983, RESNA.

16. Margolis S: Lumbar support issues. Presented at the Eighth International Seating Symposium, Vancouver, BC, February 1992.

17. Margolis SA, Wengert ME, Kolar KA: The subASIS bar: no component is an island: a five-year retrospective. Presented at the Fourth International Seating Symposium, Vancouver, BC, February 1988.

18. Reid DT, Rigby P: Towards improved anterior pelvic stabilization devices for paediatric wheelchair users with cerebral palsy, *Can J Rehabil* 9(3):147, 1996.

19. Carlson SJ, Grey TL: The semi-rigid pelvic stabilizer for seating control. Presented at the Fourth International Seating Symposium, Vancouver, BC, February 1988.

20. Noon JH, Chesney DA, Axelson PW: Development of a dynamic pelvic stabilization system. In *Proceedings of the 21st annual conference on rehabilitation engineering,* Arlington, Va, 1998, RESNA.

21. Evans MA, Nelson WB: A dynamic solution to seating clients with fluctuating tone. In *Proceedings of the 19th annual conference on rehabilitation technology,* Arlington, Va, 1996, RESNA.

22. Orpwood R: A compliant seating system for a child with extensor spasms. In *Proceedings of the 19th annual conference of rehabilitation engineering,* Arlington, Va, 1996, RESNA.

23. Trefler E, Angelo J: Comparison of anterior trunk supports for children with cerebral palsy, *Assist Technol* 9(1):15, 1997.

24. Carlson SJ, Ramsey C: Assistive technology. In Campbell SK, editor: *Physical therapy for children,* ed 2, Philadelphia, 2000, Saunders.

25. Brubaker CH, Sprigle SH: Seating and wheelchairs, *Curr Opinion Orthop* 1(3):445, 1990.

26. Bednarczyk JH, Sanderson DJ: Kinematics of wheelchair propulsion in adults and children with spinal cord injury, *Arch Phys Med Rehabil* 75:1327, 1994.

27. Kermoian R: Locomotion experience and psychological development in infancy. In Furumasu J, editor: *Pediatric powered mobility: developmental perspectives, technical issues, clinical approaches,* Arlington, Va, 1997, RESNA.

28. Deitz J, Swinth Y, White O: Powered mobility and preschoolers with complex developmental delays, *Am J Occup Ther* 56(1):86, 2002.

29. Butler C: Effects of powered mobility on self-initiated behaviors of very young children with locomotor disability, *Dev Med Child Neurol* 28:325, 1986.

30. Butler C, Okamoto GA, McKay TM: Powered mobility for very young disabled children, *Dev Med Child Neurol* 25:472, 1983.

31. Berry ET, McLaurin SE, Sparling JW: Parent/caregiver perspectives on the use of power wheelchairs, *Pediatr Phys Ther* 8(4):146, 1996.

32. Carlson D, Myklebust J: Wheelchair use and social interaction, *Top spinal cord inj rehabil* 7(3):28, 2002.

33. Paulsson K, Christoffersen M: Psychological aspects of technical aids: how does independent mobility affect the psychosocial and intellectual development of children with physical disabilities? In *Proceedings of the 2nd international conference on rehabilitation engineering,* Washington, DC, 1984, RESNA.

34. Schiaffino S, Laux J: Prerequisite skills for the psychosocial impact of powered wheelchair mobility on young children with severe handicaps, *Developmental Disabilities Special Interest Section Newsletter* 9(2):1, 1986.

35. Wright-Ott C: The transitional powered mobility aid: a new concept and tool for early mobility. In Furumasu J, editor: *Pediatric powered mobility: developmental perspectives, technical issues, clinical approaches,* Arlington, Va, 1997, RESNA.

36. Field D: Powered mobility: a literature review illustrating the importance of a multifaceted approach, *Assist Technol* 11(1):20, 1999.

37. Hasdai A, Jessel AS, Weiss PL: Use of a computer simulator for training children with disabilities in the operation of a powered wheelchair, *Am J Occup Ther* 52(3):215, 1998.

38. Hays RM: Childhood motor impairments: clinical overview and scope of the problem. Presented at the Fourth International Seating Symposium, Vancouver, BC, February 1988.

39. Jones CK: In search of power for the pediatric client, *Phys Occup Ther Pediatr* 10(2):47, 1990.

40. Barnes KH: Training young children for powered mobility, *Developmental Disabilities Special Interest Section Newsletter* 14(2):1, 1991.

41. Kangas KM: Clinical assessment and training strategies for the child's mastery of independent powered mobility. In Furumasu J, editor: *Pediatric powered mobility: developmental perspectives, technical issues, clinical approaches,* Arlington, Va, 1997, RESNA.

42. Oregon Research Institute/Applied Computer Simulation Labs (website): http://www.ori.org/~vr/. Accessed October 15, 2007.

43. Reid DT: The effects of the saddle seat on seated postural control and upper extremity movement in children with cerebral palsy, *Dev Med Child Neurol* 38:805, 2002.

44. Buning ME, Angelo JA, Schmeler MR: Occupational performance and the transition to power mobility: a pilot study, *Am J Occup Ther* 55(3):339, 2001.

RESOURCES

The Alliance for Technology Access

2173 E. Francisco Boulevard, Suite L
San Rafael, CA 94901
Phone: 415.455.4575
Fax: 415.455.0654
TTY: 415.455.0491
www.ataccess.org
(Provides a list of Alliance for Technology Access Centers in the United States and distributes a newsletter.)

Rehabilitation Engineering and Assistive Technology Society of North America (RESNA)

1700 Moore Street, Suite 1540
Arlington, VA 22209-1903
Phone: 703-524-6686
Fax: 703-524-6630
www.resna.org

Christopher and Dana Reeve Paralysis Resource Center

Short Hills Plaza
636 Morris Turnpike, Suite 3A
Short Hills, NJ 07078
1-800-539-7309
(Information on understanding paralysis and other conditions.)

American Academy of Cerebral Palsy and Developmental Medicine

www.aacpdm.org
(Information on cerebral palsy and other developmental disorders.)

Oregon Research Institute/Applied Computer Simulation Labs

1715 Franklin Blvd.
Eugene, OR 97403-1983
Phone: 541-484-2123
TDD: 800-735-2900
Fax: 541-484-1108
www.ori.org/~vr/

APPENDIX

Answers to Discussion Questions

CHAPTER 1

1. An increased likelihood of acquiring asthma, diabetes, morbid obesity, high lead levels, depression, or becoming a victim of violence; (a) suboptimal and infrequent healthcare; (b) exacerbation of chronic conditions; and (c) risky/unsafe living environments.
2. Some examples include offering park district programs that focus on overall wellness, health, and nutrition; neighborhood health centers that focus on entire family issues, including social and emotional status of the family; resources available to families to improve their quality of life; and before- and after-school programs that offer supportive and safe environments, relevant and age-appropriate health education and nutritional information, and extracurricular programs (sports, clubs, support groups).
3. Central nervous system, peripheral nervous system, visceromotor nervous system.
4. Cephalocaudal; proximal to distal; flexion to extension. Thus a young baby tends to develop head control and then trunk control, control of shoulders and hips prior to finger control, and works out of flexion, increasing the strength of the extensors before refining the strength of the flexors.
5. (a) Difficulty eating, difficulty maintaining head and eyes in midline; (b) difficulty with ADLs and IADLs (including feeding, dressing, washing), difficulty completing two-handed midline tasks, difficulty in crawling, cruising, and walking; (c) may develop scoliosis due to paraspinals overfiring unevenly, left compared to right.
6. Low tone, child appears floppy.
7. Hypertonia/hypotonia: difficulty sitting in classroom furniture and on floor, difficulty with walking, potential difficulty with language and communication. Athetosis: will need personal assistance and significant level of help in the classroom; child may have difficulty sitting in standard chairs at the table, participating in ambulation activities.
8. Central nervous system consists of the brain and spinal cord.
9. In the CNS the pathways and tracks tend to descend from the brain to their synapses in/near the spinal cord. The PNS information travels from the periphery to the spinal degree. The central nervous system may be referred to as *gray matter* and *white matter*. This nomenclature indicates which structures are myelinated and which are not. Myelinated structures are considered to be white matter, whereas nonmyelinated structures are considered to be gray matter. The peripheral nervous system consists of the nerves that connect the central nervous system and the peripheral muscles of the body. The peripheral nervous system has sensory fibers and innervates glands and skeletal, cardiac, and smooth muscles. The peripheral nervous system can regenerate after an injury, but the central nervous system cannot.
10. By the 6th week of gestation.

CHAPTER 2

1. Reliability determines if the tool is an accurate measure of what it claims to measure. An unreliable test cannot be used for clinical measurements.
2. No, a raw score is meaningless when comparing groups. The standardized score should be used to measure change over time.
3. Assessments can be used to screen for delays or abnormalities, provide a diagnosis, evaluate outcomes and progress, develop goals, collect data, and determine a prognosis. In the school setting the therapist uses assessment tools to help justify the number of minutes of services a child is receiving, especially if the number is uncharacteristically high.
4. The age-equivalent score is useful when assessing and describing developmentally delayed children who cannot achieve a developmental index score.
5. Test validity determines if the assessment tool accomplishes its intended purpose.
6. *Face validity* is the concept that the test strongly measures what it claims to measure. Thus is the face value of the assessment valid and true? *Content validity* requires that the assessment sample a reasonable range of target behaviors. Is the content of the assessment measuring what it claims to measure? *Concurrent validity* correlates the child's performance on an assessment to another valid assessment. Will the child achieve the same age level or developmental level on two different assessments given in the same time period? *Construct validity* requires that the test explain the child's achievement within a theoretical framework. *Predictive validity* describes how well the assessment tool predicts the child's performance at a future date.
7. The therapist may gain a richer understanding of the child.
8. Both assessment tools can be standardized. On the evaluation side, in a criterion-referenced exam, the child's performance is measured by the number of criteria the child has mastered on certain tasks. In the norm-referenced assessment tool, the child's performance is compared to standards set by a sample of children from the general population.
9. Two possible answers are:
The Pediatric Evaluation of Disability Inventory (PEDI) is a norm-referenced tool that assesses functional skills of children ages 6 months to 7.5 yrs. The PEDI measures capability and performance of functional activities in three content areas: self-care, ability, and social function. The Peabody Developmental Motor Scales, Second Edition (PDMS-2) uses a stratified sample relative to the U.S. Census criteria. The PDMS-2 is designed to assess the gross and fine motor skills of children from birth through 6 years of age. Items are scored on a three-point scale. Age equivalents, motor quotients, percentile rankings, and standard scores can be calculated for each child.
10. A therapist might choose to use a qualitative assessment style when studying student interactions at an inclusive fifth grade. The qualitative assessment will allow themes to develop over time, and the researcher will be able to record these themes and ask more questions. A researcher may use a quantitative measure when measuring motor quotients or assessing a child for eligibility purposes. In these cases, numbers are needed to determine the prognosis of the child.

CHAPTER 3

1. Work around/in the refrigerator on opening the door (child has to step and move as door opens); child can work on squat-to-stand activities by picking objects off

floor and placing on refrigerator shelves or removing things from shelves; child can practice choice making by selecting things from the refrigerator; child can practice standing and weight shifting while playing wash the dishes/rinse the dishes at the sink.

2. Use snack time to work on squat to stand, sit to stand, or the reverse. Have the child play dress-up with oversized clothes and practice sitting or standing balance skills and sit-to-stand activities while donning or doffing clothes.

3. Children with more advanced skills can be seen as motor/language and/or cognitive models for children with less advanced skills. Typically developing peers receive exposure to children with delays or disorders.

4. Park district programs such as swimming, dancing, and gym.
Public library programs: Story time can be used to practice time on task and attention to task. Early literacy will also help communication and cognition. The local YMCA or YWCA may offer motor activities that will help improve strength and coordination.

5. Recognizes the influence of motor control and investigates the effects of postural control as a result of several interactions between complex neurologic and physiologic systems.

6. The main goal of PNF is to strengthen muscles within functional movement patterns, including rotation. These movement patterns are known as *diagonals*. PNF is based on the developmental sequence and the sequential mastery of motor milestones. Spiral and diagonal movements are extremely important, because these movements take strength, coordination, and control.

7. Group intervention, rhythmic intention, the conductor/teacher leading the group, and rhythmic intention.

8. Strengthening programs do not cause a direct illness or injury to children. Exercise will help to reduce loss of bone, minerals, and muscle mass.

9. Both have the potential to facilitate movement by increasing input or decreasing input to a region. Each require some training to apply correctly.

CHAPTER 4

1. If a goal or outcome is not important to the family, it will not be incorporated into the family's activities. If the activity is not part of a routine, then the child will have little time to practice and gain improvement toward mastering the goal/outcome. Additionally, the family/caregiver may be one of the few people who have seen the child across several environments and over a given time span; thus the family/caregiver can relay historical information that will be relevant to a current treatment plan.

2. With an interdisciplinary team: Goals are discipline-specific, families may not be central to team functioning, team members implement their portion of the plan.

3. Therapists on a transdisciplinary team will cross-treat and work on goals that may not necessarily be related to their specific discipline. They will also treat the child in a variety of environments, so that the child has the opportunity to practice several skills in a variety of environments.

4. School-based therapy must focus on educationally relevant outcomes/goals. The goal of any therapeutic treatment is to allow the child to function better in the school environment.

5. The IFSP outcomes should be transdisciplinary and require that the goals are family priorities. The IFSP also dictates in what environment/setting the therapy

services will occur. The IFSP is the therapeutic plan for children ages 0-3. The IEP outcomes are educationally relevant, and the therapy setting is an educational setting. The IEP is in place for children 3-21 years of age.

6. Children with more advanced skills can be seen as motor/language and/or cognitive models for children with less advanced skills. Typically developing peers receive exposure to children with delays or disorders.

7. Park district programs such as swimming, dancing, and gym.
Public library programs: Story time can be used to practice time on task and attention to task. Early literacy will also help communication and cognition. The local YMCA or YWCA may offer motor activities that will help improve strength and coordination.

8. Multidisciplinary team—strength: quality services provided; weakness: little communication between team members, and perhaps redundancy or conflicting services are being offered.
Interdisciplinary team—strength: shared responsibility for team, regular collaboration between service providers and family, co-treatment opportunities may exist; weakness: family may not be considered an integral part of the team.
Transdisciplinary—strength: specialty area role release, cross training and cross treatments occur, family at center of team; weakness: confusion for families about who is delivering what services to the child, requires a team that is in sync and works well together.

CHAPTER 5

1. Hallmark signs include reduced quality of movements, spasticity, muscle weakness, ataxia. These signs typically appear before the age of 3 years if the child experiences birth trauma.

2. Causes of CP include: low birth weight, infection in utero, jaundice, Rh incompatibility, oxygen shortage, stroke, toxicity. Classification: Several ways to classify—by muscle tone, movement pattern, impairment or severity.
Tone: hypertonia, hypotonia, ataxia, athetoid; pyramidal or extrapyramidal; Gross Motor Function Classification System.

3. Level 1 describes the child who can move without devices before the age of 2. A child at level 1 will experience difficulties with higher-level gross motor skills, balance, and coordination.
Level 2 describes a child who will gain floor mobility by 2 years of age. As a youngster, the child at level 2 will ambulate short distances independently, but uses assistive devices to ambulate within the community and may have difficulty on steps and in running and jumping. He may ambulate independently in later childhood.
Level 3: Children develop sitting skills with support; they use atypical movement patterns typically without reciprocal movements for mobility. These children ambulate with assistive devices but tend to use wheelchairs for community mobility.
Level 4: Children develop head control and can roll by 2 years of age. As they age, the children develop supported sitting skills and nonreciprocal movements. Children at level 4 typically need trunk support to sit and assistive devices for mobility.
Level 5: Children at level 5 develop limited volitional control and antigravity movements. They require extensive equipment and assistance for mobility and self-care.

CHAPTER 6

1. Motor vehicle accident, shaken baby syndrome, near drowning, sports injuries, tumors/neoplasm, child not restrained properly in a motor vehicle.
2. Typically classified with the Glasgow Coma Scale or the Rancho Los Amigos Cognitive Recovery Scale.
3. Long-term impairments include decreased cognitive abilities; long- and short-term memory loss; and deficits in attention, reasoning, abstract thinking, judgment, problem solving, and/or information processing. Child may also experience speech and language disorders, psycho-social behavioral issues, sensory deficits, perceptual motor disabilities, and decreased physical functioning.
4. Increase in scores reflect improved observable function in a particular area.
5. If a person receives a score of 3 in the sub-domain of verbal response, this indicates that the person is verbal but may not be using appropriate words. However, sounds are consistently words and not just sounds or utterances.
6a. He should be classified as a Level IV. At this stage, individuals are confused, agitated and alert, very active, aggressive, perform motor actions, but behavior is nonpurposeful; person will have an extremely short attention span.
6b. Limited ability to follow verbal and nonverbal direction, limited communication using yes/no inconsistently, limited wheeled mobility, limited ambulation. Strategies would include implementing a communication board with simple text and color organization—morning activities in red, afternoon activities in green, evening activities in blue, for instance. Break down activities into smaller tasks, and order them with text or pictures so child can use as guide in completing activity. Use a smiley face with YES under it and a frown face with NO under it so that child can point and indicate choice. Honor choice of yes or no, even if it seems inaccurate, to reinforce concepts. For example, if child indicates he does not want a snack, even though he really does, then deny snack at that time. Also, verbal commands need to be clear and concise. Limit commands to one to two steps, gradually building in complexity as child's understanding and memory improve. May need to get a chair lift or bilateral railings to assist child in getting to bedroom, or perhaps relocate bedroom to a first floor area temporarily.

CHAPTER 7

1. Retinal hemorrhages; subdural and/or subarachnoid hemorrhages with little or no sign of external head trauma.
2. Babies and children often go untreated because of the subtle onset of symptoms and slow, progressive changes of mood, alertness, and/or function. The diagnosis is made with a CT scan or MRI scan demonstrating subdural and retinal hemorrhages.
3. The therapist must keep in mind that often families are separated due to long hospitalizations and/or guardianship issues. The child may live in an alternative housing situation. The child will have significant physical and cognitive changes post-injury. The child may have symptoms of posttraumatic stress syndrome.
4. Areas that may be affected by injury include arousal, attention, communication skills, mobility, muscle performance.
5. Shaken baby syndrome is a form of child abuse and a result of uncontrolled stressors and triggers.
6. Neurologic deficits, blindness, cognitive limitations.

7. Treatment should include range of motion, splinting, positioning to protect skin integrity and control atypical tonal influences.
8. One third will have permanent disability (paralysis, cognitive limitations, blindness), one third will die from sustained injuries, one third will recover.
9. Male in his early 20s, known to child, aware of his actions, shakes child in lieu of spanking because of less noticeable marks on child.
10. A highly specialized multidisciplinary team that can support the medical, social/emotional, and physical needs of the child and caregivers.

CHAPTER 8

1. JRA is an autoimmune disease in which the body mistakenly identifies some of its own cells and tissues as foreign.
2.

	PAUCI-ARTICULAR	POLY-ARTICULAR	SYSTEMIC
Subtypes	3	2	0
Joints involved	4 or fewer	5 or more	All and internal organs
Gender prevalence	5 times more in girls	3 times more in girls	0

3. Children with JRA often develop uveitis (iridocyclitis), which is inflammation of the iris and ciliary body.
4. Nonsteroidal antiinflammatory drugs (NSAIDs); disease-modifying antirheumatic drugs (DMARDs); biologic response modifier; and corticosteroids.
5. Pain relief, maintaining and gaining PROM and AROM, maintaining and increasing strength and endurance, improving the child's mobility and independent functioning.
6. **C**alcinosis, **R**aynaud phenomenon, **E**sophageal dysmotility, **S**clerodactyly, and **T**elangiectasias.

7. Localized scleroderma may display different types of skin involvement. Systemic juvenile scleroderma involves the internal organs and occurs less frequently in children than localized scleroderma.
8. Hard skin.

CHAPTER 9

1. Muscle atrophy, insufficient room within the uterus for normal fetal movement, central nervous system and spinal cord deformities, atypical development of tendons, bones, joints, or joint linings.
2. In one type of AMC the child presents with abducted and laterally rotated hips, flexed knees, clubfeet, medially rotated shoulders, extended elbows, and wrists in flexion with ulnar deviation. In the other type the child presents with flexed and dislocated hips, extended knees and clubfeet, medially rotated shoulders, flexed elbows, and flexed and ulnarly deviated wrists.
3. The members of the team typically include the child, family, orthopedic surgeon, and physical and occupational therapy.
4. Since muscle disuse and atrophy are hallmark characteristics of AMC, intensive therapy aims to get as much strength, endurance, and motor control as possible. Intensive therapy helps the child learn to move using different muscle groups than the child has used prior to therapy.
5. Work to achieve flexion in one UE and extension in the other UE.
6. Infant intervention will incorporate ways for the caregiver to hold the child and position the child when sleeping and feeding that will assist in gaining range, but also can occur as part of the typical family routine and interactions with the child.
7. Strengthening should be system-wide, but focused on increasing and maintaining abdominal, hip, and knee strength.
8. When one hip is dislocated.

9. Kicking balls of varying weights; repetitive squat-to-stand activities, such as getting a sponge wet and then painting the wall with it; stepping activities/obstacle courses; jumping on a trampoline; riding a bike with adaptations if needed.
10. Swimming, horseback riding, and dance/movement classes.

CHAPTER 10

1. Cardiac involvement, cognitive delays, atlantoaxial instability.
2. Prone on elbows, supported sitting, support child over their shoulder.
3. Using sign language and verbal commands, limit immediate choice to two or three opportunities to choose from at a time, use pictures to help child understand the order of activities and which activities are going to occur.
4. Ascending and descending steps, jumping rope, swimming, rising up and down on tiptoes. The child may benefit from orthotics to help maintain foot position and balance.
5. Swimming, dance/movement class, bike riding, jumping on a mini trampoline.
6. Individual states' early intervention programs, National Association for Down Syndrome, local support groups, library, educational system.
7. Atlantoaxial instability, extreme joint laxity, hypotonia.
8. PTAs are an integral member of the therapy team and must help the child and family be involved members of the team as well. The PTA can help to motivate the child by making the exercises fun and functional. Therapeutic exercise should be embedded as much as possible into the child's daily routines.
9. Hypotonicity, ligament laxity, hearing loss, cardiac limitations.
10. She could roll the ball instead of kicking it. Susie could use a peer to kick the ball, and then she could run the bases.

CHAPTER 11

1. Headaches, irritability, lethargy, difficulty keeping eyes open, vomiting, seizures.
2. Bilateral AFOs and a reverse walker. This child maybe able to progress to Lofstrand crutches.
3. Juan might consider using a walker or a manual wheelchair to conserve energy for the fieldtrip.
4. Washing dishes at the sink, organizing/rearranging the refrigerator contents, washing things that are up high so she needs to stretch to achieve.
5. Let him sit for 20 minutes and see if the redness diminishes, add padding to the lateral calcaneus area, contact Jackson's parents/guardian and suggest they make an appointment with the orthotist as soon as possible
6. Latex-free supplies and equipment should be considered in the therapy gyms (e.g., equipment built from wood, metal, or other nonlatex materials).
7. Joe's program should include teaching Joe how to perform skin checks, strengthening exercises for the upper and lower extremities and trunk, and instruction in donning and doffing braces appropriately. He will need to practice the transfers in different settings: cafeteria, classroom, bathroom, etc. His program should also include activities to improve standing balance and weight shifting while using the braces. Joe's walker may be more cumbersome than he was used to. He will need to increase his awareness about where the walker is in relation to other people walking by and adjust his movements while using the walker.
8. She will require the use of a rental power wheelchair for school until she is able to resume using her manual wheelchair. Tess may be able to use forearm platform crutches, depending on her postsurgical instructions.

CHAPTER 12

1. Many autistic children do have highly developed "splinter skills." Individuals with autism often demonstrate poor eye contact when interacting with others; demonstrate marked impairment in facial expressions, body postures, and gestures; typically fail to form successful peer relationships; and exhibit limited or no joint attention. Odd or exaggerated responses to sensory stimuli are common in autistic children. Autistic children often rigidly adhere to routines or rituals with no apparent functional purpose.
2. The Children's Health Act of 2000, the New Freedom Initiative of 2001, and the Combating Autism Act of 2006.
3. Children with autism also frequently use stereotyped or repetitive language. They often may have standard rote responses to certain questions or situations, or may perseverate (uncontrollably repeat) a word or phrase.
4. Autistic children generally do not engage in spontaneous or imitative play. A child with autism often will demonstrate abnormally intense interest in unusually narrow areas of interest. Autistic children often rigidly adhere to routines or rituals with no apparent functional purpose.

CHAPTER 13

1. Children at this age are inquisitive and may pull scalding liquids onto themselves; children are also susceptible to abuse scald injuries secondary to their inability to escape the perpetrator or the situation.
2. First-degree burn: also known as *superficial burn*; painful but self-limiting; no scarring typically; due to overexposure to the sun. Second-degree burn: partial-thickness burns, including superficial or deep. Superficial partial-thickness include damage to the epidermis; deep partial-thickness include the epidermis and deep portion of the dermal layer; both cause increased sensitivity to pain and temperature in the area of the burn. Superficial partial-thickness burns appear red with large, thick-walled blisters; deep partial-thickness burns have a marbled, white edematous appearance with large, thick-walled blisters. Third-degree burn: known as *full-thickness burns*; total destruction of the epidermis and dermis and may include deeper tissues such as fascia, muscle, subcutaneous fat. Pain and temperature sensation is destroyed. Skin appears white, brown-black, charred, and leathery, and blistering does not typically occur.
3. Total burn surface area measures the percent of body tissue affected by the burn injury. There are three common methods used to measure TBSA: rule of nines, the palm of the child's hand, and the Lund-Browder chart.
4. They are both chemical burns. Acid burns produce coagulation necrosis, whereas alkalis cause liquidation necrosis (tissue is liquefied). Alkali burns tend to penetrate more deeply and are more dangerous.
5. Shock, edema, heterotrophic ossification, amputation, peripheral nerve involvement.
6. Tissue may form scar tissue secondary to the laying down of highly disorganized collagen; hypertrophic and keloid scarring may also occur. Itching may cause severe discomfort as the tissues heal.
7. Maintain range of motion, restore function.
8. Primarily for easy donning and doffing and for the cosmetic appearance of the mask.

CHAPTER 14

1. Hands, limbs, feet.
2. None.
3. Congenital and acquired.
4. Above knee = transfemoral; below elbow = transradial.

5. *Amelia* refers to the occasion where an entire bone/segment is missing; *hemimelias* refer to a longitudinal anomaly where all or part of one bone is missing; *phocomelia* refers to the congenital absence of the proximal section of the limb.

6. PFFD is a longitudinal deficiency where the femur is malformed and shortened. Typically the remaining femoral segment is held in flexion, abduction, and external rotation. This deformity is classified into four types: Class A, B, C, or D. *Class A:* normal hip joint with intact and well-seated femoral head and acetabulum, shortened femoral segment with subtrochanteric varus angulation. *Class B:* femoral head present, acetabulum is adequate but defective, capital fragment within acetabulum. *Class C:* femoral head and acetabulum absent, short femoral fragment, no articulation between femur and acetabulum. *Class D:* femoral head and acetabulum absent, no relation between femur and acetabulum. Several surgical intervention strategies are available to the child with PFFD, depending on the length of the remaining limb.

7. A baby should be fitted with a passive prosthetic device before the age of 3 months.

8. Children will require an adaptation to allow them to achieve mobility. If the child has a transfemoral amputation, he or she may be fitted with a device that will allow 4-point rocking and crawling. If the child has a transtibial amputation level, the child should be fitted for a prosthetic device when beginning to pull to stand.

9. This child requires a stable base of support. This child would benefit from a prosthesis with a single-axis knee hinge that manually and intentionally can be locked or unlocked. The knee is locked, usually via a webbing strap, in extension. The child ambulates with the knee locked in extension. The child should be encouraged to unlock the knee when returning to a sitting position.

10. Wear the prosthesis consistently. Pick up two objects and place them in their correct containers so that he can play with his toys.

CHAPTER 15

1. Physical activity, allergens, chemicals, smoke, respiratory coughs and colds.

2. Low income children of color.

3. Child's asthma history, triggers and symptoms, ways to contact parent/guardian and healthcare provider, medications, physician and parent/guardian signatures, peak flow reading.

4. This device measures how well air is flowing into and out of a person's lungs. The person must be over 5 years old.

5. It is better to have a higher number/reading on the monitor.

6. Preventive medication is used to help decrease the inflammation of the airways or to decrease the triggers. Rescue medication helps to quickly open a person's airway during an asthma attack.

7. The person may take a dose of rescue medication prior to exercise. Modify routine if child has had a recent asthma attack.

8. Wheezing, shortness of breath, tightness of the chest, coughing, increased respiratory rate.

9. Stop exercising immediately.

10. High temperature, high barometric pressure, and the fall season were the most highly correlated factors associated with severity of symptoms.

CHAPTER 16

1. The child has a smaller heart size, which results in less stroke volume.

2. Strength improvements are due to improved coordination and neuromuscular recruitment.

3. Greenstick fractures and growth plate fractures.

4. Salter-Harris I: fracture along the entire growth plate without involving surrounding osteology. Salter-Harris V: Compression fracture in the mid-substance or the growth plate.

5. This is an avulsion of the bone where the patellar tendon attaches to the tibia. Children involved in jumping sports are most susceptible to Osgood-Schlatter disease.

6. Rehab programs should begin conservatively. Surgery is recommended rarely; more commonly rest is recommended. The rehabilitation program should consist of strengthening and flexibility, focusing on functional activities.

7. Stress fractures are not common in children. When they occur, they usually occur in the same spot in the foot. There are a large number of epiphyseal plates in a small area in the metatarsals, which is the most common site for stress fractures. These occur more often in females than males, especially during adolescence because of hormonal changes. Delayed menarche or amenorrhea increases the incidence of stress fractures.

8. Child experiences pain around the medial aspect of the elbow, possibly due to medial epicondylitis. Typically caused by overuse and most commonly seen in throwers.

9. This is caused by a proximal humeral growth plate fracture. This injury occurs primarily due to poor technique and underdeveloped musculature.

10. When the child is able to understand and follow detailed instructions on proper technique and progression.

CHAPTER 17

1. Extremely premature, very low birth weight.
2. Typical preterm profile.
3. PROM (premature rupture of membranes), PTL (preterm labor), fetal heart rate decelerations, cesarean section, VLBW, 1315 grams.
4. Low Apgars, Grade III IVH, PDA, first-time parents with long commute.
5. Speech-language pathologist, lactation consultant. She suggested prone swaddling as the best position for G.M. and suggested feeding time was the best time to attempt to interact with the baby. She provided parent education regarding reading baby's stress indicators, decreasing stress, and modifying the environment. She also recommended a gel pillow and frequent position changes to address concerns about head shape. She assured the family she would be available to answer questions and would provide a home program and referral to early intervention prior to discharge.

CHAPTER 18

1. Linear/planar, contoured, custom molded.
2. Power and manual.
3. It is best to consider the least amount of intervention, depending on the environment. At home the child may be able to cruise and take steps while holding onto furniture. At school the child may opt to use Lofstrand crutches in order to reduce fatigue and maintain balance. Some children prefer Lofstrand crutches to axillary crutches, because the Lofstrand cuffs allow the child to maintain control of the Lofstrand and use his hands for motor skills. For instance, the child can push his tray through the cafeteria line with his hands while the Lofstrand crutch is kept from falling by the cuff. Depending on distances needed to travel and the child's speed and fatigue, it may be prudent to consider a walker for longer distances.
4. This child would benefit from a linear seating system that offered minimal pressure relief and positioning. The child

would benefit from a lightweight manual wheelchair.

5. In a rear-wheel-drive chair, the steering and acceleration is generated in the rear wheels. This causes the sensation of the wheelchair user being pushed from behind. The midwheel-drive steering and acceleration is directly under the user's center of gravity. This gives the effect of the user moving as one with the chair. The midwheel drive chairs have a smaller turning radius, and they more closely mimic the turning performance of a typically developing child.

6. PL 101-476: Education of All Handicapped Children Act; 1986-2004 Amendments (IDEA); PL105-394: TRAIDA (Tech Act); PL 93-112: Rehabilitation Act; and PL 101-336: Americans with Disabilities Act.

7. The purpose of the seating system is to provide external postural support for the child in sitting when the child has functional limitations as a result of impairments in musculoskeletal alignment, postural control, muscle tone, or strength.

8. The custom-molded seating system will support her skeletal deformities well. A midwheel-drive power chair will allow her to maneuver more easily around campus, utilize public transportation easily, and it will integrate with the customized seating system.

9. A tilt-in-space system maintains the hip and knee angles as it tips on an axis. This system is recommended for individuals who need to tip back but have difficulty repositioning within the seating system. The reclining system allows flexion and extension of the lower extremities. This system is ideal for individuals who require frequent pressure-relief assistance and range of motion throughout the day.

10. The therapist should inquire about the ability of the child/family to transport and store the power system. The therapist should also inquire about accessibility issues at home/school/work. The therapist must also advise the child/family that they should complete a daily exercise regimen, because caloric needs may drop significantly.

GLOSSARY

Acceleration dependent injury Related to the effects that occur when a force is applied to a movable head; may be either translational or rotational in nature.

Acquired limb deficiency Amputations caused by trauma, vascular disease, tumors, infections, or burn injuries.

Adjusted age (AA) Refers to the child's age after adjusting for prematurity. It is the age the child should be if they had been born full term, or the chronological age (CA) minus the weeks premature.

Age-equivalent score The mean chronological age represented by a certain developmental index score.

Amelia The occasion where an entire bone/segment is missing.

Amniotic band syndrome (ABS) The cause of several varying birth defects, including amputation of the arms, legs, and digits when the fetal parts are entrapped in a fibrous amniotic band in utero.

Asperger syndrome A neurobiological disorder in which children often demonstrate many autistic symptoms, including elevated sensitivities to certain sounds, tastes, textures, or light. Individuals with Asperger syndrome generally seem normal, but often have difficulties with pragmatic language and can be overly literal or have problems with idiom and language use in a social context.

Assistive technology device (ATD) Defined by legislation to include any item, piece of equipment, or product system that increases, maintains, or improves an individual's functional status.

Assistive technology service Defined as any service, such as physical therapy, occupational therapy, or speech therapy, that directly assists someone with a disability in the selection and acquisition of an ATD or training in its use.

Asthma management plan A plan that includes the child's asthma history, triggers and symptoms, ways to contact the parent/guardian and healthcare provider, physician and parent/guardian signatures, the child's target peak flow reading, and a list of asthma medications. It also includes the child's treatment plan for medications, based on symptoms and peak flow readings.

Atlantoaxial instability Is characterized by excessive movement at the junction between the atlas (C1) and axis (C2) and is due to either a bony or ligamentous abnormality.

Autism The most common of a series of related neurobiological disorders known collectively as *autism spectrum disorders* or *pervasive developmental disorders*.

Autism spectrum disorders Other forms of autism that include Rett syndrome, Asperger syndrome, childhood disintegrative disorder, and pervasive developmental disorder not otherwise specified.

Autoimmune disease One large group of diseases characterized by altered function of the immune system of the body, resulting in the production of antibodies against the body's own cells.

Blastocyte An undifferentiated embryonic cell.

Central nervous system One of the three systems the human nervous system is made of. It consists of the spinal cord, brainstem, and two cerebral hemispheres.

Cerebral palsy A permanent, nonprogressive neurologic disorder of motor function; describes a group of chronic conditions impairing control of posture and movement. CP appears in the first few years of life and generally does not worsen over time.

Chemical burn A burn injury that is divided primarily into two groups, acid and alkali. Acids produce coagulation necrosis by denaturing proteins upon tissue contact, and the development of this area of coagulation limits any extension of the injury. Alkalis cause a liquefaction necrosis, meaning the tissue is liquefied by contact with the alkali and then necroses as a result.

Child abuse Mistreatment of a child by a parent, guardian, or other caregiver.

Childhood disintegrative disorder A condition occurring in 3- and 4-year-olds who have developed normally to age 2. Over several months, a child with this disorder will deteriorate in intellectual, social, and language functioning from previously normal behavior. An affected child shows a loss of communication skills, regression in nonverbal behaviors, and significant loss of previously acquired skills.

Chronological age (CA) Refers to the age of the child in days, weeks, or months from the time of birth.

Club foot deformity A birth defect in which the foot is turned inward, is stiff, and cannot be brought to a normal position.

Computerized tomography A medical imaging method that employs tomography, a process in which digital geometry processing is used to generate a three-dimensional image of the internal structures of an object from a large series of two-dimensional x-ray images taken around a single axis of rotation.

Conductive education An integrated system for children with cerebral palsy, spina bifida, and other motor disorders. Conductive education allows the child to learn to move within functional skills and is based on four primary principles: a conductor, the group setting, rhythmic intention, and a specific task series for each functional skill.

Congenital limb deficiency Amputations that occur in utero.

Contoured system One of three postural support systems that provides external postural control by increasing the points of contact, especially laterally. The seat and back surfaces are rounded by shaping layers of firm foam, air, or gel to correspond to the curves of the body.

Contrecoup injury The secondary reaction of the brain after initial force/injury.

Coup injury An injury in which the brain does not decelerate, rather it continues to move laterally until it is stopped by the lateral aspect of the skull.

Criterion-referenced measures Based on milestones of motor skills performed by typically developing clients; are more useful when developing a treatment plan or curriculum for a patient.

Custom-molded system One of three postural support systems and the third level of intervention that provides an intimate fit by closely conforming to the shape of the client's body, thereby giving the most postural support.

Developmentally supportive care Based on the belief that infants are vulnerable to sensory overload and overstimulation.

Diplegia A condition caused by cerebral palsy in which a child's functional problems occur primarily in the legs, with little or no involvement in the arms.

Disablement model (NAGI model) Widely used to describe a patient and the effect of injury or pathology on the patient's livelihood.

Down syndrome A genetic disorder caused by the presence of all or part of an extra chromosome 21.

Electrical burn Burn injuries are attributable to a variety of household mechanisms. Low-voltage injuries have very low morbidity and mortality. Both morbidity and mortality increase proportionally as voltage increases.

Embryonic stage Stage occurs during weeks 2 to 8 of gestation, in which rapid growth and development of the major body systems, including the respiratory, digestive, and nervous systems, occur.

Enablement model (ICF WHO model) The World Health Organization's model of enablement; describes how the patient's injury or pathology impacts his or her activities and participation in society, based around the body structure and function, activity limitations and participation restrictions, and environmental factors.

Escharotomy Incisions through burns that may be necessary to reduce the pressures within the burns caused by the ever-increasing edema during the initial stages of burn progression. This is done to restore circulation when the tissue pressures compromise blood flow.

Fetal stage Constitutes the time 8 weeks postconception until birth. Rapid growth continues, organs and body systems become more refined. Fingernails, toenails, and eyelashes develop. The fetus actively moves within the uterus.

Full-thickness burn A third- or fourth-degree burn that involves the destruction of all the epidermal and dermal layers and extends down into the subcutaneous tissue.

Germinal stage Stage from fertilization until roughly 2 weeks gestational age in which the zygote implants into the uterine wall and divides.

Gestational age The age of a child expressed in number of weeks postconception.

Glasgow Coma Scale Aims to give a reliable, objective way of recording the conscious state of a person for initial and continuing assessment.

Gross Motor Functional Classification A classification system that categorizes children by degree of severity or functional capability. This system provides a qualitative, objective measure of prognosis of gross motor skills; a child can be classified at one of five levels, depending on the child's skill level.

Growth plate fracture A fracture in a long bone most commonly found near a joint; a common fracture among growing children.

Hemimelia Refers to a longitudinal anomaly where all or part of one bone is missing.

Hemiparesis A condition caused by cerebral palsy in which the child has weakness and poor motor control of one arm and one leg on the same side of the body.

Heterotopic ossificans The formation of real bone within soft tissue, which often causes pain, decreased range of motion, and swelling of the joint. This is a common risk for children who experience brain injury or spinal cord injury.

Homunculus A small anatomic model of the human form.

Hydrocephalus The enlargement of the ventricular system in the brain due to an increase in cerebrospinal fluid.

Hypertonia Increased rigidity, tension, and spasticity of the muscles caused by cerebral palsy; can sometimes lead to functional limitation, disability, or in severe cases reduced quality of life.

Hypertrophic scar Takes the form of a red, raised lump on the skin, but does not grow beyond the boundaries of the original wound; often improves in appearance after a few years.

Hypotonia Reduced tension or pressure.

Individualized educational plan Describes the goals for the school year an educational team sets for children with delayed skills.

Individualized family service plan Establishes outcomes and related strategies, based on the caregiver's priorities, concerns, and professional assessments. The team, which includes the family and all evaluators, determines the amount of services to be provided and how best to meet the needs of the child in a natural environment.

Interdisciplinary A mix of practitioners from different disciplines who maintain their own professional roles and use a cooperative approach that is very interactive and centered on a common problem to solve.

Intracranial pressure The pressure exerted by the cranium on the brain tissue, cerebrospinal fluid, and the brain's circulating blood volume.

Iridocyclitis An inflammation of the iris and ciliary body.

Joint contractures A chronic loss of joint motion due to structural changes in non-bony tissue.

Joint inflammation A localized protective reaction of tissue in the joints to irritation, injury, or infection; characterized by pain, swelling, and sometimes loss of function.

Kinesio taping Used to support weakened muscles or prevent muscle overuse. Kinesio tape is flexible and has elastic properties that can strengthen a weakened muscle to prevent cramping or overcontraction.

Leukotaping Rigid strapping used to support a joint in a normal alignment. Muscle facilitation for appropriate firing can be achieved by laying the tape parallel to the muscle fibers.

Longitudinal deficiencies Unilateral or bilateral deficiency in which one of the bones in the segment is missing or malformed along the long axis of the segment.

Magnetic resonance imaging (MRI) Primarily used in medical imaging to visualize the structure and function of the body. It provides detailed images of the body in any plane.

Meningocele One of the levels of spina bifida in which the neural arches do not connect, and there is a sac covering the child's spinal column containing the herniation of the meninges. The spinal cord is not trapped, and these children often do not show any symptoms.

Micrognathia An abnormally small jaw.

Mosaicism Denotes the presence of two populations of cells with different genotypes in one individual who has developed from a single fertilized egg.

Multidisciplinary A mix of practitioners from multiple disciplines who work together in a common setting but without an interactive relationship.

Muscle atrophy Refers to a decrease in the size of skeletal muscle.

Myelomeningocele One of the levels of spina bifida in which the spinal cord and tissue protrude through the vertebral defect into an open area in the back. The spinal cord is malformed and defects may extend below the level of the primary herniation. The defect can occur at any spinal level, but is often seen in the lumbosacral area.

Neonatology An area of pediatric medicine that seeks to optimize the infant's potential for development and measure the limits of viability for premature infants.

Neural tube defects Birth defects in the brain and spinal cord. The two most common neural tube defects are spina bifida and anencephaly.

Neurodevelopmental treatment Embraces knowledge of motor control and looks at the effects of postural control as a result of interactions between many neurologic and physiologic systems. Therapy that is meant for children with cerebral palsy or other motor disorders and enhances the individual's capacity to function.

Norm-referenced measures An assessment standardized on a normal population; allows standard scores, percentiles, and age-equivalent calculations to be made.

Osteochondritis dissecans An injury to the articular cartilage and the corresponding bone.

Partial-thickness burn A second-degree burn that penetrates more deeply; involves destruction of all the epidermal layers and extends into the dermis.

Pauciarticular JRA A pauciarticular (involving only a few joints) disease in which children test positive for antinuclear antibodies and have a high risk for iridocyclitis. Pauciarticular JRA can affect the spine, although possibly not until the late teens, and the children may test positive for the gene identified with adult ankylosing spondylitis.

Peak flow monitoring A monitoring system that employs a simple device that measures how well air is moving out of a patient's airways.

Percentage score Expresses the percent of items passed on a scale.

Percentile score *Percentile* means "per hundred." A percentile score gives an individual's ranking in a group. If a child scores in the 80th percentile on a test, the score is equal to or higher than the scores of 80% of the children who took the test.

Peripheral nervous system Connects nerves to the central nervous system; is built from sensory fibers that innervate glands and skeletal, cardiac, and smooth muscle.

Pervasive Developmental Disorder—Not Otherwise Specified (PDD-NOS) A subthreshold condition in which the individual meets some but not all of the diagnostic criteria necessary for a diagnosis of autism. Children diagnosed with PDD-NOS demonstrate issues with socialization and behavior similar to but less severe than those evidenced by persons with autism; they have fewer if any language issues.

Phocomelia Refers to the congenital absence of the proximal section of the limb.

Planar system One of three postural support systems; it is the least intensive and consists of a flat seat and back.

Polyarticular JRA An arthritis in children that involves five or more large joints. Includes two subtypes. In the first subtype, children identified with a special kind of antibody in their blood known as *rheumatoid factor (RF)* often have a more severe form of JRA. In the second subtype, children only experience joint involvement.

Postconceptual age (PCA) Child's chronological age (CA) plus the gestational age (GA). For example, a child with a CA of 4 weeks who was born at 28 weeks gestation has a PCA of 32 weeks.

Preventive medication One of two types of medication. Can be oral or inhaled; used to help decrease inflammation of the airways or to decrease the response to a trigger such as an allergen.

Primitive reflexes Any reflex normal in an infant, including grasp reflex, Moro reflex, and sucking reflex.

Proprioceptive neuromuscular facilitation Intervention for children with muscle imbalances to strengthen muscles within diagonal and rotational movement patterns. PNF is based on developmental sequence and the sequential mastery of motor milestones.

Prosthesis A device, either external or implanted, that substitutes for or supplements a missing or defective part of the body.

Quadriparesis A condition caused by cerebral palsy in which some children have problems in all four extremities.

Qualitative assessment Assessment that interprets the phenomenon of performance, often in context of performance and presented as a descriptive narrative. This assessment will frequently be open-ended, with no forced choice. Anecdotal observations and self-reports are examples of qualitative assessments.

Quantitative assessment Performance or achievement information or description made with objective, measurable data. Often this assessment is standardized and structured. Behavior occurrence as measured by behavioral objectives, task achievement, and specific values achieved (such as pounds lifted) is an example of a quantitative assessment.

Rancho Los Amigos Levels of Cognitive Functioning Multi-level scale of cognitive recovery that ranges from 1 to 8; used for assessment of recovery, for communication between medical professionals and facilities, and to measure change and progress during the rehabilitation course.

Raw score Actual points earned on an assessment, or the number of items passed on a certain test.

Reliability Determines if the tool is an accurate measure of what it claims to measure.

Rescue medication One of two types of asthma medications, usually in the form of an inhaler (e.g., albuterol). This medication quickly helps to open the airways to help a person breathe easier.

Residual limb The part of the limb that remains after amputation.

Responsiveness The ability to detect minimally significant clinical change.

Retinal hemorrhage Hemorrhage inside the intraocular space caused by a sudden increase in venous pressure in the head. The rise in pressure is communicated by the optic nerve sheaths, causing blood to leak through damaged vessels; accompanied by retinal edema. Severe damage to the eyes may cause permanent, partial, or total blindness.

Rett syndrome An early-onset (prior to age 4) genetic condition associated with an abnormality on the X chromosome. Children develop normally through the first few months of life, then lose hand function and develop stereotyped hand movements that resemble hand wringing or hand washing around 5 months of age. Head growth slows, and social impairments similar to those in autism emerge.

Rigidity Significant resistance to movement.

Rotational injury Occurs when the brain remains stationary in a moving, rotating skull. Rotational injuries are related to shearing trauma and also have been associated with diffuse axonal injuries.

Rule of nines A method of measuring the extent of a burn; divides the body surface into areas, each of which is considered to be 9% or a multiple of 9% of the total body surface area.

Scaled score Provides an estimate of the child's ability level along a continuum of items. Scores range from 0 to 100; 0 is low capacity, and 100 is highly capable.

Scheuermann disease A wedge-shaped fracture that has an overuse, postural cause.

Scleroderma Also known as *systemic sclerosis*, a connective tissue disease involving the skin, blood vessels, and immune system.

Secondary injury Occurs due to processes induced in response to the initial trauma. Secondary injuries account for a significant portion of the overall damage that occurs with TBI.

Sensory integration Therapy that assists children by using controlled sensory input to help those with sensory processing difficulties. Three major components: normal sensory function, sensory integration dysfunction, and a programmatic guide for using sensory integration techniques.

Shaken baby syndrome A highly preventable disorder in which the brain is jolted back and forth inside the skull, creating first acceleration then deceleration movements inside the skull.

Spacer A large chamber fitted to an inhaler; useful in dispensing a dose of medication more effectively. Spacers increase the amount of medication that reaches the lungs instead of being deposited in the mouth and throat.

Spastic quadriplegia A condition caused by cerebral palsy in which a child experiences symptoms from both triplegia and diplegia.

Spasticity Pertaining to sudden, abnormal, involuntary muscular contraction consisting of a continued muscular contraction.

Spina bifida occulta Describes the condition where the neural arches do not connect, but there is no neural material located outside the spinal canal. This is the most common form of spina bifida, characteristically involving the lower lumbar spine. It is also the most benign, with typically no resultant neurologic effects or abnormalities.

Standard scores Describe deviations from the mean, or average, score for the group. Standard deviations are used to describe the divergence.

Standard tests Tests that include a set of tasks or questions that are intended to assess a particular type of behavior when presented under standardized conditions.

Strength training The use of resistance to muscular contraction to build the strength, anaerobic endurance, and size of skeletal muscles.

Superficial burn First-degree burns that are limited to the epidermis.

Systemic JRA Also known as *Still disease*, a type of JRA accompanied by high spiking fevers off and on for weeks and a rash on the chest and thighs. In addition to joint involvement, internal organs such as the heart, liver, spleen, and lymph nodes can be affected.

Tethered cord syndrome Occurs when the spinal cord is fixed caudally because of pathology. The tethered spinal cord becomes stretched, distorted, and ischemic. The child with tethered cord may show atypical neurologic signs, including decreased strength, increased spasticity in the lower extremities, changing urologic patterns, back pain, or scoliosis.

Therapeutic taping Therapy for children with muscle weakness, joint instability, joint malalignment and postural asymmetries; uses rigid or flexible taping to support and influence muscle groups.

TheraTogs An orthotic product that is designed to capture the benefits of taping without directly adhering to the skin.

Thermal burn Thermal burn injuries are the most likely to occur to infants and children; extremely common in young children and can occur from spilled food and beverages, including grease spills, hot tap water, clothes irons, curling irons, space heaters, and ovens/ranges.

Tone The normal tension found in muscles.

Total body surface area (TBSA) The amount of body surface over which a burn injury extends.

Transdisciplinary A team of practitioners from different disciplines in which members cross over professional boundaries and share roles and functions.

Translational injury An injury that causes a reaction to a force applied to the side of the skull with lateral movement of both the skull and the brain. This can cause significant brain damage.

Transverse amputation Occurs in the transverse plane of the extremity through the shaft of the involved bone.

Traumatic brain injury A traumatically induced physiologic disruption of brain functioning, resulting in partial or total impairments of one or more areas of functioning.

Triplegia A condition caused by cerebral palsy in which one arm and hand are virtually uninvolved, while all other limbs are involved.

Trisomy 21 One of the three types of chromosomal abnormalities that can lead to Down syndrome. Trisomy 21 occurs in 95% of Down syndrome cases and results in an extra chromosome 21. Individuals with trisomy 21 have 47 chromosomes instead of the typical 46. Translocation occurs when the long arm of the extra chromosome 21 attaches to chromosome 14, 21, or 22.

Validity Determines if the assessment tool accomplishes its intended purpose.

Wheeled mobility Segment of the assistive technology available to individuals with disabilities.

Zygote The result of fertilization, when the sperm and the ovum combine to form a new cell.

INDEX

A

About.com· Physical Therapy, 158
Acceleration-dependent injuries, 69
Acids, burns caused by, 150
Acromioclavicular joint separation, 181
Activities, and risk of traumatic brain injury, 70
Activities of daily living (ADLs)
   and amputation, 152
   in rheumatoid disorders, 100
   in spina bifida child, 126
Activity limitations
   in arthrogryposis multiplex congenita, 111
   for autistic child, 140
   for burn patients, 157
   for child with cerebral palsy, 64
   for child with limb deficiencies, 166
   for child with traumatic brain injury, 79
   in Down syndrome child, 117
   in rheumatoid disorders, 101
   in shaken baby syndrome, 88, 90
   for spina bifida child, 128
Adjusted age (AA), 191, 192
ADLs. See Activities of daily living.
Adolescents
   strength training for, 177
   weightlifting program for, 176-177
Aerobic exercise, in spina bifida, 127
Afferent fibers, function of, 4
AFP. See Alpha-fetoprotein.
Age-equivalent score, defined, 19
Ages and Stages Questionnaire (ASQ), 137
Agonist, in proprioceptive neuromuscular
   facilitation, 33
Air pollution, and asthma, 170, 173
Alberta Infant Motor Scale (AIMS), 21t, 22-23
   for child with CP, 59
   purpose of, 22
Albuterol, for asthma, 172, 172t
Alkalis, burns caused by, 150
Alliance for Technology Access, 227
Alpha-fetoprotein (AFP), in spina bifida, 122
Ambulation. See also Mobility.
   in autistic child, 139
   of child with arthrogryposis multiplex congenita,
     109, 110

Ambulation. See also Mobility. (Continued)
   in child with shaken baby syndrome history, 89
   for infants, 11, 11t
   in intervention plan, 30
Ambulation aids, 206
AMC. See Arthrogryposis multiplex congenita.
Amelia, 160
American Academy of Allergy, Asthma, and
   Immunology, 175
American Academy of Cerebral Palsy and
   Developmental Medicine, 227
American Academy of Pediatrics, Committee on
   Sports Medicine and Fitness of, 177
American Burn Association, 146
American National Standards Institute (ANSI), 221
American Physical Therapy Association (APTA), 45
Americans with Disabilities Act (ADA), 205
Amniotic band syndrome (ABS), 160
Amniotic fluid, AFP levels in, 122
Amputations
   acquired, 160
   in burn injuries, 152
   congenital, 160
   transverse, 160
   traumatic or surgical, 162-163
   types of, 160, 161t
Anemia, in NICU infants, 201
Angelo, J., 213
Ankle
   injury of, 184-185
   osteochondritis dissecans of, 178
Ankle-foot orthosis (AFO)
   in child with shaken baby syndrome history, 89
   in spina bifida, 125
Antagonist, in proprioceptive neuromuscular
   facilitation, 33
Anthropometric characteristics, in rheumatoid
   disorders, 100
Antinuclear antibodies (ANAs), in pauciarticular
   JRA, 96
Anti-seizure medications, in shaken baby
   syndrome, 89
Anti-spasticity medications, in shaken baby
   syndrome, 89
Antithrust seats, 211

Note: Page numbers followed by *f* indicate figures; *t*, tables; and *b*, boxes.

Edwards Brothers Malloy
Thorofare, NJ USA
November 17, 2015